POSTGRADUATE MEDICINE

OTHER PUBLISHED WORK

By the same Author:
The Clinical Significance of the Essential Biological Metals

With D. S. Hopton:
Practical Hints for Housemen

Postgraduate Medicine

I. J. T. DAVIES

M.B.(Lond.), M.R.C.P.(Lond. and Edin.)

Consultant Physician (Highland Health Board);
Regional Director of Postgraduate Medical Education,
Raigmore Hospital, Inverness

Third edition

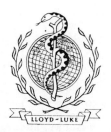

LLOYD-LUKE (MEDICAL BOOKS) LTD
49 NEWMAN STREET
LONDON
1977

FIRST EDITION . . . 1969
Spanish translation . . 1971
SECOND EDITION . . . 1972
Reprinted 1972
Italian translation . . . 1974
THIRD EDITION . . . 1977

PRINTED AND BOUND IN ENGLAND BY
HAZELL WATSON AND VINEY LTD
AYLESBURY, BUCKS

ISBN: 0 85324 123 6

FOR
JOYCE, EDWIN, BENJAMIN AND ELEANOR

PREFACE TO THIRD EDITION

I have revised the whole book bearing in mind continuing changes of emphasis in current views and management and I have tried to add new information which is likely to be of lasting relevance. I have continued to try to cater for candidates for the MRCP examination as well as other postgraduates who require a reasonably concise overview of current and orthodox medicine. The book should be of value to an increasing number of candidates for the MRCGP as well as for Vocational Trainees doing their period of hospital medicine. Foreign medical graduates sitting the TRAB examination should find the book useful for acquainting them with current medical phraseology.

I have added a new chapter on metabolic bone disease and renal stones—this reflects a personal interest as well as an attempt to explain a subject made unnecessarily difficult in many standard texts.

In this edition I have omitted the chapter on adverse drug reactions. When this chapter was first written knowledge and awareness of the subject was in its infancy but now the problems are so well recognised that their inclusion in *Postgraduate Medicine* is no longer appropriate.

I am most grateful to Dr. George Morrice who prepared the Index for the edition. In conclusion, I hope the third edition of *Postgraduate Medicine* continues to be read.

IEUAN DAVIES

Lentran House
Lentran,
By Inverness IV3 6 RL
June, 1976

PREFACE TO FIRST EDITION

Medical textbooks fall into two main groups: those intended for medical students and those which are large, comprehensive and intended mainly for reference purposes. It seemed to me that there was need for a book intended to be read from cover to cover which served the needs of those engaged in general medicine and which attempted to bridge the gap between the theoretical knowledge of the final year medical student and the practice of sound, safe and orthodox medicine.

Medical education has now achieved the status of a distinct discipline with the increasing recognition that the haphazard, do-it-yourself system of undergraduate and postgraduate medical education should be replaced by co-ordinated, well taught and applicable courses of instruction. These courses require a great deal of enlightened thought, clear analysis of the problems, energy and expertise in their construction and delivery. I am grateful for the countless fruitful discussions I have had with friends and colleagues experienced in the problems of medical education who have given considerable thought to the difficulties in overcoming the knowledge, experience and interest gaps.

Concepts, facts and ideas which I know are often ill-understood by those working for the membership diploma of one of the Royal Colleges of Physicians have been explained and amplified. I hope I have given some guidance to the important practical considerations in general medicine as well as crystallising some of the current problems.

Into one compact and convenient volume I have tried to distil the basic requirements of current postgraduate medicine which will be useful, not only to general and specialist physicians but also to final year medical students, to interested general practitioners, and to those working for surgical, anaesthetic and obstetrical postgraduate degrees.

In order to make the book as viable and useful as possible I would be pleased to hear from any reader who has views about other information that might have been included and grateful for guidance which would clarify any of the explanations.

I wish to express my sincere thanks to those who have given me so much encouragement; to the medical secretaries who have typed the manuscript and to the staff of the photographic department of Llandough Hospital who prepared the illustrations.

My thanks are due to the Editor of the *British Journal of Hospital Medicine* for permission to use the section on Shock which has been revised but appeared originally in that journal.

I am grateful for the assistance of Doctors Jeremy Cobb, Sam Davies and Neville Hodges who helped in the preparation of the index. Mr. Douglas Luke, the publisher, has been most helpful, courteous and understanding and it is a joy to express my gratitude to him.

Finally, I have received from my kind and patient wife, Dr. Joyce Davies, M.R.C.P., such help and encouragement that without her I would never have contemplated, let alone complete, the work.

IEUAN DAVIES

Llandough Hospital,
Penarth,
Glam. CF6 1XX
October, 1968

CONTENTS

1

CARDIOLOGY

Complicated new investigations have not replaced the need for careful clinical assessment of the heart. Most of the specialised techniques are based on simple physiological principles; knowledge of their application and limitations is of value in the full assessment of a patient.

DYSPNOEA

The grading of dyspnoea is helpful in recording the progress of symptoms and in briefly communicating the degree of disability. The accepted convention is:

Grade 1. Dyspnoea on severe exertion such as running up two flights of stairs.
Grade 2A. Dyspnoea on moderate exertion such as walking normally up two flights of stairs.
Grade 2B. Dyspnoea on mild exertion such as walking slowly up one flight of stairs.
Grade 3. Dyspnoea on minimal exertion such as walking from room to room.
Grade 4. Dyspnoea at rest.

It is of value to record the extent of interference with the patient's way of life, for example, dyspnoea which prevents a housewife from doing the family shopping or a husband from driving the family car is usually severe. It is helpful to record the exact disability which breathlessness imposes on a patient. For example can a housewife make one, two or three beds "on the trot" without having to rest in between each, can she sweep out one room without resting, can she carry the week's shopping home or can she run downstairs to answer the door? The number of flights of stairs that can be climbed at a normal pace is a useful guide; or if the patient has only tried one flight—does he think he *could* climb a second flight if there was one?

Dyspnoea is a subjective, uncomfortable awareness of breathing. It is mainly due to excessive use and fatigue of the respiratory muscles. The pulmonary venous congestion which occurs with left-sided heart failure results in congestion of the interstitial lung tissue and airways diminishing the elastic properties of the lungs and increasing the ventilatory effort needed to transfer air through the airways. Normal expiration is probably triggered by a number of reflexes of which the best known is the Hering[1]-Breuer[2] in which stretch receptors in the alveolar walls are stimulated during inspiration, and impulses pass via the vagus to the respiratory centre which initiates relaxation of the inspiratory muscles. Expiration is a passive process due to the inherent elastic properties of the lungs. The normal rate and depth of breathing at rest are probably mainly due to the inherent rhythmicity of the respiratory centre secondarily modified by afferent reflexes from the lungs and, during exercise, by alterations of the gas tensions in the blood (Sleight, 1964). Congestion of the alveolar walls will accelerate the afferent reflexes (increasing the rate of breathing). Later, breathing becomes further accelerated because of anoxia of the respiratory centre due to alveolar wall oedema interfering with the diffusion of oxygen from the alveoli into the blood. Early cardiac failure is accompanied by dyspnoea before there is any alteration in pH, oxygen or carbon dioxide content of arterial blood perfusing the respiratory centre. The rapid relief of cardiac dyspnoea by morphia is probably due to decrease in awareness of breathing as well as depression of the respiratory centre, slowing the rate of breathing thereby reducing fatigue of the respiratory muscles.

Paroxysmal nocturnal dyspnoea when lying flat at night and ortho-pnoea (Gk. orthos: straight) are due to reduced mechanical advantage of the diaphragm, redistribution of oedema fluid from dependent parts, reduced sensitivity of the respiratory centre during sleep leading to failure of early compensatory mechanisms and increase in cardiac output and venous return in the recumbent position.

Occasionally, patients who are dyspnoeic due to a pulmonary embolus prefer to lie flat; the reason for this is that they feel faint if they sit upright because they have a low cardiac output.

Breathlessness which is present when the patient lies in a particular position is seen in the uncommon occurrence of a pedunculated tracheal or bronchial polyp.

CARDIAC PAIN

Ischaemic cardiac pain arises from pain receptors in the myocardium and is transmitted via the sympathetic nerves to the upper thoracic sympathetic ganglia and thence to the upper five thoracic spinal nerves. This explains the radiation of cardiac pain in the distribution of T 1–5 and the relief of pain by division of these sympathetic ganglia. These nerves supply the upper oesophagus, accounting for the frequent

1. KARL EWALD KONSTANTIN HERING (1834–1918). Vienna and Leipzig physio-logist.
2. JOSEF BREUER (1842–1925). Vienna psychiatrist.

similarity of oesophageal pain and angina, they also supply some of the muscles and ligaments surrounding the shoulder joints, accounting for the reflex spasm and disuse of the left shoulder which may occur following cardiac infarction. Disuse of the joint may be accompanied by a periarthritis and calcification. The left joint is much more frequently involved than the right but the converse is true when periarthritis is due to excessive use, because most people are right-handed. The first thoracic nerve supplies sensation to the inner side of the upper arm and occasionally to the lower arm and little finger accounting for the radiation of cardiac pain down the arm. Distinction between oesophageal and cardiac pain may sometimes be made by infusing dilute hydrochloric acid or dilute sodium bicarbonate through an oesophageal tube and noting whether this induces the patient's pain. Following a large meal, T wave changes may occur in the ECG in the absence of ischaemic heart disease, and are due to slight alteration in the position of the heart. Occasionally, pain due to reflux oesophagitis, motor incoordination and hiatus hernia may induce ischaemic ECG changes, and may be relieved by trinitrin.

The pain of pericarditis is occasionally confused with angina. The lower part of the parietal pericardium alone is pain-sensitive and is supplied by the phrenic nerve (C 4–5). Gross distension of the pericardium with fluid gives rise to a dull ache in the front of the chest which may be referred to the back of the neck and shoulder in the distribution of C 4–5. Usually the occurrence of a pericardial effusion in acute pericarditis leads to a lessening of pain because of separation of the inflamed visceral and parietal pericardium. The characteristic pain of pericarditis is usually sudden in onset and frequently pleuritic in nature due to involvement of contiguous diaphragmatic parietal pleura. Acute pericarditis is accompanied by superficial inflammation and necrosis of the myocardium which is responsible for the accompanying ST elevation in the ECG and for any similarity between the pain of pericarditis and myocardial ischaemia. However no pathological Q waves occur in the ECG in pericarditis.

Dissection of the aorta may be similar to myocardial infarction as shock is a common accompaniment in both. The pain of dissection is unlike that of myocardial infarction in that it is usually "tearing" and it is maximal at its onset and gradually wanes, whereas the pain of myocardial infarction is frequently preceded by premonitory pain. The pain of dissection usually radiates to the back and abdomen; following aortic dissection occlusion of peripheral arterial pulses is less common than is generally believed. Dissection involving the aortic valve leads to severe aortic incompetence. The dissection may continue over several days and if the abdominal aorta is involved abdominal pain is usually severe and continuous; bleeding into the peritoneum gives rise to paralytic ileus and signs of peritonitis. The clue may be the presence of a pathological arterial bruit. Occasionally bleeding is into the gut. An unexplained and puzzling feature of dissection of the thoracic aorta is a gap of several days between the onset of the tearing pain of dissection and enlargement of the aortic knuckle on the chest x-ray.

Other causes of chest pain which may simulate the pain of myocardial ischaemia include pain of musculo-skeletal origin, Tietze[3] syndrome (tenderness and swelling of upper costochondral junctions), pleuritic pain and bronchial carcinoma, especially if it causes rib erosion.

In the assessment of chest pain which is believed to be musculo-skeletal in origin the insertion of muscles into the thorax is diagnostically important if excessive use or strain of the muscles is responsible for chest pain, viz:

1. External oblique—inserted in a line from fourth costal cartilage to the tip of the twelfth rib.
2. Rectus abdominus—inserted into the fifth, sixth, and seventh costal cartilages.
3. Pectoralis major—inserted into the front of the sternum.
4. Serratus anterior—inserted into the same line as the external oblique.

THE PULSE

It is traditional for doctors to feel the radial pulse; however, the character and rhythm of the pulse are best assessed in the more proximal pulses—the carotids and brachials are the most convenient. Occasionally the radial pulses are most suitable for detecting pulsus paradoxus and the femorals for detecting a collapsing pulse.

The normal peripheral arterial pulse is made up of three components. The first, known as the percussion wave, is due to a forward moving column of blood expanding the peripheral arteries as a result of the relatively high resistances it meets in the arterioles as compared with the main arteries. The second is the tidal wave and is probably caused by two separate mechanisms—one is reflection of a pressure wave from the high-resistance arterioles back up the column of blood, and the other is transmission of a wave along the wall of the arteries, beginning at the aorta with the ejection of blood from the left ventricle. The third wave—the dicrotic wave—is due to transmission down the column of blood of a wave resulting from bulging downwards, into the ventricle, of the cusps of the closed aortic valve (Fig. 1).

In aortic stenosis the ejection of blood from the ventricle is prolonged and there is delay in arrival of the full percussion wave at the periphery. The tidal wave is less affected. If the stenosis is severe, the per-

3. ALEXANDER TIETZE (1864–1927). Breslau surgeon.

cussion wave is delayed beyond the tidal wave which is felt as a notch on the upstroke of the pulse tracing—the anacrotic notch (*Gk.* ana—up; krotos—stroke). The tighter the stenosis, the more delayed will be the percussion wave and the lower on the upstroke will be the anacrotic notch.

The collapsing pulse of aortic incompetence or arteriovenous shunting is due to disappearance of the dicrotic wave since leaking valves will not abruptly stop retrograde flow and will not reflect a pressure wave towards the periphery. The bisferiens pulse (*L.* to beat twice) of combined stenosis and incompetence has two easily palpable impulses, the first due to the tidal wave, as in the anacrotic pulse, and the second due to an apparently forcible percussion wave due to disappearance of the dicrotic wave. The dicrotic pulse of widespread peripheral arteriolar dilatation, usually due to fever, is a combination of a rapid upstroke due to early run-off into the arterioles, and an easily palpable dicrotic notch on the downstroke (*Gk.* dictrotos—twofold beating). The characteristic pulses of hypertension and atherosclerosis of the major vessels are similar in that there is a rapid and strong upstroke due in the one case to a high arteriolar resistance and in the other to loss of elasticity of the aorta.

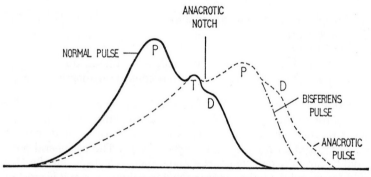

FIG. 1.—Components of the normal and abnormal peripheral pulse.
P—Percussion wave
T—Tidal wave
D—Dicrotic wave

Other abnormal pulses are:

1. **Pulsus alternans,** in which *regular* alternate beats are diminished in volume. It is specially easy to appreciate this by palpating the radial pulse while deflating a sphygmomanometer cuff around the upper arm—as the pressure falls there will be a sudden doubling of the pulse rate.

2. **Pulsus bigeminus** (or coupling), in which every alternate beat is an extrasystole and therefore of diminished volume *but* following this extra-

systole there is a long compensatory pause; unlike pulsus alternans every beat is not equidistant (*L*. geminus—a twin).

3. **Pulsus paradoxus** occurs in constriction of the heart, whether by thickened pericardium, pericardial effusion, or, rarely, in severe asthma when there is a gross trapping of air within the chest. During inspiration there is a fall in pulse volume. It is important to note that this is not paradoxical but it an exaggeration of the normal. During inspiration the pulmonary vascular bed increases in size due to traction on the vessels by the expanding lung. If the heart is constricted the volume of the right ventricle is fixed during inspiration and expiration, therefore, the increased volume of the pulmonary vascular bed cannot be accommodated by increased output from the right ventricle. The left ventricle is underfilled and the pulse volume falls. Also, if the pericardium is tethered to the diaphragm by adhesions, as the diaphragm descends the heart elongates and decreases in volume, reducing the filling of both ventricles.

PERIPHERAL ARTERIAL INSUFFICIENCY

Relative ischaemia of a limb is suggested on inspection by:

1. Atrophic shiny skin with loss of hair.
2. Brittle deformed nails.
3. Persistent skin infections.
4. Skin which looks permanently red, or cyanosed due to chronic anoxia, causing the superficial vessels to become permanently dilated.

The skin of the ischaemic limb is cooler than the normal side; before deciding for certain about differences in temperature between the two sides make sure that the limbs are in the same position and that they have been exposed for the same length of time. The peripheral pulses should be carefully palpated at rest and if there is a suspicion of arterial insufficiency and the pulses appear equal in volume at rest it is most important to exercise the limbs and palpate the pulses again. Occasionally peripheral pulses appear equal at rest but after exercise the pulse on one side may disappear due to blood being diverted by the exertion to the leg with the most patent arteries.

Simple Confirmatory Tests of Arterial Insufficiency

1. With the limbs horizontal press the skin of both limbs in corresponding positions. After removing the pressure blanching will be seen; the blanched area should normally begin to flush in 5 seconds. If the circulation is completely obstructed and the skin permanently cyanosed blanching will not occur. This situation exists in early gangrene.

2. Elevation of both limbs to 45 degrees normally does not result in much change of colour of the limbs. If part of the limb becomes pale the arterial supply is impaired With the limbs in this position the skin compression test can be carried out as above—flushing of the blanched area should occur within 10 seconds.

3. If elevation of the limbs to 45 degrees results in pallor the patient should be asked to hang the legs over the couch so that they are below the level of the body. In this position the pink colour should return to the skin within 10 seconds. At 10 seconds the veins on the dorsum of the feet should also have filled when the legs are in a dependent position.

Reactive hyperaemia test.—A blood pressure cuff is inflated to the systolic pressure around the limb when it is elevated. The limb then rests in the horizontal position for 5 minutes and the cuff deflated. Flushing gradually extends down from the level of the deflated cuff to the foot; this is followed by progressive fading. If the arterial supply is good the whole process—flushing plus fading—should be complete in 2 minutes. Inflating the blood pressure cuff occludes the arteries and temporarily paralyses the sympathetic supply to the cutaneous vessels which become maximally dilated so that when the cuff is removed blood immediately enters the dilated cutaneous vessels, if it reaches them.

THE JUGULAR VENOUS PULSE (JVP)

The internal jugular vein runs in a straight line from the angle of the jaw to the medial end of the clavicle. It lies *deep* to the sternomastoid and platysma; when the internal jugular vein is examined it is mandatory that the patient's head be resting comfortably on the back-rest and the head be slightly flexed so that the platysma and sternomastoid are relaxed. The *vertical* height of the top of the venous pulse above the sternal angle should be measured by placing a ruler on the sternal angle. If the venous pulse cannot be seen, pressure on the abdomen may cause it to be visible above the clavicle for one or two heart beats; if the level remains more than 4 cm above the sternal angle for more than two beats the filling of the right atrium is impaired and mild heart failure is present.

The simplest way of appreciating the mechanism of the jugular venous pulse is to consider it in relation to ventricular contraction (Fig. 2). The two main waves of the JVP are *a* and *v*. The *a* wave is due to atrial contraction ejecting the last portion of blood from the atrium into the ventricle at the end of the diastole. As well as forcing blood into the ventricle atrial contraction causes reflux into the superior vena cava and jugular veins. The *x* descent, following the *a* wave is due to the atrium expanding (atrial diastole) and accommodating the blood which has refluxed up into the veins. As the ventricle begins to contract the tricuspid valve closes, blood returning to the right atrium gradually fills it and once it is full further blood is accommodated in the veins, causing the *v* wave. As the ventricle relaxes the intraventricular pressure falls and as soon as the hydrostatic pressure of blood in right atrium and veins exceeds the intraventricular pressure the tricuspid valve opens and blood enters the ventricle. Any blood entering the heart during diastole can flow direct into the ventricle.

The *a* wave will be elevated (giant *a* wave) in conditions which prevent normal filling of the ventricle, e.g. tricuspid stenosis and right ventricular

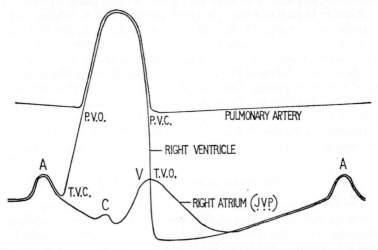

FIG. 2.—Pressure in pulmonary artery, right ventricle and right atrium during systole and diastole.

A—A wave.
C—C wave.
V—V wave.
T.V.C.   Tricuspid valve closes.
P.V.O.—Pulmonary valve opens.
P.V.C.—Pulmonary valve closes.
T.V.O.—Tricuspid valve opens.

failure (most commonly due to pulmonary hypertension and pulmonary stenosis). If the right atrium contracts while the ventricle is also contracting and the tricuspid valve is closed all the blood in the atrium will reflux up the veins causing a big *a* wave. In complete heart block the atria and ventricles are beating independently; atrial systole will sometimes occur during ventricular systole and sometimes during diastole. This results in irregular big *a* waves of varying height called cannon waves.

In tricuspid incompetence part of the force of right ventricular contraction is transmitted to the atrium—this occurs during ventricular systole and causes the giant *v* wave. Atrial fibrillation will abolish the *a* waves but may be associated with some elevation of the *v* wave even in the absence of heart failure—the fibrillating atrium is unable to accommodate as much blood as the normal atrium. In constrictive pericarditis the walls of the ventricle are held apart by the adherent pericardium so that when the ventricle is filling there will be an initial rapid flow, this is reflected in the JVP as a rapid *y* descent (Friedreich's[4] sign). A rapid *x* descent also occurs because the walls of the atrium are similarly held apart, this rapid *x* descent occurring during ventricular systole is responsible for the so-called "systolic collapse of the JVP" in constrictive pericarditis. Conditions which obstruct venous filling of the heart (congestive failure and constrictive pericarditis) will cause an elevation of the JVP during inspiration (Kussmaul's[5] sign).

The Blood Pressure

Recently it has become conventional to take as the diastolic pressure the point at which the sounds entirely disappear rather than the point at which there is an abrupt change of sound. This method of taking the blood pressure correlates best with direct intra-arterial measurement of the pressure (Bordley *et al.*, 1951).

The blood pressure in the legs is best measured by an occluding cuff around the thigh and palpation or auscultation of the popliteal artery, or foot pulses: if the foot pulses are used the patient can remain in the supine position and the ordinary arm band can be used around the lower leg (Hocken, 1967). By this method the systolic pressure is usually 20 mm higher than in the arm; in coarctation the systolic pressure in the femoral artery is less than 20 mm higher than in the brachial. The circumference of the arm has an effect on the blood pressure. If the circumference is more than 25 cm the ordinary sphygmomanometer will register a diastolic pressure above the true value.

The Apex Beat

The apex beat is normally defined as the lowest, outermost point at which the cardiac impulse is palpable. Some people prefer the point of maximum impulse (PMI) as the best method of detecting displacement or enlargement of the heart. The outward displacement of the chest wall during systole at a time when the heart itself is getting smaller is due to the fact that the base of the heart is anchored by the great vessels but the apex is mobile. The outward movement during ventricular contraction occurs because of partial rotation of the heart. In constrictive peri-

---

4. NIKOLAUS FRIEDREICH (1825–1882). Heidelberg physician.
5. ADOLF KUSSMAUL (1822–1902). Strasbourg physician.

carditis there is retraction of the apex during systole because the pericardium is adherent to the chest wall so that decrease in size of the ventricle will be transmitted to the chest wall and the thickened pericardium will not allow forward movement of the apex. The apical impulse may be double if atrial contraction is forcible as in hypertrophic obstructive cardiomyopathy (palpable 4th sound).

Hypertrophy of either ventricle may often be assessed by the character of the precordial impulse. Left ventricular hypertrophy characteristically causes a sustained apical impulse palpable over a small area if only hypertrophy is present; if dilatation of the left ventricle is present as well as hypertrophy the heaving sustained impulse is felt over a wider area. Right ventricular enlargement causes a tapping apical impulse which is short and poorly sustained. Right ventricular hypertrophy may also cause a palpable impulse at the left sternal edge—"the parasternal heave." Mitral stenosis may cause a tapping apex beat even though the right ventricle is *not* hypertrophied—the tapping apex beat of uncomplicated mitral stenosis is due to rapid and forceful closing of the mitral valve and is, therefore, a "palpable first heart sound". If the apex beat is not palpable the patient should be asked to turn on the left side and a further attempt made to locate it. It is often not palpable in obesity, emphysema, pericardial effusion, pleural effusion and pneumothorax. The apex beat will be found on the right side in dextrocardia, whether congenital or acquired (from fibrosis of the lower lobe of the right lung).

The various types of apical impulse are:

1. Normal.
2. Left ventricular.
3. Right ventricular (usually with a "parasternal heave").
4. Displaced.
5. Retractile (i.e. moving *inwards* during systole) as in constrictive pericarditis.
6. Paradoxical—outward movement of some part of the precordium other than over the apex of the heart during systole. This occurs when there is a ventricular aneurysm which fills and expands during systolic contraction of the ventricle.

Percussion of the heart does not accurately delineate its borders but the "cardiac dullness" is abnormally extensive with a pericardial effusion or large aortic aneurysm. Dullness occurs to the right of the midline in dextrocardia.

The apex beat may be recorded graphically by an apex cardiogram (ACG), which records in addition to the ventricular contraction a preceding *a* wave due to atrial contraction and succeeding "rapid" and "slow" filling waves attributable to rapid and slow passive filling of the ventricles which occurs before the atria contract. The main value of the apex cardiogram is in timing events in records of other parameters such as phonocardiography.

HEART SOUNDS AND MURMURS

The mechanisms of production of sounds within the cardiovascular system are:
1. Turbulence of the blood; this occurs when there is rapid flow through narrowed tubes or when there is a sudden change in size of a tube. At high flow rates turbulence produces high-pitched sounds and at slow rates low pitched sounds.
2. Vibration of vessels and valves. Rapid distension of the chambers of the heart causes vibration of their walls. Vibration of valves occurs when blood is flowing rapidly over them, or when they open or close forcefully.

HEART SOUNDS

The first sound is due to a combination of mitral and tricuspid valve closure. In mitral stenosis the first sound is loud because prolonged flow of blood through the narrowed valve means that the valve is wide open at the beginning of ventricular systole resulting in more forceful closure of the valve when the ventricle contracts. In the normal the cusps of the mitral valve have time to "float" into the closed position before the onset of ventricular systole. The first sound will vary in intensity if the valve is sometimes fully open and sometimes nearly closed when ventricular systole starts. This is the situation in complete heart block (when atria and ventricles are beating completely independently) and in ventricular tachycardia which is always slightly irregular so that the cusps of the mitral valve are in a slightly different position at every ventricular systole. The second heart sound consists of two components, the first is due to closure of the aortic valve and the second to closure of the pulmonary valve. During inspiration, blood is drawn into the chest increasing the load on the right ventricle. The increased volume of blood takes longer to expel resulting in prolongation of right ventricular systole during inspiration and closure of the pulmonary valve occurs after the aortic valve.

Conditions prolonging systole of one ventricle will result in delaying the component of the second sound produced by that ventricle. Right bundle-branch block, pulmonary stenosis and atrial septal defect will delay the pulmonary component of the second sound resulting in audible aortic and pulmonary components widely separated, furthermore, the splitting may already be maximum in expiration so that increasing the volume of blood entering the right ventricle by inspiration will not result in any further splitting (fixed splitting). Conditions which increase the pressure in the pulmonary artery result in a narrowed split but a loud pulmonary second sound because of the rapidity with which the valve shuts. Pulmonary stenosis, in which there is a lowered pressure in the pulmonary arteries, results in a quiet pulmonary second sound, as the lowered pulmonary artery pressure does not shut the valve so abruptly and it causes a delay in the sound because of prolongation of right ventricular systole. In the case of the aortic valve, left ventricular systole is prolonged in aortic stenosis and in late activation of the left ventricle (left bundle-branch block). The aortic component may be so delayed that it occurs after the pulmonary component; if the pulmonary component is delayed normally during inspiration the two sounds may be superimposed so that only one sound is audible. This means that during inspiration only one sound is heard but in expiration two components are heard; this is the reverse of normal and is, therefore, called reversed or paradoxical splitting. Reversed splitting may occur in the absence of left bundle-branch block; it is then a sign of left ventricular dysfunction and occurs commonly following myocardial infarction. High systemic pressure or reduced elasticity of the aorta will result in forceful closure of the aortic valve and a loud aortic component to the second sound.

The third heart sound occurs during the period of rapid filling of the ventricles (at least 0·12 sec. after the second sound), it is caused partly by sudden distension of the ventricular walls—mainly the wall of the left ventricle—and partly by turbulent flow at the mitral valve. Conditions which cause early rapid filling of the ventricles will produce a pathological third sound: heart failure (in which venous pressure is elevated causing rapid flow into the ventricle), mitral incompetence, ventricular septal defect and constrictive pericarditis (by holding the ventricular walls apart and thus allowing a sudden influx of blood). A third sound is physiological in youth (up to the age of 40).

The fourth sound is due to contraction of the atria—this occurs at the end of the diastole and is responsible for ejecting the remaining small volume of blood into the ventricles (the ventricles fill mainly due to hydrostatic pressure of blood in atria and great veins). The occurrence of the fourth sound at the end of the diastole is the reason for its alternative name—presystolic triple rhythm (the rhythm that occurs with a third sound is sometimes called protodiastolic). The fourth sound will be heard in conditions which hinder the filling of the ventricles at the end of diastole, the most usual causes are left ventricle failure and myocardial infarction or ischaemia in which the fibrotic or necrotic myocardium is more resistant to distension than normal. In tachycardia the third and fourth sounds cannot be identified separately and are heard as one sound—summation gallop.

The opening snap is a high pitched sound, best heard at the left sternal edge; it occurs in mitral stenosis. The sound is due to sudden rapid opening of the mitral valve because of the elevated left atrial pressure—the higher the atrial pressure the quicker the valve will open. The height of the left atrial pressure is related to the severity of the valve stenosis. Hence, the earlier the opening snap occurs in diastole the more severe the stenosis. If the valve is heavily calcified it is unable to open as quickly as if it is supple, therefore an opening snap is unusual in calcific mitral stenosis (this is not an absolute rule—there are exceptions). The opening snap does not usually occur if there is associated mitral incompetence.

At the beginning of ventricular contraction the aortic and pulmonary valves open and blood is ejected into the aorta and pulmonary arteries. Dilatation or rigidity of these vessels will result in turbulence of blood or in excessive vibration of their walls leading to a high pitched sound called an "ejection click". Hypertension, atherosclerosis and post-stenotic dilatation may cause early systolic ejection clicks. Clicks also occur in pulmonary and aortic valve stenosis (without post-stenotic dilatation) and are due to vibration of valve cusps resulting from the high rate of flow (because of the narrowing) across them. The importance of clicks is that they do not occur in stenosis other than at the valve. Occasionally pulmonary and aortic "stenosis" is due to narrowing below the valve, this may be muscular narrowing (hypertrophic obstructive cardiomyopathy) or more rarely fibrous narrowing. Narrowing above the valves is exceptionally rare.

MURMURS

The loudness of murmurs depends on the quantity of blood flowing past the lesion which causes them. During ventricular systole blood is pumped into a high pressure system (the aorta)—the speed of flow increases as ventricular pressure increases and then decreases as the high pressure system becomes full. If outflow from the ventricle is narrowed a murmur is produced whose loudness increases to a maximum and then declines; because they occur during ejection of blood such murmurs are called "ejection" murmurs (*synonyms:* "diamond shaped" murmurs and crescendo-decrescendo murmurs). If the flow of blood from the ventricle is into a low pressure chamber of large volume, blood will begin to flow at the beginning of ventricular contraction and will continue to the end of systole unabated, such murmurs are, therefore, called pansystolic (holosystolic) and occur in incompetence of the atrio-ventricular valves (separating high pressure ventricles from low pressure atria). The definition of an ejection murmur is, therefore, one whose maximum intensity is near mid-systole and a pansystolic murmur is one more or less equally loud throughout systole.

Diastolic murmurs occur when blood is flowing into a ventricle during diastole either from the aorta or pulmonary artery because of incompetence of their valves, or from the atria through a narrowed atrioventricular valve. Like systolic murmurs their loudness will depend on the volume of blood flowing. In the case of aortic incompetence the pressure is higher in the aorta at the beginning than at the end of diastole (the pressure falls off as blood is distributed to the arterioles). In the case of mitral stenosis the murmur will be loudest during the period of maximum ventricular filling which is towards mid-diastole and during the ejection of the last portion of blood from the atria (i.e., during atrial systole). The murmur of aortic (and pulmonary) incompetence begins early in diastole and then gradually wanes, whereas the murmur of mitral stenosis begins towards mid-diastole (after the opening snap), wanes and then rises again as the atrium contracts. The longer blood takes to enter the ventricle from the left atrium the tighter is the stenosis, hence, the severity of the stenosis can be judged by the length of the murmur. The auscultatory methods of assessing the severity of uncomplicated mitral stenosis are:

1. Length of the mid-diastolic murmur.
2. Closeness of the opening snap to the second sound.
3. Loudness of the first heart sound.

The site and radiation of a murmur is often as important as its character in deciding its origin. Sounds arising from the cardiovascular system seem to be better conducted to the surface through blood than through tissues; murmurs from the aortic valve will, therefore, be heard best when blood in contact with the valve is nearest the surface, i.e., over the ascending aorta (second right intercostal space), and over the left ventricle (i.e., apex). Murmurs originating from the mitral valve will be heard over the left ventricle but the left atrium is too deep to conduct sound to the surface. This phenomenon gives rise to one of the most useful rules in cardiology, namely murmurs arising from the base of the heart (aortic and pulmonary valves) are often heard at the apex, but murmurs arising from the apex (mitral and tricuspid valves) are never heard at the base. The main use of this rule is in distinguishing a long aortic ejection systolic murmur (which sounds like a pansystolic murmur) from a true pansystolic murmur arising from the mitral valve or a ventricular septal defect. Murmurs arising from the right side of the heart will generally be louder during inspiration due to increased blood entering the right side of the heart.

The effect of various drugs on murmurs is of little value in practice. Amyl nitrate causes vasodilatation and increases venous return leading to an increase in the murmur of pulmonary stenosis. After a few more seconds the murmur of aortic stenosis will increase (when the increased venous return reaches the left side of the heart). Vasopressor drugs such as phenylephrine which increase peripheral resistance and hence left ventricular pressure increase the intensity of murmurs arising from mitral incompetence and left-to-right shunt such as ventricular septal defect. In practice these drugs may also affect the pulmonary vascular resistance and so are not used widely.

Grading of murmurs.—In order to communicate in a shorthand way the intensity and duration of murmurs their loudness and length can be graded. There are two conventions of grading; one has six grades of loudness and length and the other four grades. It is good practice always to record *graphically* the auscultatory findings.

Innocent and Functional Murmurs

Functional murmurs are murmurs which arise in the absence of organic disease at their site of origin, e.g. the ejection systolic murmur at the pulmonary area in an ASD or the diastolic murmur at the mitral valve in a VSD. The aortic and/or pulmonary systolic murmurs which are present in anaemia, thyrotoxicosis and pyrexias are also examples of functional murmurs.

Innocent murmurs are a common source of confusion and considerable experience is sometimes required in deciding whether a murmur indicates underlying heart disease or not and whether further cardiac investigation is indicated. As a rule all innocent murmurs are systolic in timing; they are heard only over a small area and do not radiate widely; they are *not* loud and often vary with the patient's posture. It is axiomatic that the ECG and chest x-ray should be within normal limits and the patient be free of cardiac symptoms if a murmur is assumed to be innocent. A previous history of rheumatic fever or a rheumatic fever type of illness (pain in the joints or confinement to bed with an undiagnosed illness during childhood) should make one very wary of diagnosing an innocent murmur.

Examples of Innocent Murmurs

1. Cardiorespiratory murmur. Most of these are due to obstruction to blood flow to a small part of the left lung overlying the heart. Some are possibly due to distortion of the pulmonary valve cusps from traction on the pulmonary artery by surrounding lung. These murmurs are nearly always systolic and are loudest in inspiration.

2. Venous hums. These are often loudest in diastole or may be continuous. They are common in childhood, pregnancy and thyrotoxicosis. They are usually best heard at the base of the heart and at the root of the neck. They are loudest in inspiration and in the upright posture because of increased venous return with these manoeuvres; the murmur

may become louder when the head is turned away from the side being auscultated because of stretching and narrowing of the jugular veins on the side being examined. Venous hums can usually be abolished by the Valsalva manoeuvre, lying down and manual compression of the jugular veins. The most difficult differential diagnosis is usually a patent ductus arteriosus.

3. Pericardial sounds—due to pleuro-pericardial adhesions. These are often very variable in their site, timing and variation with respiration. They can sometimes be increased by firm pressure of the diaphragm of the stethoscope on the precordium.

4. Carotid and arterial bruits are fairly common in normal people.

5. Chest deformity may cause a short systolic murmur.

6. Still's murmur is any high-pitched, innocent, systolic, apical murmur occurring during childhood.

7. Mammary souffle—due to dilated arteries and veins in the breast during pregnancy.

ELECTROCARDIOGRAPHY

Muscular contraction of the myocardium is associated with a change in the surface charge on individual muscle cells (depolarisation). The electrocardiogram measures the summation of the surface charges of all muscle cells in the myocardium. It is convenient to place the electrical contacts for recording these changes at a number of sites on the body which have been found empirically to reflect either electrical activity of a known part of the heart or flow of electricity in a known direction. The limb leads reflect the amount of electricity flowing in their direction and the chest leads (V leads) show the electrical activity in the part of the heart which they overlie.

It is conventional to describe the flow of electricity during ventricular contraction in terms of the predominant direction of flow (a system which describes both direction and strength of flow is known as a vector system). The Einthoven[6] triangle is a convenient mnemonic for remembering which ECG leads are attached where and in what direction electricity is flowing when one limb lead shows a bigger deflection than another (Fig. 3a).

Example: if the biggest QRS deflection of any of the limb leads is in lead II then the QRS vector is said to be $+60°$. This is the direction of flow of the largest amount of electricity when viewed from the front; it is, therefore, the mean frontal QRS vector.

The direction of flow of electricity could be viewed from other sites, e.g., from the side or from above, however, these other sites are not as useful as considering the flow of electricity from in front. From Fig. 3b

6. WILLEM EINTHOVEN (1860–1927). Leyden physiologist.

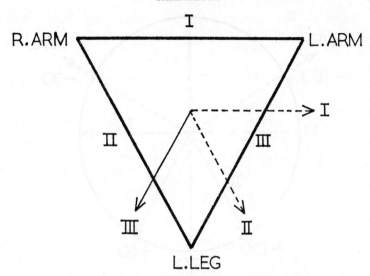

FIG. 3(*a*).—Einthoven triangle showing the direction of the three limb leads parallel to the sides of the triangle.

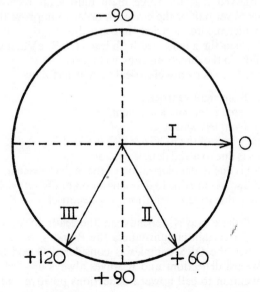

FIG. 3(*b*).—Direction of limb leads viewed from the front.

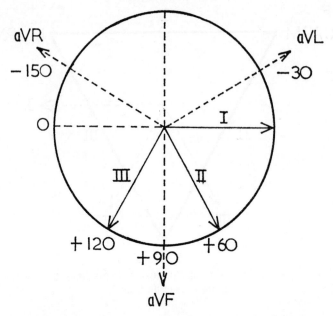

FIG. 4.—Direction of standard and augmented limb leads viewed from the front.

it will be observed that the three main limb leads record electricity flowing in the lower half of the circle; in order to improve the "pick up field" leads which record electricity in other directions are introduced— these are known as the augmented limb leads (aVR, aVL, and aVF) and they record flow in the directions shown (Fig. 4).

The chest or V leads record electrical activity as follows:

V1 + V2—from right ventricle.
V3 + V4—from interventricular septum.
V5 + V6—from left ventricle.
The normal waves of the ECG are P Q R S and T.
The P wave is due to atrial depolarisation.
The Q wave is due to depolarisation of the interventricular septum.
The R and S waves are due to depolarisation of the ventricles.
The T wave is due to repolarisation of the ventricles.

The size of these waves depends on the leads in which they are recorded. Under certain circumstances the P and T waves may be inverted but when the QRS complex is considered Q and S waves are always downward deflections and R waves always upward deflections. It is the convention to call upward deflections positive and downward deflections negative.

(Note this may give rise to confusion because in the frontal plane vector reference circle directions below the horizontal are positive and above the horizontal are negative.)

The Normal Direction of the QRS Vector

The lead in which the positive deflection is greatest is taken as the direction of the QRS vector. Usually it is accurate enough to note the height of the R wave but strictly speaking the depth of any negative deflection (Q or S) should be subtracted from the height of the R wave to determine the lead in which the true positive deflection is the greatest.

Noting the lead in which the negative deflection is maximum is a useful method of checking the direction of the vector (which will be in a direction diametrically opposite the lead with the greatest negative deflection). The lead in which the sum of the positive and negative deflections is zero is the lead at right angles to the vector.

In normal adults the mean frontal QRS vector should be between $0°$ and $+110°$. Vectors of $0°$ to $-90°$ are known as left axis deviation and vectors more than $+100°$ as right axis deviation. Conditions which alter the mechanical position of the heart may also alter the direction of the vector. For example left axis deviation may be caused by a high diaphragm due to ascites or pregnancy as well as hypertrophy of the left ventricle. Right axis deviation is normal in young children and occurs in right ventricular hypertrophy.

Examples of frontal QRS vectors.—(i) Figure 5: the frontal QRS vector is $+105°$. The leads with the largest positive QRS complexes are leads II, III and aVF which means that the vector lies between $+60°$ and $+120°$. The leads in which the total of the QRS complexes most nearly approaches zero are leads I and aVR; these are the leads which are nearly at right angles to the vector. Lead aVF is at right angles to lead I (see Fig. 4). On close inspection it will be seen that the negative deflection in lead I is slightly more prominent than the positive deflection, i.e., the vector is almost at right angles to lead I but is pointing slightly away from the direction of lead I; it lies around $+100°$. Applying the same rules to lead aVR (which records electricity at $-150°$), again the negative deflection is slightly more prominent, therefore, the vector is slightly less than $+120°$ (which is the direction at right angles to aVR), i.e., around $+110°$. We have now located the vector between $+100°$ and $+110°$ which for practical purposes we call $+105°$.

(ii) Figure 6: the frontal QRS vector is $+25°$. The leads with the biggest deflection are leads I and II, hence the vector lies between $0°$ and $+60°$. The size of the QRS complexes in aVL and aVF are more or less the same (slightly more in aVL). The direction midway between aVL $(-30°)$ and aVF $(+90°)$ is $+30°$. In fact the positive deflection is slightly more in aVL than aVF, therefore the direction is nearer aVL, i.e. less than $+30°$, say $+25°$. This is confirmed by the fact that the sum of the QRS complexes in lead III ($+120°$) is almost zero; in fact the negative deflection is slightly more than the positive, hence the vector is directed slightly away from lead III, more or less at right angles to it, i.e. at $+25°$.

MYOCARDIAL DAMAGE

A damaged myocardial cell loses its ability to pump out sodium and it becomes persistently electrically negative. At rest this results in the remainder of the myocardium having a slight negative charge. With contraction and depolarisation the remainder of the myocardium becomes electrically negative but the injured area cannot take part in this depolarisation so that although it is negatively charged it is not as much so as the remainder of the myocardium. This positivity as compared with the remainder of the myocardium causes elevation of the ST segments in the leads which face the area of damage. It is important to note that there is no experimental proof for this so-called current of injury away from a damaged area, it is really an ingenious explanation for an entirely empirical but extremely useful observation that when myocardial fibres are damaged there is elevation of the ST segments of some leads and depression of ST segments of other leads. The current of injury is found with damaged muscle but if the muscle dies then it is electrically silent and the ST segments revert to normal. If myocardial infarction involves the whole thickness of the wall of the ventricle it is electrically "silent" and any lead overlying the infarcted area will record electricity seen through the "window" of the infarcted area; in practice the electricity recorded through the "window" arises from the septum and is thus seen in the overlying lead as a Q wave. Thus, an area of myocardial ischaemia near the surface (subepicardial) is seen as elevation of ST segments and an area of complete infarction of the ventricular wall (transmural infarction) is seen as a Q wave in the appropriate leads.

Myocardial infarction of the right ventricle is very rare, all infarcts involve some part of the left ventricle. The distribution of the coronary arteries is variable, nevertheless it is possible to localise anatomically the site of the infarction as well as the likely blocked artery. The left coronary artery divides a few centimetres after its origin into left anterior descending which supplies the anterior surface of the left ventricle and the left circumflex which supplies the lateral part and the lower posterior (inferior) part of the left ventricle. The remainder of the posterior wall of the left ventricle is supplied by the right coronary artery. The order of frequency of occlusion is anterior descending (anterior and anteroseptal infarcts), right coronary (true posterior infarct) and left circumflex (anterolateral and inferior infarcts).

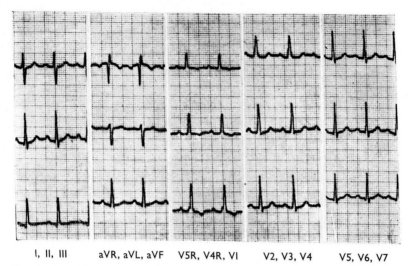

I, II, III   aVR, aVL, aVF   V5R, V4R, VI   V2, V3, V4   V5, V6, V7

FIG. 5.—ECG showing right ventricular hypertrophy. Note frontal plane QRS vector of $+105°$, tall R waves in V1, small S waves in V5 and 6 and T wave inversion in V1.

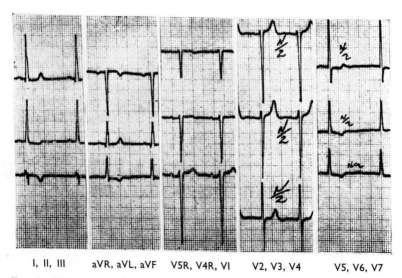

I, II, III   aVR, aVL, aVF   V5R, V4R, VI   V2, V3, V4   V5, V6, V7

FIG. 6.—ECG showing severe left ventricular hypertrophy. Leads V2 to V6 are recorded at half the normal sensitivity. Note QRS frontal plane axis of $+25°$, deep S wave in V1, tall R in V6 and inverted T waves in leads V6 and V7.

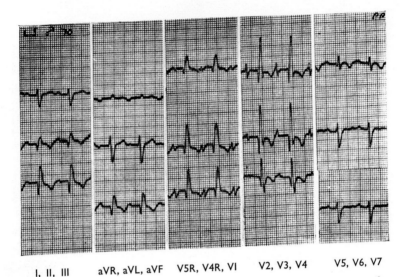

| I, II, III | aVR, aVL, aVF | V5R, V4R, VI | V2, V3, V4 | V5, V6, V7 |

FIG. 7.—ECG showing right bundle-branch block. Note widened QRS complexes beyond 0·12 sec., tall R wave in V1 and deep S wave in V6.

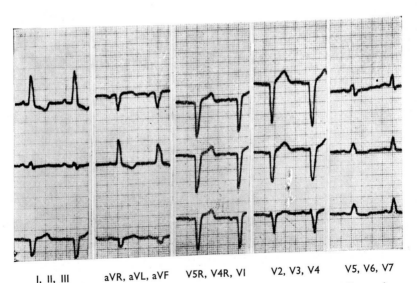

| I, II, III | aVR, aVL, aVF | V5R, V4R, VI | V2, V3, V4 | V5, V6, V7 |

FIG. 8.—ECG showing left bundle-branch block. Note widened QRS complexes but relatively normal shape and direction.

Patterns of infarction.—Subepicardial infarcts will have elevation of appropriate ST segments and transmural infarcts will have additional Q waves. Subendocardial infarcts can only be appreciated if they involve the anterior surface (they cause symmetrical inversion of the T waves).

Anterior infarcts:
    Changes in lead I, aVL and V1, 2 and 3

Anteroseptal infarcts:
    Changes in lead I, aVL, and V3, 4 and 5

Anterolateral infarcts:
    Changes in lead I, aVL and V4, 5, 6 and 7

Posterior infarcts:
    Tall R waves only in leads V1 and 2

(Q waves do not occur because the "window" is at the back of the heart and ST segment changes do not occur because none of the leads lies over the infarcted area.) The reason for the tall R waves in the right ventricular leads is that with loss of the posterior wall of the heart the leads record straight from the anterior wall without the effect of some neutralisation from electricity arising from the opposite side of the heart.

Inferior infarcts:
    Changes in lead II, III and aVF.

All the above changes indicate acute infarction.

As fibrosis and healing occur the Q waves usually remain but the ST depression and T inversion return to normal. These changes start after about seven days; the speed with which they occur is variable but usually the ST segments are isoelectric in three weeks after an acute infarct. The development of a ventricular aneurysm is suggested by persistent ST elevation.

It is important to note that Q waves are not always pathological, they are caused by normal septal depolarisation and are only abnormal in certain leads or if they are more than a certain size. They are usually normal in lead III but should be considered abnormal if they:

1. Exceed 0·04 second.
2. Exceed a quarter of the height of the R wave.
3. Are present in several leads.

Exercise electrocardiogram.—An ECG taken during and after exercise is sometimes helpful in deciding whether atypical chest pain is due to myocardial ischaemia. It is important to be aware of the limitations of the exercise ECG. The only *certain* sign of myocardial ischaemia on the exercise ECG is ischaemic elevation or depression of the whole of the ST segment of more than 1 mm—this alteration only occurs if the lumen of the coronary arteries is reduced to less than half the normal (Mattingly, 1962). A negative exercise ECG does not exclude myocardial ischaemia—approximately 25 per cent of patients with classical *angina* have a *normal resting* and *exercise* ECG. Other abnormalities are often seen in the exercise ECG and undoubtedly occur more frequently when there is myocardial ischaemia; however, these same abnormalities are also seen commonly in normal people so that these changes occurring in an individual patient with atypical chest pain must *not* be taken as evidence that the patient's pain is due to myocardial ischaemia. These changes are:

1. Frequent ectopic beats.
2. Widening of the QRS complexes.
3. T wave inversion.
4. Depression of the beginning of the ST segment.

Myocardial Ischaemia

(Coronary artery disease, coronary insufficiency, ischaemic heart disease or coronary heart disease.)

The ST elevation and Q waves described above imply actual infarction of myocardium; nevertheless, the myocardium may become transiently ischaemic due to narrowing of the coronary arteries. These are the signs of myocardial ischaemia, without infarction:

1. Divergence of QRS and T vectors of more than 60°. Transient T wave inversion may occur in the absence of ischaemia in a large number of conditions such as a heavy meal, hypoglycaemia, head injuries, exercise, smoking and hiatus hernia. Deep persistent inversion of the T waves is usually pathological.
2. Flat T waves in several leads.
3. Abnormally tall T waves.
4. Inverted U waves.
5. Depression of the ST segment.
6. An abnormally sharp angle between ST segment and T wave.
7. Left bundle-branch block.
8. QRS vector more than −30°.

Bundle-branch Block

The bundle of His[7] divides into right and left branches after leaving the atrioventricular node.

7. WILHELM HIS, jr. (1863–1934). Göttingen and Berlin physician.

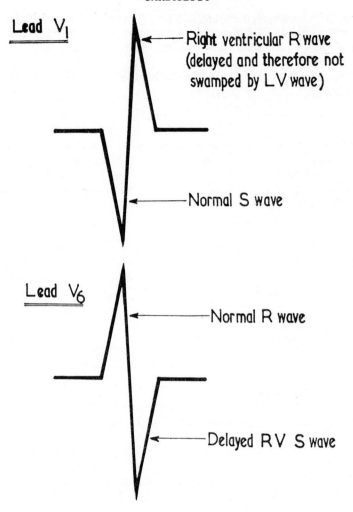

Lead V₁

Right ventricular R wave (delayed and therefore not swamped by LV wave)

Normal S wave

Lead V₆

Normal R wave

Delayed RV S wave

Prolongation of the QRS complex more than 0·12 seconds (3 small squares on the ECG paper) implies that there is delay in the spread of depolarisation—this is due to injury to either the right or left branches of the bundle of His. Lead V1 records electrical activity over the right ventricle, however, because the left ventricle is so much thicker than the right the electricity picked up by V1 is due to left ventricular activity as "seen by" a right ventricular lead. The electricity arising from the right ventricle is "swamped" by that from the left. In right bundle-branch block activation of the right ventricle is delayed but left ventricular activity is normal, therefore, in V1 right ventricular electricity is seen after the normal V1 deflection—it is seen as a positive R wave. Conversely in V6 right ventricular activity is seen after the normal R wave as an S wave. The characteristic patterns of right bundle-branch block are shown on page 23.

Figure 7 shows these patterns in an ECG.

In the chest leads left bundle-branch block is seen as prolongation of the QRS complexes but without alteration of their general shape and direction (Fig. 8).

In the limb leads right bundle-branch block is frequently accompanied by right axis deviation and left bundle-branch block by left axis deviation.

Ventricular Hypertrophy

In the limb leads hypertrophy of either ventricle is usually seen as right or left axis deviation. The increase in size of the hypertrophied ventricle causes an increase in the voltage recorded by leads over that ventricle. In the case of left ventricular hypertrophy (Fig. 6) the R wave is taller than normal in V6 (this is accompanied by a deep S and V1—since the S in V1 is also due to left ventricular electricity). In right ventricular hypertrophy (Fig. 5) the normally "hidden" right ventricular R wave in the S of V1 may appear and be more powerful than the LV S wave so that right ventricular hypertrophy is accompanied by a positive R wave in V1. If right ventricular hypertrophy is severe there may be delay in activation, i.e. the appearances may be those of right bundle-branch block. In addition there may be T wave inversion in leads recording the appropriate ventricle (lead I and V6 for the LV and lead III and V1 for the RV).

Hypertrophy of the atria, the left in mitral stenosis and the right in cor pulmonale, may also be appreciated in the ECG. The best lead is limb lead II; right atrial enlargement causes a tall P wave (P pulmonale) and left atrial enlargement causes a wide bifid P wave (P mitrale).

Arrhythmias

Atrial fibrillation.—This is the commonest. P waves are always absent and the ventricular rate is always totally irregular. *Atrial tachycardia* occurs when the sinus node or an ectopic atrial focus fires off impulses and the ventricles contract very rapidly. Some of the atrial impulses may be blocked at the atrioventricular node and the ventricles only respond to the impulses which are not blocked (atrial tachycardia with block). The ventricles usually respond to atrial impulse with a normal QRS complex; sometimes, however, conduction of the impulse in one of the branches of the bundle of His is disturbed and the ventricular QRS complex is abnormal or "aberrant".

At a normal rate an atrial ectopic focus may discharge prematurely, giving rise to an atrial extrasystole, in which case the P wave is abnormal in shape and the P-R interval abnormally short.

Atrial flutter.—This consists of regular rapid atrial discharges some of which are regularly blocked by the atrioventricular node so that the ventricular rate is slower. Because of the difficulty in distinguishing different types of tachycardia arising from the atria or atrioventricular node such tachycardias are frequently called "supraventricular" tachycardias.

Atrioventricular (A-V) nodal rhythms.—The shape of the ventricular QRS complex is usually normal. Electrical impulses may be conducted upwards towards the atria from the A-V node giving rise to an inverted P wave. This P wave may precede, be lost in, or follow the ventricular QRS complex.

Ventricular ectopic beat.—Conduction of the QRS complex is always abnormal and usually resembles the complexes of either right or left bundle-branch block. They may occur singly or in groups as a ventricular tachycardia; there are no preceding P waves.

Distinction between Supraventricular and Ventricular Tachycardias

1. No P waves in ventricular tachycardia.
2. Supraventricular tachycardia is usually perfectly regular whereas a ventricular tachycardia is usually slightly irregular.
3. In ventricular tachycardia the first heart sound varies in intensity due to the slight irregularity causing variations in length of the diastolic pause.
4. Shape of QRS complexes will be normal in supraventricular tachycardia unless there is associated aberration.
5. The shape of the complexes in ventricular tachycardia will resemble any previous ventricular ectopic beats—if a previous ECG is available.
6. Carotid sinus compression may show a supraventricular tachycardia but not a ventricular tachycardia.

A-V block.—First degree: prolongation of the P-R interval. Second degree: some "dropped" beats, i.e. every P wave is not followed by a QRS complex. The Wenckebach[8] phenomenon is a particular type of second degree block in which the P-R interval becomes progressively longer before one beat is "dropped". The P-R interval then becomes short and the cycle is repeated.

Third degree A-V block occurs when none of the P waves trigger off ventricular complexes (complete heart block).

8. KAREL FREDERIK WENCKEBACH (1864–1940). Dutch physician who practised in Vienna.

Other Important ECG Abnormalities

Digitalis effect.—Shortened QRS complex, prolongation of P-R interval, T wave inversion, and coupling (alternate normal and ectopic beats). It is important to remember that almost every known arrhythmia may be caused by digitalis so that if a patient has been taking digitalis this should be considered as a possible cause. Characteristically digitalis slows the heart rate when given in therapeutic doses; nevertheless, if the dose exceeds the patient's needs a tachycardia may be produced which will aggravate pre-existing heart failure (which may lead to the mistaken conclusion that the patient is underdigitalised).

Hypocalcaemia causes prolongation of the Q-T interval, the normal Q-T interval varies according to the heart rate. The upper limits of normal with different rates are given in tables. The Q-T interval is also prolonged in any condition which delays repolarisation of the ventricles, such as myocardial ischaemia, myocarditis and procainamide.

Hyperkalaemia causes tall, pointed T waves and widening of the QRS complex.

Hypokalaemia causes flattening of the T waves, prominent U waves and prolongation of the P-R interval.

The Effect of Drugs on the Electrocardiogram (Surawicz and Lasseter, 1970)

The main mechanisms of action of drugs in altering the electrocardiogram are:

1. Direct effect on myocardial fibres.
2. Direct effect on conducting tissue affecting rate, rhythm and conduction.
3. Alterations of general haemodynamics or metabolism.
4. Structural damage to myocardium.
5. Combinations of 1–4.

Digitalis.—The effects of digitalis on ventricular repolarization cause:

1. Depression of the ST segments.
2. Decreased amplitude of the T wave often with reversed polarity.
3. Shortening of the Q-T interval.
4. Increase in amplitude of the U wave.

The characteristic sharp downward curve of the ST segment running into the inverted T wave gives rise to the so-called reversed correction mark configuration (i.e. ∨ instead of √). The effects of digitalis toxicity are often most marked in leads II, III, and aVF and in the right chest leads in contrast to the changes of left ventricular hypertrophy. Occasionally digitalis can produce elevation of the ST segment, pointed, inverted or upright T waves. It is essential to realize that the effects of digoxin on the ECG may last up to 6 weeks. Effects of digitalis on rhythm and rate include bradycardia, nodal rhythm, ectopic beats, supraventricular tachycardia, coupling and ventricular tachycardia.

Quinidine and procainamide.—Therapeutic doses usually slow the sinus rate and increase the P-R interval. In atrial fibrillation the rate is slower and atrial flutter may develop with an increase in the ventricular rate which may then slow if more quinidine is given; eventually sinus rhythm may be restored. These drugs in higher doses increase the duration of the QRS complex and causes lowering and widening of the T waves so that they resemble those seen in hypokalaemia. Toxic dose of these drugs cause gross widening of the QRS complexes, a high degree of A-V block and bradycardia.

Lignocaine.—Therapeutic doses of lignocaine do not produce any effects on the rate or form of the normal ECG although it may slow or abolish ventricular ectopic beats.

Phenytoin.—The most common affect of phenytoin is to slow the sinus rate and to produce some A-V block.

Propranolol. The main effect is to prolong A-V conduction and to reduce ventricular slowing. There is normally no change in the QRS complexes and T waves.

Suxamethonium.—This may produce hyperkalaemia in the presence of soft tissue injury.

Phenothiazines.—The main effects are prolongation of the Q-T interval with widening and lowering of the T waves.

Imipramine.—The effects are similar to those of phenothiazines. Supraventricular and ventricular tachycardia may also occur.

Emetine, chloroquine and antimony compounds.—These may produce non-specific T wave changes which are usually transitory and best seen in the right chest leads.

RADIOLOGY OF THE HEART

The heart size and silhouette as well as a number of other diagnostic features may be gleaned from a routine P-A film of the chest. The usual rules for inspection of chest x-rays should be observed (see p. 96). The size of the heart is best expressed as a percentage of the maximum diameter of the chest (the cardiothoracic ratio or CTR); this should normally be below 50 per cent. Care should be taken to exclude conditions which may increase the apparent size of the heart. These include:

Too short a distance between x-ray tube and plate (as in a portable x-ray).

Film not taken with the patient taking a full inspiration.

High diaphragm.
Bradycardia.
Pericardial effusion.
Depressed sternum.
Kyphoscoliosis.

Increase in the CTR in the absence of any of the above means enlargement of one or both ventricles. It is usually not possible to say with certainty on a P-A film which ventricle is enlarged, but left ventricular enlargement is said to produce a round apex which encroaches on the diaphragm. Right ventricular enlargement is said to produce a straight left border to the heart. In the lateral views it may be easier to distinguish isolated ventricular enlargement. When the left ventricle enlarges the cardiac silhouette is seen overlapping the spine in the left lateral view and in right ventricular enlargement the retrosternal translucency is encroached upon. It is generally thought that pure hypertrophy of either ventricle does not cause cardiac enlargement; if the heart is enlarged it implies dilatation as well as hypertrophy.

Left atrial enlargement is seen as an abnormal shadow below the left pulmonary artery in the plain film and in a barium swallow lateral film the barium filled oesophagus will be indented. The left main bronchus may be lifted upwards by a giant left atrium so that it comes off from the trachea at an angle of more than 45° from the vertical. Enlargement of the right atrium is seen on the right lower border of the cardiac silhouette.

Descriptions of the cardiac silhouette should begin at the left border of the upper mediastinum where a left-sided superior vena cava or subclavian artery may be seen. The normal structures seen in the silhouette should be described in order: the aortic knuckle may be enlarged, calcified, double as in coarctation or small in conditions with a low cardiac output such as mitral stenosis. Next, the left pulmonary artery, left atrium, left border of the heart (left ventricle), right atrium, right pulmonary artery and superior vena cava should be described. An overpenetrated film of the heart may show calcification in one of the valves or coronary arteries, it may also show left atrium, descending aorta or an abnormal shadow behind the heart such as a hiatus hernia, paravertebral abscess or collapsed left lower lobe. Calcification may occur in the coronary arteries (particularly the left), a ventricular aneurysm or pericardium. It is not possible to say for certain from a P-A film whether calcification is in the mitral or aortic valve—a working rule is to draw a line between the right cardiophrenic angle and the junction of pulmonary artery and left atrium—calcification above this line is probably in the aortic valve and below the line is probably in the mitral valve. Screening of the heart gives a much better idea of the site of the calcification: screening should also demonstrate the degree of pulsation of the cardiac silhouette, which is reduced in the presence of pericardial effusion, and any paradoxical (i.e., expanding during systole) pulsation suggestive of a ventricular aneurysm. Conditions associated with an increased pulmonary blood flow (such as an ASD) cause excessive movement of the pulmonary arteries ("hilar dance") which will be seen on screening.

The proximal pulmonary arteries may be enlarged in pulmonary hypertension, increased pulmonary blood flow or in post-stenotic dilatation due to pulmonary stenosis. The disal pulmonary arteries will be prominent ("pulmonary plethora") if there is increased flow. In pulmonary hypertension there is often an abrupt decrease in size of the pulmonary arteries ("peripheral pruning"). In Eisenmenger's syndrome the dilatation of the proximal pulmonary arteries is often gross. Haziness of outline of enlarged proximal vessels may be due to pulmonary oedema.

The upper lobe veins are prominent if there is an elevated left atrial pressure as in left ventricular failure or mitral stenosis. Anomalous pulmonary veins may be seen draining into the superior vena cava.

The lung fields should be carefully inspected for evidence of pulmonary oedema which may be manifested by:

1. Kerley's[9] "B" lines (septal lines) which are small, horizontal, parallel lines 1–2 centimetres in length occurring at the costophrenic angles. They are due to dilated lymphatics within the interlobar septa.
2. Pleural effusions either in the costophrenic angles or in the transverse or oblique fissures.
3. Ill-defined homogeneous opacities radiating out from the hila.
4. Bilaterial lower zone haziness.
5. Haziness over the whole of the lung fields.
6. Dilation of the upper lobe veins.
7. Hazy outline to the hilar vessels.

Rarely pulmonary oedema may occur in one lung only, the explanation for this is not known. Other abnormalities in the lung fields which may occur with heart disease are:

1. Deposition of haemosiderin which may calcify or ossify.
2. Pulmonary infarcts.
3. Notching of the under surface of the upper ribs may occur in coarctation of the aorta.

Occasionally pulmonary oedema occurs when the heart size is not increased. These are the main conditions to think of:

9. Peter James Kerley. Contemporary radiologist, Westminster Hospital, London.

1. Constrictive pericarditis.
2. Mitral stenosis.
3. Constrictive type of cardiomyopathy.
4. Blocked lung lymphatics (e.g. in pneumoconiosis and silicosis) preventing normal drainage of fluid from the lungs.
5. Viral pneumonias.
6. Inhalation of toxic fumes.
7. Head injury or cerebrovascular accident.

CARDIAC CATHETERISATION

The purposes of catheterising the heart are to sample blood, to measure pressures and to inject radio-opaque contrast material. The right heart is catheterised via a peripheral vein, usually the saphenous or median basilic in the antecubital fossa. The aorta and left ventricle are catheterised by inserting the catheter into the femoral artery by the Seldinger[10] technique. This is ingenious and simple: a needle is inserted into the femoral artery through which a fine guide wire is fed into the artery, the needle is withdrawn over the wire which is left in the artery. The intra-arterial catheter is then threaded onto the wire and when the end of the catheter is near the artery both the wire and catheter are advanced together; when the catheter is in the lumen of the artery the guide wire is withdrawn.

The pressures and wave forms of every chamber entered are recorded. The ventricular and atrial pressures are necessary in order to know the extent to which a lesion may be putting a strain on the appropriate chamber. The gradient across the aortic or pulmonary valve during systole is a measure of the narrowing of the valve. Normally the systolic pressure in the left ventricle and aorta is the same but if the valve is narrowed the pressure in the aorta will be low and in the ventricle high, this difference in pressure is the gradient. The same is true of the pulmonary valve. The site at which the gradient occurs indicates the site of the stenosis; this is important if it is anticipated that the stenosis is below the valve (subvalvar or infundibular) as in hypertrophic obstructive cardiomyopathy. Mitral stenosis causes an elevation of left atrial pressure, this can be indirectly recorded by "wedging" a catheter into a distal pulmonary artery. The left atrial pressure is transmitted to the pulmonary veins and back to pulmonary arterioles. Thus, it is possible to know left atrial pressure without catheterising the left heart.

If a shunt is suspected the oxygen saturation of the blood at known sites is estimated; the site at which there is an increase of oxygen saturation in the right heart will indicate the level of a left-to-right shunt. The extent of the step up in oxygen saturation will indicate the size of the

10. S. I. SELDINGER. Contemporary Swedish radiologist.

shunt. The cardiac output can be calculated if the mixed venous (right atrial) and arterial oxygen saturations and the amount of oxygen consumed in a given time are known (Fick[11] principle). Another method of demonstrating a shunt is by dye dilution curves. An instrument which can detect the presence of a dye in the blood is attached to the lobe of the ear. Dye is injected in the right side of the heart; if a right-to-left shunt is present, the dye will appear early at the ear ("early appearance time") because it has not had to go through the lungs to enter the left heart. In a left-to-right shunt with the dye injected into the right heart, it traverses the lungs and enters the left heart; some will return to the right heart via the left-to-right shunt and will again pass through the lungs into the left heart. The instrument will, therefore, record a normal peak and a second smaller peak ("recirculation peak").

Angiocardiograms taken during the injection of radio-opaque material will delineate the heart chambers. To demonstrate the extent of leakage of a valve a cine-angiogram is preferable; to demonstrate disordered anatomy of a valve or chamber a series of bi-plane "stills" are better.

RHEUMATIC FEVER

The incidence of rheumatic fever is declining in highly developed countries but it is still common in the underdeveloped countries. The diagnosis of rheumatic fever is facilitated by application of the diagnostic criteria formulated by Ducket Jones and known by his name (American Heart Association, 1956). The major criteria are the cardinal features of rheumatic fever. The minor criteria are non-specific evidence of a systemic disorder which gives an indication of the progress of the disease or evidence of previous streptococcal infection.

DUCKET JONES[12] CRITERIA FOR THE DIAGNOSIS
OF RHEUMATIC FEVER

Major Criteria	Minor Criteria
1. Carditis (unexplained murmurs, congestive heart failure, cardiac enlargement).	1. Fever.
	2. Raised ESR or leucocytosis.
	3. Previous attack of rheumatic fever.
2. Arthritis.	
3. Rheumatic nodules.	4. Arthralgia.
4. Sydenham's[13] chorea.	5. Prolonged P-R interval on the ECG.
5. Erythema marginatum.	
	6. Raised ASO titre, or streptococcal sore throat.

11. ADOLF FICK (1829–1910). German physician.
12. THOMAS DUCKET JONES (1899–1954). American physician.
13. THOMAS SYDENHAM (1624–1689). English physician.

At least one major and two minor or two major and one minor criteria must be present to make the diagnosis.

In practice difficulties of diagnosis arise in children who develop polyarthritis due to other causes. These are frequently associated with fevers, raised ESR and often with a raised ASO titre. Since these fulfil the necessary criteria they may be diagnosed as rheumatic fever. Common causes of a febrile polyarthritis in children are Henoch[14]-Schönlein[15] purpura, Still's[16] disease, arthralgia of German measles and Reiter's syndrome in teenaged boys.

Treatment of Rheumatic Fever

The most important factor in assessing the prognosis is the state of the heart when the patient is first seen. If there is no evidence of carditis when first seen subsequent valve lesions are unlikely to develop. Evidence of mild carditis (prolonged P-R interval and pericardial friction rub) is associated with a low incidence of valve lesions. Recurrent attacks of rheumatic fever follow the same pattern as first attacks; carditis in a first attack is likely to be associated with carditis in subsequent attacks.

Several controlled trials have not shown that corticosteroids have a long-term advantage over salicylates in the treatment of acute attacks (Bywaters and Thomas, 1962; Combined Rheumatic Fever Study Group, 1965). However, other observers believe that steroids given early in the attack do prevent valve damage (Dorfman et al., 1961; Wilson, 1960). Attacks of rheumatic fever associated with severe carditis should be treated with corticosteroids. Salicylates will relieve the fever and joint pain. The duration of treatment is variable; in the absence of carditis six weeks' treatment will usually be sufficient. If there is carditis twelve weeks' treatment is the rule with a gradual reduction of the dose provided the ESR and fever do not rise and the child continues to gain weight.

Prophylaxis

Following an attack of rheumatic fever associated with carditis patients should be kept on long-term antibiotic prophylaxis against subsequent streptococcal infections, either with oral penicillin taken *twice* daily or (more effectively) with monthly injections of benzathine penicillin. A previous attack of rheumatic fever not associated with carditis warrants continuous oral prophylactic penicillin. The age of 15 is the arbitrary age at which prophylaxis is stopped provided there has not been an attack of rheumatic fever for five years. As to the treatment of sore throats in children who have not had rheumatic fever, mild sore throats should probably not receive routine penicillin unless there is

14. EDUARD HEINRICH HENOCH (1820–1910). Berlin paediatrician.
15. JOHANNES LUCAS SCHÖNLEIN (1793–1864). Berlin physician.
16. SIR GEORGE FREDERIC STILL (1868–1941). London paediatrician.

bacteriological evidence of streptococcal infection or the sore throat is likely to be part of an epidemic of streptococcal sore throats or there are severe toxic manifestations (high fever, headaches, vomiting and difficulty in swallowing).

VALVE LESIONS

Mitral Stenosis

The mitral valve consists of two cusps, the larger is the aortic cusp and is situated close to the aortic valve, the smaller is the septal cusp. The cusps are prevented from inverting by the cordae tendinae which are anchored to the ventricular wall by the papillary muscles. Narrowing of the valve orifice is due to inflammation of the cusps causing them to fuse. The normal size of the mitral orifice is 5 sq. cm. The area must be more than halved before there is any significant haemodynamic effect. In the presence of stenosis the left atrium has to contract more forcibly to pump blood into the left ventricle leading to the presystolic murmur during atrial contraction. However, most blood enters the ventricle passively in the middle of diastole; as blood flows through the narrowed orifice turbulence is produced which results in the mid-diastolic murmur. Other associated signs are the loud first sound and the opening snap.

The elevated left atrial pressure is transmitted back to the pulmonary veins, this causes reflex vasoconstriction of the pulmonary arterioles which may become fixed and irreversible. This happens in about 20 per cent of mitral stenotics and may occur when the stenosis is mild—it does not depend on the severity of the stenosis. The pulmonary artery pressure becomes elevated resulting in right ventricular hypertrophy. Intermittent pulmonary oedema may occur due to the raised pulmonary venous pressure. As the disease progresses the left atrium dilates and fibrillates; this may be responsible for a sudden deterioration of symptoms; if the atrium contains clot the onset of fibrillation may cause a systemic embolus.

Haemoptysis is a common symptom of mitral stenosis and may be due to:

Rupture of a pulmonary vein.
Rupture of a bronchial vein.
Pulmonary infarction.
Associated chronic bronchitis.
Pulmonary haemosiderosis.
Rarely, rupture of a pulmonary arteriole.

The assessment of a case of mitral stenosis involves consideration of symptoms, auscultatory findings, chest x-ray, electrocardiogram (whether there is any evidence of right ventricular hypertrophy), screening of the heart (to detect valve calcification) and occasionally right heart catheterisation.

The purpose of right heart catheterisation is to measure the pulmonary artery pressure, this is normally done before and after exercise. The pressure may be normal at rest but in the presence of increased pulmonary vascular resistance there is a sharp rise on exercise. The pulmonary artery pressure of normals does not rise more than a few millimetres of mercury after exercise. It is also important to measure the height of the left atrial pressure—this is possible by "wedging" the catheter firmly in a pulmonary arteriole; this will accurately reflect left atrial pressure changes. The rate of decline of the x and y descent are noted. There is a slowing of the rate of descent analogous to the appearances of the jugular venous pulse in tricuspid stenosis (see page 7).

In the plain x-ray of the chest pulmonary hypertension is seen as increase in the size of the heart, and dilatation of the proximal pulmonary arteries. The peripheral pulmonary arteries end abruptly—"peripheral pruning". Elevation of left atrial pressure is suggested by left atrial enlargement, increased venous markings in the upper zones and decreased markings in the lower zone due to changes in regional pulmonary blood flow. Septal or Kerley's "B" lines at the bases are due to distended septal lymphatics associated with an elevated pulmonary venous pressure. Later pleural effusions, pulmonary haemosiderosis and pulmonary fibrosis may occur.

Mitral valvotomy is technically a simple operation; it is usually performed where there are facilities for open heart surgery because there is a risk that the valve will not split "cleanly" and torrential mitral incompetence may be produced which can only be treated by replacement with a prosthetic valve. The transventricular mitral valvotomy is performed by clamping the left auricle, making a small incision in it through which the surgeon passes a finger; the clamp is slowly released so that he can insert his finger into the left atrium and touch the mitral valve without any blood being lost. Through an incision in the wall of the left ventricle he passes a finger (and valve dilator) towards the mitral valve, guiding it with the finger in the left atrium. The incidence of re-stenosis following valvotomy used to be high, often necessitating a second and third valvotomy. The speed with which re-stenosis occurs increases with each valvotomy; the incidence following a first valvotomy was about 5 per cent after 5 years and as high as 40 per cent after 7 years (Lowther and Turner, 1962).

It is important to realise that the auscultatory methods of assessing mobility of the valve cusps are sometimes misleading. The first heart sound may be loud and an opening snap present in a few cases in which the valve is calcified or very sclerotic. Furthermore mitral incompetence may be present with a loud first sound and an opening snap—it used to be thought that these two auscultatory findings excluded significant mitral incompetence (Turner, 1968).

Mitral Incompetence

The mitral valve may become incompetent as a result of (i) damage to the valve cusps either by rheumatic fever or bacterial endocarditis, (ii) dilatation of the fibrous valve ring, and (iii) distortion of the cusps by malfunction of the papillary muscles by which the cordae tendinae are attached to the ventricles. The papillary muscles are part of the ventricular muscle and may be involved in any disease affecting the myocardium, particularly myocardial infarction in which one papillary muscle may be infarcted. They are also affected in congestive heart failure, in which the papillary muscles may not function adequately in common with the remainder of the myocardium. The functional mitral regurgitation which occurs in left ventricular failure is probably due to papillary muscle dysfunction, as it usually rapidly disappears when the failure is controlled. The alternative suggestion that the functional incompetence is due to dilatation of the valve ring is less likely because the fibrous ring is stiff and hard and is unlikely to be able to decrease rapidly in size. The murmur which occurs with dysfunction of one papillary muscle may occur in any part of systole; it is often high-pitched and ejection in type. Damage to a papillary muscle can occur in myocardial infarction—particularly posterior infarcts.

A murmur similar to that of mitral incompetence may also be produced by myocardial infarction causing rupture of the interventricular septum; this is commoner with anteroseptal infarcts. In this case the murmur is usually pansystolic, best heard at the left sternal edge and frequently accompanied by a thrill and features of right heart failure if there is a significant left-to-right shunt.

Myxomas.—Clinical features which should alert one to the possibility of a left atrial myxoma simulating mitral valve disease are:

1. No history of rheumatic fever.
2. Female patients in the second half of life.
3. Unexplained episodes of severe congestive heart failure.
4. Short history of "mitral stenosis" with an intermittent murmur.
5. Absence of valve calcification.
6. Attacks of syncope, particularly related to alterations of position.
7. Systemic manifestation (fever, leucocytosis, raised ESR, anaemia and raised gamma globulin).
8. Systemic emboli in the presence of sinus rhythm.

Left atrial myxomas are much commoner than right; when myxomas do occur in the right atrium they may simulate lone tricuspid stenosis or constrictive pericarditis by causing signs of severe right-sided failure with a normal sized heart.

Aortic Stenosis and Coarctation

Narrowing is commonest at the level of the valve (valvar stenosis) and is either congenital (bicuspid valve) or due to rheumatic fever. Narrowing below the valve is much rarer and is either due to a fibrous diaphragm or due to abnormal muscular hypertrophy—hypertrophic obstructive cardiomyopathy. Narrowing above the valve (supravalvar stenosis) is extremely rare, it is congenital and often associated with idiopathic hypercalcaemia and a characteristic facies.

Aortic sclerosis consists of atherosclerotic hardening and irregularity of the cusps of the aortic valve without gross narrowing. Clinically, the character of the pulse is vital in diagnosing the cause of an ejection murmur at the aortic area. Valvar aortic stenosis is associated with an anacrotic pulse; aortic sclerosis with a normal pulse; and hypertrophic obstructive cardiomypopathy with a "jerky" pulse with a rapid upstroke. Severe aortic stenosis is accompanied by angina, which does not usually improve with trinitrin, syncope, particularly during exertion, and left ventricular failure. The murmur is conducted to the carotid vessels and to the apex and is accompanied by a diminished and delayed aortic second sound; excessive delay of the aortic second sound results in reversed or paradoxical splitting. Valvar stenosis is usually associated with an ejection systolic click, whether post-stenotic dilatation is present or not. Valvar stenosis of congenital origin does not usually cause calcification of the aortic valve whereas rheumatic valvar stenosis frequently causes valve calcification.

Indications for surgery.—Aortic stenosis in children and young adults may cause sudden death before any symptoms or ECG evidence of ventricular hypertrophy have developed. Operation on the aortic valve is usually considered if there is a systolic gradient of more than 50 mm Hg across the valve. In patients who have developed aortic stenosis later in life operation is not usually advised until moderate symptoms have developed or there is evidence of rapid deterioration of left ventricular function. There is evidence that calcific aortic stenosis developing in middle age affects valves which have been abnormal from birth.

Hypertrophic obstructive cardiomyopathy should be suspected if the pulse is "jerky", the murmur does not radiate into the neck, there is no ejection systolic click and the valve is not calcified. It is worth emphasising that aortic sclerosis is accompanied by the murmur of aortic stenosis but a normal pulse form.

Congenital aortic stenosis due to a bicuspid valve is frequently associated with coarctation of the aorta. Coarctation may occur at any level and may be multiple; however, by far the commonest site is immediately after the origin of the ductus arteriosus (adult type), narrowing above the ductus is usually more severe and is not often seen in adults (childhood type). The childhood type of coarctation is associated with a well-known but extremely rare feature, viz. cyanosis of the legs and clubbing of the toes with normal upper extremities. This is due to associated pulmonary hypertension, causing unsaturated blood to enter the lower aorta from the pulmonary artery through a patent ductus arteriosus. If the left subclavian artery originates below the patent ductus the left arm and hand will be cyanosed whereas the right will be normal.

Coarctation is much commoner in men and in Turner's syndrome than in otherwise normal women; it is frequently accompanied by other congenital abnormalities such as bicuspid aortic valves, mitral stenosis and berry aneurysms of the cerebral arteries. Berry aneurysms are due to congenital defects in the walls of the arteries which are usually situated at the bifurcation of the vessels; they do not usually enlarge until associated hypertension and atherosclerosis cause critical weakening.

The collateral arterial circulation which develops in severe coarctation results in palpable arterial pulsation on the back which is best seen with the patient leaning forward. The collateral arteries may cause a murmur which is indistinguishable from that of coarctation itself. Sometimes pressure on a palpable collateral artery will abolish the murmur if it is originating from the collaterals. Rib notching seen on the plain chest x-ray on the under surface of the upper ribs is due to enlarged intercostal arteries eroding the ribs.

Other causes of rib notching are:

1. Neurofibromatosis and enlargement of nerves (amyloidosis and congenital hypertrophic polyneuropathy).
2. Inferior vena cava obstruction.
3. Following a Blalock operation (left-sided only).
4. Rarely, congenital.

Coarctation may be associated with post-stenotic dilatation of the aorta and subacute bacterial endocarditis which usually affects the bicuspid aortic valve. The site of the coarct or the site where the stream of blood impinges on the arterial wall may be the seat of subacute bacterial aortitis.

The causes of elevated blood pressure in coarctation has not been established with certainty. The simplest explanation is that the narrowed aorta and collaterals provide a greater resistance to flow to the lower limbs than the upper, however, in many cases of coarctation the diastolic pressure is the same in both upper and lower limbs. Another suggestion is that reduced renal blood flow or pulse pressure is responsible for generalised hypertension of renal origin but the lower limbs are protected by the narrowed aorta. A third suggestion is that the arterioles of the upper limbs have developed differently from those of the lower (Pickering, 1968).

The usual causes of death in patients with coarctation are bacterial endocarditis, ruptured aorta, congestive cardiac failure and ruptured cerebral aneurysm. 25 per cent of patients survive to old age (Gross, 1950). Malignant hypertension is said never to occur. The operative mortality of uncomplicated cases is low and, if discovered during childhood, surgical correction of uncomplicated coarctation is usually advised around the age of 15.

The real dilemma arises in patients who have coarctation which is not discovered until adult life and who are entirely free of symptoms. Having reached adult life they could so easily belong to the 25 per cent of *all* cases which survive to old age, furthermore there is no guarantee that correction of the coarctation will reduce the blood pressure, and thirdly, the commonest cause of death is subacute bacterial endocarditis (SBE). If the patients are carefully observed and follow the precautions against SBE the chances of developing subacute bacterial endocarditis are reduced. If the patient is entirely free of symptoms, operation in the adult is normally performed only if hypertension is severe and difficult to control, or if there is cardiac enlargement or left ventricular hypertrophy. I think there is a strong case for performing carotid angiograms on such patients and advising operation if a cerebral aneurysm is found.

Aortic Incompetence and Aortic Aneurysms

Aortic incompetence in the absence of any other valve lesions is likely to be due to syphilis. This is even more likely if there is coronary ostial stenosis which causes angina not relieved by trinitrin or if there is dilatation of a calcified ascending aorta. None the less, the commonest cause of aortic incompetence is rheumatic fever and it is usually associated with mitral stenosis. Severe aortic incompetence from any cause may be associated with a mitral diastolic murmur if the regurgitant jet causes roughening of the aortic cusp of the mitral valve (Austin Flint[17] murmur). Mitral incompetence may occur if left ventricular failure causes papillary muscle dysfunction or dilatation of the mitral valve ring.

Other causes of aortic incompetence are:
1. Bacterial endocarditis.
2. Ruptured sinus of Valsalva.[18]
3. Atherosclerosis.
4. Marfan's syndrome.

17. AUSTIN FLINT (1812–1886). New York physician.
18. ANTONIO MARIA VALSALVA (1666–1723). Bologna surgeon and anatomist.

5. Aortic aneurysm.
6. Lathyrism.

Aortic incompetence causes an increase in the stroke volume, and this increased volume of blood usually produces an ejection murmur of functional aortic stenosis; on rare occasions this functional aortic stenosis can cause a systolic thrill even though there is no organic narrowing at the valve.

Patent ductus arteriosus causes signs which can be similar to those of aortic incompetence. In patent ductus the systolic murmur occurs late in systole, is usually accompanied by a thrill, is often heard posteriorly and is loudest anteriorly on the left side.

Aortic aneurysm.—Aneurysm of the ascending aorta is known as the "aneurysm of signs" because compression of the superior vena cava is marked. Compression of the right main bronchus may cause collapse of the right lung. Aneurysm of the arch of the aorta is known as the "aneurysm of symptoms" (compression of trachea, oesophagus, recurrent laryngeal nerve and stellate ganglion resulting in cough, dysphagia, hoarseness and Horner's[19] syndrome). Dissecting aneurysms are associated with a tearing pain which may mimic ischaemic cardiac pain but unlike myocardial infarction hypertension is usual in the early stages. Enlargement of the aorta as seen on the chest x-ray may not occur for several days after the dissection. Dissection may occur anywhere along the length of the aorta and occlusion of any of the branches of the aorta may occur including the coronary, carotid, spinal, renal and mesenteric arteries, although it is exceptional in cases of dissection to be able to detect any difference between the femoral pulses.

Dissection of the aorta should be suspected if severe chest pain is accompanied by any neurological signs, hypertension, evidence of bleeding, or abdominal pain. There may even be a rise in serum transaminases and ECG changes of ischaemia.

Pulmonary Stenosis

Like aortic stenosis the narrowing may be valvar, subvalvar or supravalvar. Valvar pulmonary stenosis is almost invariably of congenital origin. The physical signs include a pulmonary ejection systolic murmur accompanied by an ejection click, wide splitting of the pulmonary second sound which is diminished in intensity. Later, severe stenosis is accompanied by signs of right heart failure. The loudness of the pulmonary systolic murmur is not a good indication of the severity of the stenosis as mild stenosis usually produces a soft murmur, moderate stenosis a loud murmur and severe stenosis a soft murmur due to right heart failure causing a diminution in cardiac output. There may be post-

19. JOHANN FRIEDRICH HORNER (1831–1886). Zurich ophthalmologist.

stenotic dilatation with valvar stenosis and an ejection click; a click is not heard in subvalvar infundibular stenosis.

Subvalvar stenosis is often associated with a ventricular septal defect which causes functional muscular hypertrophy of the infundibulum (or outflow tract) of the right ventricle.

Stenosis of the main pulmonary arteries and branches occurs but is very rare. Peripheral pulmonary artery stenosis causes a murmur which is heard in systole and diastole over a large part of the chest and is, therefore, one of the rare causes of a continuous murmur.

Indications for surgery.—If the patient has pulmonary stenosis alone then symptoms and evidence of right ventricular hypertrophy are sufficient indications for resection even if the systolic gradient across the valve is small. In the absence of symptoms a systolic gradient approaching 100 mm Hg is the accepted indication for resection.

Pulmonary Incompetence

This is most frequently due to severe pulmonary hypertension—the resulting murmur is called the Graham Steell[20] murmur and is often surprisingly loud.

Tricuspid Incompetence

This is nearly always associated with lesions of other valves. However, lone tricuspid incompetence is being seen more frequently in drug addicts who develop bacterial endocarditis as a result of intravenous injection of unsterile drugs. It occurs in right-sided heart failure and is accompanied by a giant *v* wave in the JVP and systolic pulsation of an enlarged liver.

Tricuspid stenosis is almost always accompanied by some degree of incompetence. Characteristically, murmurs originating from the right heart increase on inspiration due to increased filling and hence output of the right heart.

Subacute Bacterial Endocarditis (SBE)

The commonest organisms responsible for SBE are *Streptococcus viridans*, *Streptococcus faecalis* and *Staphylococcus aureus*. Other rare causative organisms are pneumococci, *E. coli*, salmonella, brucella, haemophilus, *Candida albicans*, Q fever and possibly some viruses and mycoplasmas.

The left side of the heart is involved in over 90 per cent of cases. The two commonest causes of involvement of the right side are intravenous injections with unsterile syringes seen particularly in drug addicts in whom the tricuspid valve is frequently involved, and ventricular septal

20. Graham Steell (1851–1942). Manchester physician.

defects in which the endocarditis occurs in the right ventricle where the jet of blood from the left ventricle impinges on its wall. The practical importance of the predominance of left-sided involvement is that it may be necessary to culture arterial blood in order to grow the causative organism.

The main symptoms and signs are referable to cardiac involvement, septicaemia and embolic complications. There are two unexplained but well documented clinical observations with regard to the cardiac manifestations: the first is that SBE is uncommon in the presence of atrial fibrillation and the second is that the disease rarely occurs for the first time in the presence of heart failure, although heart failure is a common late complication.

Associated septicaemia is responsible for the fever, raised sedimentation rate, splenomegaly, clubbing, positive blood culture and anaemia. The anaemia is usually the anaemia of infection in which there is toxic depression of the bone marrow resulting in a normocytic normochromic anaemia. A Coombs positive haemolytic anaemia occurs occasionally. Leucocytosis usually occurs but is not invariable; occasionally there is a leucopenia. The gamma globulins are often raised and sometimes the rheumatoid and LE latex tests are positive in the absence of rheumatoid arthritis or SLE (Williams and Kunkel, 1962).

As a result of the septicaemia mycotic aneurysms may occur in any artery and abscesses in any organ. The embolism of fragments of the vegetations gives rise to some of the more exotic manifestations of SBE. Emboli are responsible for small renal infarcts ("flea-bitten kidney") which give rise to microscopic haematuria. In the skin emboli are seen as petechiae which characteristically occur in crops and have a white centre. Similar lesions occur in the conjunctivae, in the soft and hard palates and in the retina of the eye where they are referred to as Roth[21] spots. Other manifestations of SBE are splinter haemorrhage under the nails and café au lait pigmentation of the skin. It is important to note that splinter haemorrhages may occur in 20 per cent of the normal hospital population.

Osler's[22] nodes are said to be pathognomonic, they consist of crops of raised reddish nodules which are always tender and usually occur in the pulp of the fingers and palms of the hands. Another lesion which occurs on the palms and soles is the Janeway[23] lesion; this is never tender and consists of an area of erythema or haemorrhage which is not usually raised.

Arthralgia is fairly common in SBE and may cause confusion with acute rheumatic fever. The nodules of rheumatic fever may be confused

21. MORITZ ROTH (1839–1914). Basle pathologist.
22. SIR WILLIAM OSLER (1849–1919). Physician, Baltimore and Oxford.
23. EDWARD GAMALIEL JANEWAY (1841–1911). New York physician.

with Osler's nodes. However, the rheumatic nodule is not tender and is not in the skin, it is subcutaneous and the skin can be rolled over it. Rheumatic nodules usually last several weeks and the overlying skin is not red, they are often symmetrical in distribution and tend to occur over bony surfaces. The nodules of rheumatoid arthritis are similar to rheumatic nodules but are permanent and are associated with the characteristic joint deformity.

SBE is sometimes one of the most difficult diagnoses to make. It is important to appreciate that over a quarter of the cases occur in patients over the age of 60, that a cardiac murmur is not always audible, that a normal valve may become infected (particularly in children), that the disease presents with neurological signs and symptoms in approximately 20 per cent of cases and that infection is especially liable to occur following childbirth or urethral instrumentation.

Treatment of SBE

Prophylactic treatment consists of surgical correction of amenable congenital heart lesions and adequate penicillin cover for dental extractions; other procedures such as cystoscopy and childbirth should be covered with penicillin plus streptomycin, as the most likely infecting organisms is *E. coli*. All the teeth should be x-rayed and any which are very carious or associated with apical abscesses should be extracted. SBE is unusual in edentulous people and total dental clearance is sometimes recommended especially after second attacks of SBE.

The site of infection in SBE is usually avascular heart valves. Bacteriostatic antibiotics prevent organisms dividing and give the body's own defence mechanisms chance to destroy organisms; however, in SBE the infection is out of reach of the host's defence mechanisms, hence as a general rule bactericidal drugs are preferable to bacteriostatic.

Streptococcus viridans is the commonest cause of SBE and is always sensitive to penicillin; however, the degree of sensitivity varies. Organisms which are highly sensitive are treated with 500,000 units of benzyl penicillin 6-hourly. For organisms which are relatively resistant to penicillin much higher doses of penicillin are required. Up to 100 mega units a day may be necessary. Streptomycin 0·75 g twice daily is combined with penicillin for treatment of relatively resistant organisms. In patients over 50 years of age streptomycin should be stopped after two weeks because of its toxic effect on the vestibular branch of the eighth nerve. It should only be started again if there is a recurrence of fever. Penicillin and streptomycin are both bactericidal and are synergistic. High doses of penicillin are best administered by continuous intravenous infusion. There are certain disadvantages of very high doses of penicillin: if the sodium salt is given the high intake of sodium may precipitate heart failure—this can be overcome by giving the potassium salt. High doses of penicillin may cause cerebral oedema and haemolytic anaemia; they may also cause a slight fever even in a patient who is not normally penicillin sensitive—this may be taken as indication that the infection is not controlled. Treatment is usually continued for six weeks or until signs of infection (fever, leucocytosis, raised sedimentation rate and weight loss) have subsided.

The dose of antibiotic should be adjusted according to the lowest concentration which is completely bactericidal for the infecting organism. As a working rule the lowest blood level of the antibiotic should be five times as high as the least concentration necessary to kill the organism *in vitro*.

If no positive blood culture is obtained and there is strong clinical evidence of SBE, penicillin and streptomycin are given, starting with 10–20 mega units of benzyl penicillin a day and increasing the dose if the patient remains febrile after 48 hours. SBE due to other infecting organisms should be treated with large doses of the most suitable bacteriocidal antibiotic to which the organism is sensitive.

Mixed infections sometimes occur and may give rise to difficulty if only one of the organisms has been grown from the blood, particularly if a fever remains when antibiotics are given in adequate amounts to control the one organism which has been isolated. Blood cultures should always be taken at the height of a spike of fever and from arterial blood if samples of venous blood are persistently sterile in the face of continuing infection.

Death in SBE most commonly occurs from heart failure due to perforation of a valve cusp or rupture of a chorda tendineae. Perforation of an aortic valve cusp causes a rise in diastolic pressure in the left ventricle and early closing of the mitral valve with consequent fall in cardiac output and disappearance of the aortic diastolic murmur. There are three indications for emergency replacement of an infected valve:

1. The presence of drug-resistant organisms.
2. The development of recalcitrant infection around a mechanical prosthesis.
3. The development of intractable heart failure whatever the infecting organism or the stage of its treatment.

ISCHAEMIC HEART DISEASE

The myocardium may become ischaemic in the absence of narrowed coronary arteries as in severe left ventricular hypertrophy in which the myocardium outgrows its blood supply, and conditions in which the cardiac output is diminished such as aortic stenosis, tight mitral stenosis and severe pulmonary hypertension. By far the commonest cause of narrowing of the coronary arteries is atheroma; however other conditions are occasionally responsible:

1. Syphilis may cause stenosis of the origin of the coronary arteries (ostial stenosis).
2. Polyarteritis nodosa and giant-cell arteritis.
3. Coronary embolism—from valve vegetations; atrial thrombi, fat and air embolism.
4. Congenital coronary artery fistula shunting blood from the myocardium into the right side of the heart or pulmonary arteries.

Narrowing of the arteries due to atheroma occurs principally within a few centimetres of their origin. Complete occlusion is due to thrombus formation in a narrowed segment, haemorrhage beneath an atheromatous plaque (intramural haemorrhage) or dislodgement of a plaque. The clinical features of narrowing of the coronary arteries sufficient to cause myocardial anoxia are:

Myocardial infarction.
Heart failure.
Angina.
Arrhythmias.
Sudden death.

Factors Predisposing to Ischaemic Heart Disease

1. *Age.*—Although atheroma is found in the coronary arteries of children it increases progressively with age.
2. *Sex.*—Ischaemic heart disease is rare in women before the menopause although in Negroes the sex incidence is the same at all ages.
3. *Hypertension.*—The incidence is increased in hypertensives, nevertheless, the disease occurs in the absence of hypertension. In Japan, where hypertension is common, severe coronary artery disease is rare.
4. *Diabetes.*—The incidence is high in diabetics and people with a family history of diabetes. The majority of young men with clinical coronary artery disease have an abnormal glucose tolerance test (Wahlberg, 1962).
5. *Obesity.*—Life insurance statistics show an association between overweight and ischaemic heart disease; nevertheless the association is probably between obesity and hypertension. Obesity in the absence of hypertension is probably not a predisposing factor.
6. *Heavy cigarette smoking.*
7. *Sedentary occupation.*
8. *Heredity.*
9. *Height of serum cholesterol and diet.*
10. *Aggressive temperament.*

Pathogenesis of Atheroma

All the factors responsible for the deposition of lipids in atheromatous plaques are not known. An enormous amount of experimental and statistical research has not produced undisputed answers. For the clinician the problem resolves itself into deciding whether the level of serum cholesterol is a predisposing factor and, if it is, what prophylactic and therapeutic steps are of value in reducing the incidence of the disease. A brief account of the evidence will help to outline the complexity of the problem.

The blood lipids include:

1. Neutral fats or triglycerides.
2. Phospholipids, i.e. triglycerides combined with phosphates.
3. Cholesterol, which exists as free cholesterol (2/3) and cholesterol esters (1/3).

None of the blood lipids is soluble in water and they all circulate combined with plasma proteins. The plasma proteins involved are alpha and beta globulins which, when combined with lipids, are called alpha and beta lipoproteins; of these the beta lipoproteins carry much more lipid than the alpha lipoproteins, which are stable and do not vary greatly throughout life. The beta lipoproteins (also called low density lipoproteins) carry 80 per cent of the cholesterol. There is almost no end to the number of variables, each of which has been claimed to be the one most responsible for the pathogenesis of atheroma. Examples of possible important variables are:

1. The relative amount of α and β lipoproteins.
2. The amount of triglyceride present.
3. The proportion of cholesterol attached to α and β lipoproteins.
4. The relative amounts of free and esterified cholesterol attached to β lipoprotein.
5. The proportion of cholesterol to phospholipid attached to β lipoprotein.

From the available evidence, it is impossible to reach a firm conclusion; however, it seems probable that one parameter of importance is the serum concentration of cholesterol (both free and esterified) and that the incidence of coronary artery disease is increased if there is a persistent rise in the serum cholesterol (Kannel et al., 1964).

DIET, CHOLESTEROL, ATHEROMA AND CORONARY ARTERY DISEASE

Several prospective trials are in progress to try and produce incontrovertible evidence that methods of reducing the blood cholesterol also lessen the likelihood of an individual's developing *recognisable* coronary artery disease. At the outset it can be said that the evidence is not yet irreproachable that lowering the cholesterol reduces the incidence of the disease; however there are strong *pointers* that a raised level of cholesterol in the blood is in some groups of people causally related to atheroma. There is enough conflicting evidence for anybody to take up a fixed position and espouse dogmatically one or other extreme, holding fast to that evidence with which he concurs and eschewing that which is inconvenient. It is an axiom of preventive medicine and *presymptomatic* diagnosis that it is wrong to detect a disease for which no treatment is available. With regard to the cholesterol problem it is possible to say that the chance of developing coronary artery disease is increased by finding that the serum cholesterol is *consistently* raised; that the disease can *probably* be delayed in some people with a raised cholesterol, by attempting to lower the cholesterol by means which *some* people find burdensome; but that the disease *usually* develops when the serum cholesterol is normal, and that other factors collectively are *probably more* important in causing the disease. This is probably about as fair a general statement about the importance of cholesterol and coronary artery disease which can be made—many careful and thoughtful people feel that in this statement there are too many words like "usually", "probably", "some", and "chance" to advise routine measuring of the cholesterol in the general population or the widespread introduction of cholesterol-lowering diets or drugs. Other equally careful and thoughtful people say—we agree proof is lacking but the pointers are strong and unless we detect (and treat) our young men we are ignoring the pointers, and that with a relatively simple alteration in daily living the incidence of the disease can be reduced. As yet there is *no proof* which set of people is adopting the right attitude to the cholesterol problem.

For the middle-of-the-roaders it is possible to make a reasonable practical statement:—A *persistently* raised serum cholesterol is *one* of the adverse factors predisposing to the development of coronary artery disease—if there is a known second adverse factor present in a particular patient then it is wise to *treat both* adverse factors. If a marginally raised cholesterol is the only identifiable adverse factor the patient should not be informed or advised to alter his diet or be given cholesterol-lowering drugs. The evidence is not yet convincing enough to recommend routine cholesterol-lowering diets or drugs in everyone or the adoption of widespread measuring of the serum cholesterol.

Second adverse factors which would warrant treating a *persistently* raised cholesterol are:

1. A strong family history of coronary artery disease.
2. Clinical evidence of coronary artery disease.

3. Diabetes.
4. Family hypercholesterolaemia.
5. Hypertension.
6. Secondary hypercholesterolaemia if the prognosis of the primary disease is reasonable.

The Controversy and Some of the Evidence

There is some common ground even between protagonists of both the extreme views of the cholesterol problem. Almost all people interested in the problem agree:

1. There is often an association between *very* high cholesterol levels and a high risk of developing clinical coronary artery disease, e.g. in patients with familial hypercholesterolaemia.

2. Treatment of a *very* high serum cholesterol with cholesterol-lowering diet or drugs can delay the onset of clinical coronary artery disease.

3. There is doubt about what is the "normal" cholesterol level.

4. Other lipids are also factors in the aertiology of coronary artery disease.

5. Other factors such as cigarette smoking, hypertension, sex, family history, sedentary occupation and an aggressive temperament are also factors important in the pathogenesis of coronary artery disease.

The main questions at issue between the two extremes are:

1. Does cholesterol cause atheroma and coronary artery disease?

2. Can coronary artery disease be prevented by lowering a slight or moderate rise in cholesterol?

3. Are other adverse factors less or more important than the cholesterol level?

4. Can coronary artery disease be prevented by cholesterol-lowering diets and drugs in people in whom the serum cholesterol is believed to be normal?

These issues can be compacted into one fundamental practical difference between the two extremes, viz: Should asymptomatic young and middle-aged men take steps to lower their cholesterol level by diet and/or other means?

The cholesterol "lowerers" say a high cholesterol is the fundamental abnormality in causing coronary artery disease—the opposition say cholesterol is only a minor factor.

The Case for the Cholesterol "Lowerers"

1. Hypercholesterolaemia and atherosclerotic plaques histologically identical to those seen in humans can be induced in a wide variety of experimental animals by feeding atherogenic diets. To some extent these atheromatous changes are reversible.

2. Cholesterol, cholesterol esters and cholesterol-lipid complexes are always present in large amounts in atheromatous plaques and the more severe the lesions the more cholesterol they contain.

3. Prolonged hypercholesterolaemia due to diabetes and familial hypercholesterolaemia is always accompanied by severe atheroma.

4. Hypercholesterolaemia and hyperlipidaemia are common in industrial countries and so is atherosclerosis. In underdeveloped countries atherosclerosis is rare and so is hypercholesterolaemia. The diet of industrial countries is rich in cholesterol and triglycerides.

5. The level of the blood cholesterol has been successfully used to predict the likelihood of developing coronary artery disease (Kannel et al., 1964; Paul et al., 1963).

6. Evidence is accumulating that lowering the serum cholesterol by diet reduces the incidence of clinical coronary artery disease. The four major prospective trials are:

    (i) Chicago Coronary Prevention Program.
    (ii) New York Anti-coronary Club.
    (iii) Helsinki Mental Hospital Study.
    (iv) Los Angeles Veterans Administration Domiciliary Center Survey (Stamler, 1969).

The Case Against the Cholesterol "Lowerers"

1. Certain populations and sub-groups within the population have a lower than average incidence of coronary artery disease despite a diet rich in fat. The serum cholesterol of these "exceptions" may be within the "normal" range.

Populations which are "exceptional", in that their fat intake is very high and the mean serum cholesterol low and the incidence of coronary artery disease low, are: inhabitants of the Swiss alpine village of Blatter (Gsell and Mayer, 1962), Masai and Samburu tribes of East Africa (Mann et al., 1964) and Navajo Indians in the U.S. (Fulmer and Roberts, 1963).

2. In certain groups the incidence of coronary artery disease is high despite a low-fat diet. Trappist monks live on a low-fat diet but their coronary arteries are as bad as those of their less abstemious brethren the Benedictines (Groen et al., 1962).

3. The incidence of coronary artery disease varies in different groups despite similarity in their diets (Keys et al., 1963).

4. In a group of institutionalised hospital patients there was no correlation between the level of the serum cholesterol during life and the degree of coronary artery atheroma found at postmortem (Paterson et al., 1963).

5. The incidence of coronary artery disease parallels the dietary intake of sucrose much more closely than that of fat (Cleave and

Campbell, 1969). This weakens the argument of a causal relationship between dietary fat and coronary artery disease.

6. Cholesterol deposition may not be the initiating factor in atheroma. Intravascular thrombosis may be more important and cholesterol deposition is only a response of the endothelium to damage (Duguid, 1948).

7. The animal experiments in which animals given atherogenic diets develop atheroma show that they do so when given vast unphysiological amounts of cholesterol and fat (Altschule, 1966).

8. Other factors such as heredity, smoking habits, aggression and sedentary occupations are undisputed additional factors in the pathogenesis of coronary artery disease. Most of the trials to evaluate cholesterol-lowering diets also control these other factors.

9. Lowering the serum cholesterol after a myocardial infarction does not give any protection against a second infarction (Oliver, 1962).

Various attempts have been made to classify the lipid abnormalities. The one most frequently used is that of Fredrickson which relates the relative concentration of pre-β lipoproteins (mainly carrying cholesterol) and β lipoproteins (mainly carrying triglycerides).

The main lipid-lowering drugs in rough order of usefulness are:

1. Clofibrate (1·5–2·0 g/day).
2. Cholestyramine 16–32 g/day) which is an ion exchange resin that binds bile salts within the gut. This prevents their ultimate conversion into cholesterol.
3. Nicotinic acid (3–6 g/day).
5. D-thyroxine (given with β blocker to prevent peripheral effects) (4–8 mg/day).

Arcus Senilis

The value of arcus senilis as a clinical sign of cardiovascular disease or a disturbance of lipid metabolism is still debatable. The fact that such a common sign is still of undecided value as a determinant of disease suggests that its value as such is small. It is undoubtedly a common sign of "old age". Two good series have shown that the incidence of arcus is higher in men under the age of 50 who have suffered from a myocardial infarction than in normal controls of the same age (Pomerantz, 1962; Rifkind and Dickson, 1965). The serum cholesterol tends to be higher in normal males with arcus senilis. Arcus is almost always present when the serum cholesterol is over 350 mg per cent; its presence does not seem to be affected by the level of the blood pressure (McAndrew and Ogston, 1965). These workers did not confirm the higher incidence of arcus in middle-aged post-myocardial infarction patients.

Myocardial Infarction

Infarction of the myocardium may occur when there is no demonstrable occlusion of the coronary artery by thrombus. When thrombosis does occur there is often evidence of a hypercoagulable state as measured by platelet stickiness, fibrinogen level and prothrombin time. Some of these factors are affected by the level of the circulating lipids.

Auscultatory Physical Signs of Myocardial Infarction

1. Pericardial friction rub.
2. Gallop rhythm.
3. Reversed splitting of the second sound (due to left ventricular dysfunction or left bundle-branch block).
4. Paradoxical systolic expansile pulsation of precordium.
5. Soft first heart sound due to prolonged PR interval.
6. Systolic murmur due to papillary muscle dysfunction or ruptured intraventricular septum.

Enzymes in myocardial infarction.—Damage to cells leads to leak of enzymes normally contained within the cells. The nomenclature and units of the commoner enzymes have been agreed by an International Convention. All enzymes are given a systematic name and a trivial name. The International Units of measurement describe the enzyme activity per litre which transforms a micromole of substrate per minute. The same figure will give the number of milliunits of enzyme per ml. Previously enzymes were expressed in spectrophotometric units.

Aspartic transaminase (glutamic-oxaloacetic transaminase).—Normal values 5–17 iu/l (or 10–35 spectrophotometric units per ml). This is the enzyme most frequently measured following myocardial infarction; the rise in serum glutamic oxaloacetic transaminase (SGOT) roughly corresponds to the size of the infarction. Following myocardial infarction the serum concentration rises to a peak after 12–48 hours and gradually falls to normal in 5–7 days; the rise does not start for at least 6 hours. Serial measurements should always be performed, for it may be the only method of identifying an extension of the infarction. A rise in enzyme concentration may be significant even though the initial value was within the normal range; for example, a rise from 10–40 spectrophotometric units may be as significant as one from 35–65. Note that there is a rise in this enzyme following pulmonary infarction particularly if the patient is shocked. It also rises in hepatocellular damage (e.g. liver congestion in congestive cardiac failure); there is also a slight rise in pancreatitis, dissecting aneurysm, and with opiates and coumarol anticoagulants. A rise in SGOT is, therefore, not diagnostic of myocardial infarction.

Alanine transaminase (glutamic-pyruvic transaminase—SGPT).—

Normal values 4–13 iu/l or 8–25 units/ml measured spectrophotometrically. Contrary to popular misconception this enzyme may rise following myocardial infarction (this may be due to associated hepatic congestion) although the rise is not so high or consistent as with SGOT. It probably does not rise in pulmonary infarction.

Lactate dehydrogenase (LDH).—There are 5 different iso-enzymes of LDH—LDH_{1-5}. LDH_1 tends to rise only in myocardial infarction. LDH_1 as well as catalysing lactate to pyruvate (hence its name) also catalyses hydroxybutyrate to oxobutyrate; hence LDH_1 measured by its effect on hydroxybutyrate is called serum hydroxybutyrate dehydrogenase (SHBD)—normal range 50–150 iu/l. The main value of LDH_1 (and SHBD) is the fact that following myocardial infarction it tends to rise more slowly than SGOT; it usually reaches a maximum at 48–72 hours and falls to normal in 7–14 days. It is important to note that LDH (even LDH_1) nearly always rises following pulmonary infarction. It also rises with damage to renal tissue, hence if it is measured in the serum it may be an indication whether urinary infection is causing renal damage.

Iso-citrate dehydrogenase (ICD). This does not generally rise following myocardial infarction although it probably does so following pulmonary infarction.

Creatine phosphokinase (CPK).—This enzyme is specific for damage to muscle (voluntary and smooth). It may be raised due to the slight muscle damage due to an intramuscular injection. This may have important practical implications if a patient with suspected cardiac pain is given an injection of analgesic before blood is taken. CPK is also raised in myxoedema.

TABLE I

EXPECTED SERUM ENZYME INCREASES IN CERTAIN CONDITIONS

Enzyme	Myocardial Infarction	Pulmonary Infarction	Hepatic Damage	Skeletal Muscle Damage
SGOT (AsT)	++	+ in the presence of shock or pneumonia	++	++
SGPT (AlT)	+ slightly	0 usually	++	++
LDH_1 (SHBD)	++	++	±	++
ICD	0	+	++	0
CPK	++	0	0	++

Other Disturbances Following Myocardial Infarction

Pulmonary congestion and reduced arterial P_{O_2} occur much more frequently than is usually appreciated; furthermore the Po_2 may remain subnormal for up to 4 weeks (Valentine *et al.*, 1966). Pulmonary congestion causing a reduced arterial Po_2 which can usually be corrected with oxygen administration or diuretics occurred in 78 per cent of patients with myocardial infarction in one series (McNicol *et al.*, 1965).

Lactic acidaemia again is commoner than expected and is present in over half of cases admitted to hospital; the acidosis results in a fall in plasma bicarbonate and a fall in the pH of the blood. There is only a poor correlation between the presence of anoxaemia and reduced bicarbonate (Kirby and McNicol, 1966).

The output of cortisol from the adrenals is increased in most cases and the level of cortisol correlates well with the rise in white cell count and cardiac enzymes (Bailey *et al.*, 1967). The high cortisol is partly responsible for the rise in blood sugar and resistance to insulin which is also common.

The effect on the blood lipids is variable; the cholesterol and triglycerides often fall particularly if they were elevated; however, there is a very close correlation between the rise in serum-free fatty acids and the incidence of dysrhythmias. The high free fatty acids are probably due to the increased output of noradrenaline, the level of which is also closely related to the incidence of dysrhythmias (Oliver *et al.*, 1968).

From these observations it is suggested that patients at highest risk following myocardial infarction can be identified when other parameters of seriousness are not present (e.g. shock, prolonged chest pain, heart failure, dysrhythmias, bundle-branch block and bradycardia). If necessary high-risk patients can be identified by:

1. Evidence of pulmonary congestion.
2. Reduced arterial Po_2.
3. Reduced bicarbonate.
4. High circulating free fatty acid.
5. Increased blood sugar.
6. Increased blood cortisol.

PROGNOSIS IN MYOCARDIAL INFARCTION

First attacks of myocardial infarction have a better prognosis than subsequent attacks. The mortality rises progressively with increasing age in men. In women the mortality is considerably greater than in men and remains relatively constant regardless of age.

Effects of Preceding Cardiovascular Disease

1. Hypertension.—The evidence is contradictory. Pell and D'Alonzo (1964) found that previous hypertension adversely affects prognosis. Beard *et al.*(1960) found that antecedent hypertension does not affect prognosis.

2. Previous angina.—Prognosis is undoubtedly worse if angina only developed a few weeks before the infarct; however, long-standing angina does not adversely affect prognosis (Rosenbaum and Levine, 1941).

3. Previous myocardial infarction.—Again the evidence is conflicting: while common sense suggests that a second attack of myocardial infarction must be more dangerous even if only because the chance of sudden death increases, Honey and Truelove (1957b) in a careful survey could not confirm that second and subsequent attacks have an increased mortality.

Prognosis of the Acute Attack

The reported series shows that the overall hospital mortality of acute attacks of myocardial infarction is 15–30 per cent, possibly varying with treatment. The true mortality of myocardial infarction is higher because an unknown number die before they can be admitted to hospital. Factors known to affect adversely the prognosis in the acute attack are:

Shock and hypotension.
Congestive heart failure or left ventricular failure.
Persistent fever and leucocytosis.
Severity and duration of cardiac pain.
Diabetes.
Dysrhythmias including sinus bradycardia, atrial and ventricular ectopic beats and conduction defects.
Systemic and pulmonary emboli.

The outcome of the acute attack is probably not related to the size or position as judged from the electrocardiogram provided that there are no dysrhythmias or conduction defects. Subendocardial infarcts probably have a better prognosis than transmural infarcts. The slightly greater danger of posterior infarcts is due to their proximity to the conducting tissue; however, provided there is no evidence of conduction defects the risks are probably the same. Rupture of the interventricular septum is more common with anterior infarcts, rupture of the chordae tendinae and ensuing mitral regurgitation are more common with posterior infarcts.

Approximately 80 per cent of deaths from myocardial infarction will occur within the first 24 hours; the majority of the remaining deaths will occur during the following two weeks.

It should be noted that the ultimate prognosis is quite independent of whether the electrocardiogram returns to normal in terms of disappearance of Q waves, abnormal ST segments or T waves (Burns Cox, 1967).

The risk of death following acute myocardial infarction is greater if the ECG shows right bundle-branch block and left axis deviation.

Coronary Prognostic Index

Using the method of discriminant analysis with a computer Norris and his colleagues have produced a list of early measurable factors which adversely affect the *hospital* mortality from coronary thrombosis. Although of some value in estimating the prognosis in individual patients the index is of greater value in the objective assessment of claims of new treatment of coronary thrombosis (Norris *et al.*, 1969). Factors which adversely affect the prognosis of *acute* myocardial infarction in order of importance are:

Hypotension.
Old age.
Pulmonary oedema.
Transmural infarction.
Cardiac enlargement.
Previous angina.

They did not find that the prognosis was adversely affected by previous diabetes, hypertension, obesity or myocardial infarction.

Factors which adversely affect prognosis *after recovery from acute* myocardial infarction are (Norris *et al.*, 1971):

Old age.
Pulmonary oedema.
Heart size.
Previous myocardial ischaemia.

Post-myocardial infarction syndrome.—Following an operation in which the pericardium has been opened a syndrome sometimes develops three weeks to six months afterwards which consists of a fever, pericardial pain, and pericardial effusion. There is a tendency to relapse for up to two years. An identical syndrome has been described following myocardial infarction and is known as Dressler's[24] syndrome or the post-myocardial infarction syndrome. The syndrome is usually treated with salicylates and steroids. Early treatment is desirable because arrhythmias and cardiac failure are frequent complications.

The Treatment of Shock (see also p. 418)

Recent experimental work on shock (Lillehei *et al.*, 1964) has suggested that generalised arteriolar constriction leads to anoxia of the capillaries of the gut, these anoxic capillaries dilate and blood pools in them. Drugs normally used in the treatment of shock such as Aramine and noradrenaline only make matters worse by increasing vasoconstriction and thus anoxia of the capillaries. The logical drug to use is one

24. W. DRESSLER. Contemporary American physician.

which prevents arteriolar constriction; the pooling of blood should be counteracted by increasing the blood volume. There is experimental and clinical evidence that an adrenergic blocking drug such as phenoxybenzamine or tolazoline together with fluid replacement may improve the prognosis in cardiogenic shock and in shock due to Gram-negative septicaemia (Davies and Davies, 1968).

Approximately half the deaths from myocardial infarction occur within the first hour and more than 65 per cent within the first 12 hours. There is some evidence which suggests that for *some* patients the survival rate is the same at home or in a coronary care unit. For practical purposes any patient with a dysrhythmia or any other complication of myocardial infarction should be admitted to a CCU but for those patients who have no symptoms or signs other than the initial pain and who are seen for the first time at least 12 hours after the pain, home management may be considered.

There is some improvement in the mortality of myocardial infarction by the use of "mobile coronary care", in which patients are monitored and if necessary treated as soon as the ambulance arrives to take them on their journey to hospital, the diagnosis and treatment often being done by non-medical personnel.

There is some evidence that exercise rehabilitation programmes after myocardial infarction improve morale and induce a feeling of physical fitness.

Recently evidence has been produced in favour of so-called early mobilization but it should be noted that the two most important trials in this respect called 7 and 10 days "early" mobilization. Other trials have suggested that early discharge from hospital may be as safe as keeping in hospital, but following early discharge there is roughly a 7 per cent readmission rate and 7 per cent mortality after discharge in the first 6 weeks and it is still debatable whether some of these deaths would have occurred if the patients had remained in hospital.

THE ANTICOAGULANT CONTROVERSY

The rationale for the administration of anticoagulants (Friedberg, 1966) is based on:

1. The probability that thrombosis is less likely to occur if clotting of blood is impaired.
2. Experimental evidence in dogs that extension of coronary thrombosis can be prevented with anticoagulants.
3. The belief that much of the mortality from coronary thrombosis is due to peripheral venous thrombosis and embolism and extension of mural thrombus within the coronary artery.

4. Statistical evidence from series of clinical cases of myocardial infarction treated with and without anticoagulants.

The antagonists of anticoagulants argue that 1. cannot be proved, 2. is not necessarily applicable to man, 3. is difficult to prove as far as extension of clot in the coronary artery is concerned. For these reasons they believe that the issue can only be resolved by controlled double-blind trials. There have been numerous controlled trials to evaluate the efficiency of anticoagulants; they nearly all suggest that anticoagulants are beneficial, but none of them is entirely free from criticism with regard to controls, allocation of patients, quality of treatment, diagnosis, follow-up and statistical analysis. Several reports have not demonstrated any improvement in mortality following an acute attack or prevention of a further attack.

Anticoagulants for the Acute Attack of Myocardial Infarction

No one denies that anticoagulants reduce the risk of venous thrombosis and death from pulmonary embolism (Jacobs, 1963) but the concept of anticoagulants preventing further thrombosis within the artery is seriously questioned. Several autopsy studies have failed to demonstrate arterial occlusion in unequivocal cases of fatal second myocardial infarcts following soon after a first infarct (Wright et al., 1954). The conclusion is that many second infarcts are not caused by further thrombosis. In a very large international collaborative series 25 per cent of deaths from myocardial infarction had no thrombotic occlusion of any of the coronary arteries (Kagan et al., 1968).

As to the treatment of acute cardiac infarction with anticoagulants mortality figures have shown a definite reduction in thrombo-embolic complications but not necessarily of mortality. To some extent it is possible to predict those cases which will be prone to deep vein thrombosis and thrombo-embolic complications. These "bad risks" cases are characterised by:

1. Prolonged shock.
2. Intractable pain.
3. Obesity.
4. Previous myocardial infarction or deep vein thrombosis.
5. Heart failure.
6. Arrhythmias.
7. Diabetes.

The mortality of these cases is probably decreased with anticoagulants. There is no decrease in mortality in "good risk" cases who are not prone to develop deep vein thrombosis and who are treated with anticoagulants (Russek et al., 1952).

In 1969 the Medical Research Council Working Party published its findings on the value of short-term anticoagulants following myocardial infarction. It concluded that there was no significant reduction in mortality with 28 days' anticoagulants although there was a marked reduction in thrombo-embolic complications some of which were serious. This survey does not completely answer the problem as to the value of short-term anticoagulants—the level of anticoagulation was not high, some patients were transferred from control to treatment group, there was a small reduction in mortality in the treated group and a marked reduction in the number of thrombo-embolic complications.

The most rational course at present is to consider treating with short-term anticoagulants those patients who fall in the "bad risk"group who do not have a definitive contra-indication to anticoagulants.

The mortality of long-term anticoagulants is 2 per cent. "Serious" haemorrhage occurs in 7 per cent (Wright et al., 1965).

In practice some physicians do not consider that the benefits of long-term anticoagulants outweigh the risks and do not employ anticoagulants in the routine treatment or prophylaxis of cardiac infarction. Other physicians treat acute "bad risk" patients with short-term anticoagulants. Some continue prophylactic treatment in men under 55 for up to two years. Others who are convinced of the efficiency of anticoagulants continue to use them in routine treatment and prophylaxis of myocardial infarction. There is no dispute about the value of anticoagulants in the prevention of fatal pulmonary emboli following deep vein thrombosis of the legs.

Value of Anticoagulants in Preventing a Further Myocardial Infarction

There are innumerable trials showing that anticoagulants are beneficial; however, most of them have defects with regard to controls, allocation of patients and quality of treatment. Up until 1955 anticoagulants were very widely used; however, some physicians remained sceptical and despite the apparent weight of evidence against them they published their views (Honey and Truelove, 1957a; McMichael and Parry, 1960). The most comprehensive survey in favour of anticoagulants was the report of the Committee on Anticoagulants to the American Heart Association (Wright et al., 1954).

In an effort to clarify the situation, further controlled trials have been conducted—one of the best and most widely accepted came from Copenhagen. This failed to show any benefit from anticoagulants (Hilden et al., 1961). In 1964 the Medical Research Council trial concluded that while anticoagulants reduce the risk of re-infarction and perhaps of death under the age of 55, this effect largely disappears by the third year of treatment. It should be noted that this influential trial did not contain enough women for proper statistical analysis. It had come to be widely believed that any protection from anticoagulants only affects men. It has been shown that women are protected to the same extent as men. Further support for a marginally beneficial effect in patients under the age of 55 is given by the International Anticoagulant Review Group (1970). The exact duration of protection is still an open question; it is probably not more than one year and could be as little as three months (Ritland and Lygren, 1969).

Conclusions

(1) Anticoagulants given in an acute attack of cardiac infarction reduce thrombo-embolic complications.

(2) To some extent it is possible to predict those who are prone to such complications.

(3) Long-term anticoagulants probably prevent recurrence of infarction in a small number of patients under the age of 55 for up to a year following an infarct.

Withdrawal of Anticoagulants

It is suspected that cessation of anticoagulant therapy is associated with an increased number of thrombic incidents. There are clinical statistical surveys which both confirm and refute this clinical impression. Nevertheless there is good laboratory evidence of increased coagulability of the blood in *some* patients when anticoagulants are stopped (Poller and Thomson, 1965). The question then arises whether this "rebound hypercoagulability" can be mitigated by more gradual withdrawal. Again the clinical statistical evidence is conflicting but there is laboratory evidence that hypercoagulability is reduced when anticoagulants are withdrawn slowly. There seems to be a special risk of thrombotic complications in patients who have been on anticoagulants for more than two years (Kamath and Thorne, 1969). From a practical point of view it is wise to "tail off" anticoagulants gradually when this is being done as an elective procedure. When patients have been controlled on anticoagulants for more than two years "tailing off" should be done very gradually.

TREATMENT OF DYSRHYTHMIAS

Many drugs have the property of slowing the heart rate. Practically all the available drugs have been used to treat all the dysrhythmias. However, certain drugs, whose effects are well known and which work in the majority of patients with a particular dysrhythmia, are generally used before other "second line" drugs.

When confronted with a patient who has a tachycardia the *first* thing to decide is whether the tachycardia is causing:

1. Heart failure.
2. Low cardiac output, poor peripheral perfusion or hypotension.

Tachycardia with Heart Failure or Hypotension

If you think the tachycardia is causing heart failure or a low cardiac output then treatment is *urgent* and is the same whether the tachycardia is supraventricular or ventricular in origin.

Lignocaine.—50 mg intravenously over 2 minutes and then observe the ECG. Bolus injections of lignocaine given over a period of 2–5 minutes can be given until a total of at least 1 g of lignocaine has been given. The ECG and the patient should be checked after each bolus has been given. If the tachycardia is still present and the patient still in cardiac failure or a state of shock after 15–30 minutes proceed to

DC shock.—Up to 6 shocks may be necessary. If the patient is alert it is kind to give heroin 20 mg before the DC shock. If DC shock is effective the patient should be given a lignocaine drip at the rate of 1–10 mg lignocaine/minute *plus* oral procainamide 250–500 mg 6-hourly. The drip can be discontinued when the heart rate remains controlled. If heart failure is present at this stage the patient should be digitalised and given diuretics—the route and rate of administration depending on the severity of the condition. It is unusual for lignocaine followed by DC shock to fail to control tachycardia. However, should DC shock and lignocaine be ineffective the following drugs should be considered in addition, and repeated if necessary.

1. Procainamide intravenously 100 mg over 2–5 minutes.
2. Phenytoin intravenously 100 mg over 2–5 minutes.
3. Digoxin 0·25 mg intravenously if the tachycardia is supraventricular in origin.
4. Intravenous administration of a β-blocking drug.

Digoxin should not be given in the first instance before DC shock; there is evidence that in the presence of digoxin DC shock is less effective.

Tachycardia without Cardiac Failure or Hypotension

If the patient has a tachycardia which is *not* causing cardiac failure or hypotension there is much less urgency and DC shock may not be necessary. First decide whether the tachycardia is supraventricular (atrial tachycardia, atrial fibrillation, atrial flutter or nodal tachycardia) in origin. If the tachycardia is supraventricular give digoxin, the rate and route depending on the severity. If the tachycardia is ventricular in origin it is wise to assume that the situation is urgent even if the patient appears to tolerate the tachycardia well and to proceed as for the urgent situation (lignocaine bolus injections plus DC shock if necessary, etc.).

If the supraventricular tachycardia does not respond to digoxin the following drugs should be considered roughly in the order given. The route and rate of administration will depend on the urgency of the situation.

1. Lignocaine (50–500 mg intravenously).
2. Procainamide (50–500 mg intravenously).
3. β-blocking drug intravenously.
4. Phenytoin (50–500 mg intravenously).
5. Antazoline, an antihistamine with anti-arrhythmic properties (100 mg 6-hourly by mouth).
6. Neostigmine (which stimulates the vagus) (0·5 mg subcutaneously).
7. Mephentermine, which increases the blood pressure and causes reflex stimulation of the vagus.

DC shock will usually abolish a supraventricular tachycardia if it does not respond to these drugs.

Useful Tips

1. Anoxia potentiates and causes dysrhythmias; ensure that the patient is given oxygen.
2. Acidosis also potentiates and causes dysrhythmias; give 8·4 per cent bicarbonate if acidosis is present.
3. Hypokalaemia potentiates the effects of digoxin; give potassium if hypokalaemia is present.
4. Digoxin can cause any dysrhythmia. If the patient has been having digoxin before admission it may be the cause of the tachycardia.
5. Practolol should be used with the greatest caution if there is *any* heart failure present.
6. If digoxin overdose seems the likely cause of the tachycardia, the digoxin should be stopped and in an urgent situation practolol should be given (the rate and route of administration depending on the urgency).
7. Frequent ventricular or supraventricular ectopic beats (more than 5 per minute) should be treated either with a lignocaine drip or oral procainamide in doses which reduce the frequency or abolish the ectopics.

Ectopic beats (extrasystoles or premature beats).—When ventricular ectopic beats occur frequently (more than 3–5 per minute) following myocardial infarction they indicate an "irritable focus" in the myocardium and they are often followed by ventricular fibrillation particularly if an ectopic beat happens to occur during the T wave of the preceding beat (R on T phenomenon). Ventricular ectopic beats following myocardial infarction should be treated vigorously because of the danger of ventricular fibrillation. They should be treated either with a lignocaine drip and/or oral procainamide; the dose of each being adjusted so that the ectopic beats are suppressed.

There is some evidence that atrial ectopic beats following myocardial infarction are as dangerous as ventricular ectopics; if frequent they should be treated in the same way as ventricular ectopics.

Patients who develop frequent ectopic beats soon after a myocardial infarction have a poorer ultimate prognosis and it is these patients who most frequently die suddenly several weeks after the infarction when all appears to be well; for this reason oral antidysrhythmic drugs should be continued for at least *three months* in patients who have frequent ectopics soon after their myocardial infarction.

Benign ectopic beats.—Occasional atrial and ventricular ectopic beats occur in normal hearts. If they are not causing symptoms no treatment is indicated. Sometimes ectopic beats produce uncomfortable and alarming palpitations; in this case reassurance and a mild sedative may be all that is required. If the patient continues to be worried by the palpitations procainamide 250–500 mg q.d.s. should be given.

Paroxysmal supraventricular tachycardia.—The onset and termination of tachycardia are usually sudden; palpitations seem to the patient to be regular and rapid in the case of atrial or nodal paroxysmal tachycardia and rapid and irregular in the case of paroxysmal atrial fibrillation.

Supraventricular tachycardias are usually accompanied by polyuria which may be due to the anxiety they cause or it may be due to stimulation of volume receptors situated in or near the right atrium by the tachycardia leading to a diuresis.

An important cause of paroxysmal tachycardias is hyperventilation leading to a mild alkalosis; the tachycardia can sometimes be controlled by making the patient breath in and out of a paper bag.

The vagus nerve conveys parasympathetic impulses which slow the heart by inhibition of the SA and AV nodes, an attempt should be made to stimulate the vagus by deep breathing, eyeball pressure, drinking iced water or carotid sinus massage. Often the patient will have learnt some trick himself for stopping an attack, such as making himself vomit, If these measures fail the patient should be sedated and given lignocaine or phenytoin 100–500 mg intravenously if the attack is prolonged or distressing, followed by a β blocker intravenously if lignocaine or phenytoin are not effective. If the attack is still present digoxin should be given; if this fails more vigorous vagal stimulation can be given by neostigmine 0·5 mg subcutaneously; if this fails it is worth trying the antihistamine antazoline 100 mg intramuscularly and if this fails DC shock is indicated.

Frequent paroxysms of supraventricular tachycardia or troublesome palpitations should be treated with a maintenance dose of procainamide 250–500 mg q.d.s.

Elective DC Conversion

Atrial fibrillation or flutter which is rapid and not causing heart failure or hypotension should be controlled initially with digoxin.

When the rate is controlled the use of elective DC conversion should be considered. The digoxin should be stopped for 48 hours before the attempted conversion of the fibrillation or flutter. It is customary to give anticoagulants for at least 3 weeks before the conversion to lessen the likelihood of dislodging a clot from the atrial wall. Anticoagulants prevent new thrombus formation in the left atrium which allows time for organisation of old thrombus to occur. If possible the period of anticoagulation should be more than three weeks—there is evidence that complete organisation of a recent atrial clot takes longer than three weeks in some patients. Inspection of the atria in patients operated on for mitral stenosis frequently shows recent and friable clot even though the patients have been fully anticoagulated for several months. It is wise if possible to anticoagulate patients for at least two months before elective DC conversion. DC conversion should always be considered for atrial flutter and for atrial fibrillation. There are some definite *contra-indications* to conversion:

1. Atrial fibrillation due to thyrotoxicosis (until the patient is euthyroid).
2. Mitral incompetence.
3. Mitral stenosis (conversion should be attempted after a successful mitral valvotomy).
4. Ischaemic heart disease.
5. Previous arterial emboli.
6. Large left atrium.
7. Fibrillation of more than 6 months' duration.

Following successful DC conversion to sinus rhythm the patient should be given oral procainamide 250–500 mg q.d.s. for one month—this lessens the likelihood of relapse. Occasionally pulmonary oedema develops after a successful DC conversion probably because of improvement in output from the right side of the heart and the left atrium being smaller and less expansile when it is functioning normally and not fibrillating. The small left atrium is probably unable to accommodate the increased venous return from the lungs, leading to pulmonary oedema.

The Sick Sinus Syndrome describes a situation in which function of the sinus node is intermittent. The patient usually has both a bradycardia and a tachycardia. On the same cardiogram the patient may have sinus rhythm, sinus bradycardia, nodal rhythm, supraventricular ectopic beats or tachycardia. If symptoms are present long-term pacing is indicated.

CARDIAC ARREST

Sudden failure of the heart to pump blood (cardiac arrest) may be due to:

1. Complete cessation of electrical and mechanical movement within the heart (asystole).

2. Rapid but ineffective electrical and mechanical movement of the heart (ventricular tachycardia and fibrillation).

The vital priority is speed in diagnosing "cardiac arrest"—establishing the cause can come later. The initial treatment is the same whatever the cause.

Diagnosis

The diagnosis of cardiac arrest is based on:

1. The history of sudden collapse.
2. Unconsciousness.
3. Absent or diminished carotid pulses and heart sounds.

In addition the patient may be cyanosed, apnoeic, have widely dilated pupils or someone may already be doing external cardiac massage.

Treatment

A. A patent airway should be ensured. The patient should be lying on his back preferably on a hard surface (either on the floor or on a mattress under which a fracture board has been placed). To ensure a patient airway the neck should be extended and the mandible drawn forwards—this stops the tongue flopping backwards into the airway.

B. A Brook airway should be inserted and mouth-to-mouth respiration started if the patient is not breathing spontaneously. If an anaesthetist is present he should insert an endotracheal tube and the patient can be inspired from an Ambu bag, and oxygen given at the same time.

C. It should be ensured that effective external cardiac massage is being performed.

D. An intravenous infusion should be set up and 100 ml of 8·4 per cent sodium bicarbonate (1 ml contains 1 mEq or mmol) run in to prevent acidosis due to accumulation of lactic acid in the anoxic tissues.

E. An ECG machine should be set up and a definitive diagnosis made. Now is the time to assess the situation fully.

Definitive diagnosis is the stage most frequently mismanaged. The number of possible diagnoses from the ECG are only 4 and the correct treatment of each is more or less agreed. The function of the heart is to pump and the function of the ECG is to record electricity—it should be emphasised that normal electrical complexes on the ECG do not mean that the heart is pumping blood; on the other hand, the heart can be effectively pumping blood even though the ECG records abnormal electrical impulses. Both the ECG electricity and the functioning of the pump must be assessed (by feeling peripheral pulses, inspecting the pupils and listening to the heart sounds, and noting whether or not the skin remains cyanosed).

The four abnormalities of the electrocardiogram and their emergency treatments are:

1. Asystole.—Only a few or no ventricular complexes are seen.

Treatment: Injection of 5 ml of 1 in 10,000 adrenaline into 1 cardiac chamber. (The needle should be inserted into the chest where it is thought the apex beat should be and a point 2 in. deep to the sternal angle aimed for.) If this fails an injection of 5 ml of 10 per cent calcium chloride given into the heart. Injection of adrenaline and/or calcium chloride should produce ventricular fibrillation.

2. Ventricular or supraventricular fibrillation or tachycardia.—Ventricular complexes occur as a series of regular or irregular troughs and peaks.

Treatment: Intravenous lignocaine or procainamide 100–500 mg followed by DC defibrillation. It should be ensured that both electrodes are well covered with contact jelly but that the jelly does not extend beyond the electrodes; one is held on the upper sternum and the other over the apex—several shocks can be delivered if necessary.

3. Heart-block.—Ventricular complexes may look relatively normal but are slower than 40 per minute. P waves may or not be present.

Treatment: Isoprenaline 1–5 μg. intravenously very slowly followed later by external or internal pacing.

4. Sinus bradycardia.—Normal-shaped complexes with preceding P waves but at a much slower rate than normal.

Treatment: Atropine sulphate 1 mg. intravenously or intramuscularly; followed by isoprenaline if necessary.

The management of the next stage, that is, whether or not to continue resuscitation and for how long, requires experience, knowledge and confidence for it depends on a number of factors which cannot be clearly defined, such as:

1. Degree of success with the methods of resuscitation already adopted.

2. Length of time cardiac arrest was present before effective cardiac massage was started.

3. Underlying disease from which the patient is suffering.

4. State of the cardiorespiratory systems before cardiac arrest.

5. The age of the patient.

6. The expressed policy of the unit.

7. The unexpectedness of the arrest. This involves preparing the relatives for the death and the question of whether it is kinder for them to be told that the patient is already dead or whether it is kinder to give

them some time to prepare themselves. There is a generally accepted convention that the most *senior* doctor present should inform relatives in the event of death.

Sometimes the decision to desist further attempts at resuscitation is easy. Some of the factors which are relative contra-indications to continuing are:

1. Old age.
2. Malignant disease.
3. Severe cardiorespiratory disease.
4. Severe coincidental disease which is potentially fatal.
5. A delay of more than 3 minutes between collapse and starting resuscitation.
6. No improvement in condition despite adequate external cardiac massage and ventilation.
7. Prolonged asystole on the ECG with dilated and unreactive pupils which are normal at the beginning of the resuscitation attempt. (It should be noted though that the pupils may be dilated and unreactive for several hours in some patients who eventually make a complete recovery from severe drug overdosage.)

Relative indications for continuing attempted resuscitation are:

1. Youth and absence of severe disease.
2. Recovery of consciousness with external cardiac massage etc.
3. Some improvement in condition, for example contraction of pupils, groaning, spontaneous movement of limbs, spontaneous breathing, palpable peripheral pulses and normal ventricular complexes on the ECG.
4. Sudden collapse when a doctor or nurse was giving an intravenous drug.

If the resuscitation is successful the patient should be carefully observed for the next 24 hours, if possible in a recovery room or intensive care unit where there are facilities for constant monitoring of the electrocardiogram and specially trained nurses, in case a second cardiac arrest occurs.

VENOUS THROMBOSIS

Over 50 per cent of patients with deep vein thrombosis have no physical signs (Browse, 1969*a*). Deep vein thrombosis and pulmonary embolism are more common than is generally realised in healthy people with no predisposing cause (Flemming and Bailey, 1966). The site of *origin* of thrombosis is frequently not the site from which a pulmonary embolus originates; thus a pulmonary embolus in the presence of unilateral signs of deep vein thrombosis is *equally* likely to have arisen from the leg *without* physical signs. The sites of *origin of venous thrombosis* in order of frequency are (Sevitt and Gallagher, 1961):

1. Deep veins of the calf.
2. Posterior tibial veins.
3. Common femoral vein.
4. Popliteal vein.
5. External iliac vein.

Although these are the sites in which deep vein thrombosis begins, the pelvic veins are by far the most frequent *source of pulmonary emboli* (Mavor and Galloway, 1967).

Physical Signs

It must be assumed that the physical signs of deep vein thrombosis are insensitive guides and that the incidence of thrombosis is more common than they indicate. However, this applies to most other diseases and is not a reason for abandoning the signs, but a spur to improving them.

The deep veins possess valves and drain from the muscles of the calf into the anterior and posterior tibial veins; these unite just below the popliteal fossa to form the popliteal vein which continues upwards to form the femoral vein which lies medial to the femoral artery under the mid-point of the inguinal ligament. Because the femur slopes inwards and forwards from the hip to the knee the vein lies behind the femur at the lower end, medial to it in its middle third and anterior to it at the top. The deep veins of the plantar surface of the foot drain mainly into the posterior tibial vein which is situated deep to the tendo-Achilles. The anterior tibial vein runs in the groove between the tibia and fibula in the lower two thirds of the lower leg and then penetrates the interosseous membrane to join the popliteal vein.

The *superficial* veins of the lower leg are in communication with the deep veins and with each other. The short saphenous vein runs up the back of the calf from behind the medial malleolus to enter the *popiteal* vein behind the knee while the long saphenous vein runs up from in front of the malleolus on the medial side of the leg to enter the femoral vein in the femoral triangle. The femoral vein becomes the external iliac vein which is situated near the rectum. The majority of the deep veins in the calf are within the soleus muscle which is deep to the gastrocnemius. These anatomical points are important because they help appreciate a number of significant signs of deep vein thrombosis which are frequently ignored.

1. Thrombosis of the plantar veins causes pain and tenderness on palpation in the soles of the feet.

2. Thrombosis affecting the posterior tibial vein causes tenderness on palpation behind the tendo Achilles.

3. Thrombosis of the anterior tibial vein causes tenderness in the groove between tibia and fibula in front of the lower leg.

4. Because the veins in the soleus muscle are more often affected than those in the more superficial gastrocnemius, palpation of the calf should be done in such a way that the *deep* muscles of the calf are palpated; this is best done using both hands. The debonair, token clasping of the calf without removing the bedclothes which passes for palpation of the calf should be deprecated.

5. Blockage of the deep intramuscular veins of the lower leg or of the tibial veins results in more blood flowing in and between both the superficial saphenous veins. Small dilated communicating veins particularly from the short to the long saphenous veins can be seen just below the knee or above the ankle—these veins slope upwards and are more pronounced on the anterior and lateral aspects of the lower leg.

6. Obstruction of the deep intramuscular veins and local inflammation cause fluid to accumulate locally. If this is severe it is seen as oedema or increase in circumference of the leg; however, it can be detected at a stage earlier than this by careful examination. The knee is flexed to the 90° position with the foot resting on the bed—this completely relaxes the calf muscles—the flat *palm* of the hand is used to lift gently those muscles up and down trying to assess two things, firstly the weight of the muscles and secondly their hardness as compared with the opposite side.

7. Careful palpation of the popliteal vein in the popliteal fossa and posterior part of the lower thigh.

8. Careful palpation of the adductor muscles on the medial side of the mid thigh.

9. Careful palpation of the femoral vein medial to the femoral artery below *and* above the inguinal ligament. Tenderness above the inguinal ligament indicates extension to the external iliac vein.

10. Rectal examination to discover whether there is tenderness of the veins within the pelvis. In a woman vaginal examination may be indicated particularly as a base-line observation.

In a case of suspected deep vein thrombosis all the above signs should be systematically looked for in addition to the more orthodox signs, viz.:

1. Oedema.
2. Increased warmth.
3. Homan's sign.
4. Difference in circumference between the two legs.
5. Diminished arterial pulsation of the affected side.
6. Superficial thrombophlebitis.
7. Slight elevation of the temperature.

Causes of Deep Vein Thrombosis

Virchow's triad of the known predisposing factors to vascular thrombosis is:

1. Damage to the vessel wall. This may be mechanical trauma such as a blunt injury or may occur if there is hypoxia of the circulating blood or if the veins are compressed when empty of blood. Damage to the endothelium can cause thrombosis even when blood flow is normal. Certain drugs, hormones and toxins also damage vascular endothelium, e.g. adrenaline, serotonin, dextran, ACTH, bacterial endotoxins and cholesterol.

2. Reduced blood flow. This is particularly important in patients who are kept in bed thus reducing or eliminating the venous pump mechanism which is partly responsible for blood flow in the veins. The movement of the diaphragm is probably an important factor in aiding venous return; this movement is of course reduced following abdominal or thoracic surgery.

3. Increased coagulability of the blood. This occurs following bed rest and operations. It may also occur following fatty meals or in the presence of hypercholesterolaemia.

Factors Predisposing to Deep Vein Thrombosis

1. Immobility and trauma.
2. Surgery, pregnancy, parturition and oestrogen contraceptives.
3. Congestive cardiac failure.
4. Age—there are conflicting reports about effect of increasing age on the incidence of deep vein thrombosis.
5. Sex—there is probably no increased risk in women if pregnancy etc. are excluded.
6. Obesity.
7. Race—the incidence is said to be low in Africans and Indians.
8. Climate—the incidence is probably increased in cold weather.
9. Malignant diseases, polycythaemia, anaemia and dehydration.
10. Pelvic tumours.

Confirmatory Investigations

1. Phlebography. Contrast dye is injected into the superficial veins of the feet. Thrombi are seen as *constant* filling defects; recent thrombus is usually only attached at one point, hence there may be a thin line of contrast between the filling defect and the wall of the vein. Complete occlusion of a vein is assumed if the filling of the veins above and below the non-opacified vein is seen.

2. ^{125}I-labelled fibrinogen. Fibrinogen is incorporated into recent and

old clots. Radioactive counts are made at fixed points on both legs. The counts overlying thrombus will be increased. This technique can only be used to detect venous thrombosis below the mid-thigh level; above this the background radiation is too high for meaningful results.

3. Ultra-sound flowmeter. This detects slowing of blood flow in partially occluded *large* veins such as the femoral and iliac veins. It is an extremely simple technique.

Treatment

1. *Analgesics* for local pain.
2. *Elastic bandaging* of the leg beginning at the feet and working upwards; care should be taken to see that the elastic bandage does not locally constrict any part of the leg. The purpose of the elastic bandage is to compress the superficial veins and so encourage increased flow through the deep veins.
3. *Positioning of the leg.*—When the legs are horizontal the veins still drain upwards (from the posterior tibial vein at the heel to the femoral vein in the front of the thigh). The rate of flow in the veins may be increased if the foot is elevated so that the blood is then flowing horizontally or even slightly downhilll; this is probably the optimum position once venous thrombosis has occurred. However, for the *prevention* of deep vein thrombosis elevation of the *head* of the bed may be better because when the feet are raised there is a tendency for the veins to collapse and this may offset any increased flow; total blood flow to the legs is *reduced* with the leg elevated. An additional advantage of raising the *head* of the bed is that the patient tends to slip to the foot of the bed and has to keep using his leg muscles to keep himself in the proper place in the bed—this constant muscular activity promotes venous return.

Prevention of further clotting.—Heparin 10,000 iu intravenously is given immediately the diagnosis is made. An intravenous drip should then be set up and heparin given at a rate which keeps the clotting time between 15–20 mins. Heparin affects every stage of the clotting process and in particular it inhibits thromboplastin generation, the action of thrombin on fibrinogen and the conversion of prothrombin to thrombin. Heparin is a cumulative drug especially in the presence of renal failure and it also has some fibrinolytic, antihistamine and anti 5-hydroxy-tryptamine properties; it also decreases platelet stickiness. All these properties are valuable in deep vein thrombosis and pulmonary embolism. Oral anticoagulants are given at the same time—usually Sinthrome (starting dose 20 mg, maintenance dose approximately 4 mg daily).

Preservation of venous valves.—Thrombolytic treatment to preserve venous valves has been successfully used. Following deep vein thrombosis recanalisation of veins usually occurs but the valves are completely disorganised by the fibrosis within the clot. Damage to the veins may have long-term unpleasant effects such as the post-phlebitic syndrome, chronic leg oedema, induration and ulceration; any measures which can preserve the valves may be of value. To be of value treatment must be started within five days of the thrombosis developing or recent non-adherent clot should be demonstrated by phlebography. A suitable regime is 600,000 units streptokinase plus 100 mg hydrocortisone in 250 ml of dextrose/saline intravenously in the first hour followed by 600,000 units of streptokinase plus 100 mg hydrocortisone in 500 ml dextrose/saline every 6 hours i.e. 100,000 iu streptokinase every hour (Browse *et al.*, 1968). The infusion should be continued for three days. The hydrocortisone is required to suppress allergic reactions to the streptokinase. If facilities are available the dose of streptokinase should be monitored according to the euglobulin lysis time, fibrinogen level and thrombin clotting time. Thrombi which show no phlebographic evidence of disappearing in 36 hours are unlikely to be lysed and are probably not recent. However the treatment is expensive and time-consuming and most physicians doubt whether it is reasonable to use it on a wide scale for deep vein thrombosis alone.

Prevention of recurrent pulmonary emboli.—There is considerable evidence that fatal pulmonary emboli nearly always arise from the ileo-femoral (proximal) veins; clinical evidence of involvement of these veins may not be present (Mavor and Galloway, 1969). In the case of recurrent pulmonary emboli which are not prevented by adequate anti-coagulation the only hope used to be vena cava ligation or plication. With the advent of pertrochanteric and pelvic phlebography it is usually possible to outline the clot in the ilio-femoral veins or to demonstrate occlusion of the veins; if a clot is seen or obstruction is demonstrated femoral and/or pelvic venotomy and thrombectomy can be performed while infusing heparin continuously through a catheter in the femoral vein (Mavor *et al.*, 1970). The phlebography should always be perform-ed on *both* sides since a fatal pulmonary embolus frequently comes from the side in which there are no clinical signs. Occasionally vena cava ligation or plication are still required when thrombectomy fails to remove all the thrombus or is followed by rethrombosis despite full anticoagulant therapy.

Following a pulmonary embolus for which the patient has been fully anticoagulated a second embolus occurs with surprising frequency. In one series 14 per cent of patients had a second and fatal embolus and 26 per cent had a second but not fatal embolus (Browse, 1969b). This is why these sophisticated methods of investigation and treatment with thrombectomy can be so important to an individual patient.

Prevention of deep vein thrombosis.—Many series have confirmed the value of anticoagulants given prophylactically in preventing venous thrombosis following major surgery (including thoracotomy, hip, abdominal and gynaecological operations). Surgeons who have experience of operating in these patients who are well controlled on anticoagulants generally affirm that bleeding during and after operation is not a problem (Sevitt, 1968). It is a shame that local N.H.S. exigencies usually preclude such time-consuming but life-saving measures as prophylactic anticoagulation. Without anticoagulants the incidence of venous thrombosis following major surgery in patients over the age of 40 is 35 per cent. This alarming incidence *cannot* be lessened by intensive prophylactic physiotherapy to the legs post-operatively (Flanc *et al.*, 1969). There is now firm evidence that 5000 iu heparin given every 12 hours subcutaneously will lessen the incidence of deep vein thrombosis following most major operations and after myocardial infarction.

CONGENITAL HEART DISEASE

The development of the heart and great vessels is completed by two months of gestation, thereafter only increase in size occurs. This is important with regard to infections or drugs known to interfere with the development of the heart and great vessels. Rubella occurring in the first two months of pregnancy is a potential cause of cardiac mal-formation (usually patent ductus arteriosus and pulmonary stenosis), when it occurs after two months there is much less danger. Other conditions known to be associated with a higher than normal incidence of congenital heart disease are mongolism (the commonest lesion is an ostium primum atrial septal defect), Turner's[25] syndrome (coarctation and pulmonary stenosis), gargoylism (fibroelastosis), Marfan's[26] syndrome (dissecting aneurysms and atrial septal defects) and drugs such as thalidomide (atrial and ventricular septal defects). The commonest congenital heart diseases in order of frequency are ventricular septal defect, atrial septal defect (secundum type), patent ductus arteriosus and Fallot's[27] tetralogy. Fallot's tetralogy is the commonest congenital heart disease of adults causing clubbing and cyanosis.

Ventricular Septal Defects (VSD)

The defect is nearly always in the membranous part of the septum. The size of the defect does not necessarily reflect its haemodynamic severity since the defect may partly close during systole due to contraction of the muscular part of the ventricular septum; spontaneous closure of small defects is the rule. When the defect is large more blood may be passing through it than is pumped into the systemic circulation. There are two mechanisms which tend to reduce the left-to-right shunt with

25. HENRY HUBERT TURNER (b. 1892). Oklahoma physician.
26. BERNARD-JEAN ANTONIN MARFAN (1858–1942). Paris paediatrician.
27. ÉTIENNE-LOUIS ARTHUR FALLOT (1850–1911). Marseilles physician.

large defects: one is an increase in pulmonary arteriolar resistance and the other is hypertrophy of the pulmonary outflow tract causing functional muscular hypertrophic subvalvar pulmonary stenosis. The characteristic murmur of a VSD is pansystolic and best heard in the third and fourth left intercostal spaces, it radiates over the precordium and is frequently accompanied by a thrill (mitral incompetence is less commonly accompanied by a thrill and the murmur radiates into the axilla). If the muscular part of the septum contracts the murmur may only be present early in systole. There is often a third heart sound due to the extra volume of blood entering the ventricle because of diversion of a portion of the stroke volume through the defect. The maladie de Roger[28] is a ventricular septal defect which is causing no symptoms and is not accompanied by any alteration of the electrocardiogram or chest x-ray. Small septal defects frequently close spontaneously.

In larger defects the output of the right ventricle may be double that of the left ventricle into the aorta (i.e. half the cardiac output passes through the defect—a 50 per cent shunt). The increased volume of blood flowing through the pulmonary and mitral valves may cause functional mitral diastolic and pulmonary systolic murmurs. This is important because a pulmonary ejection systolic murmur does not necessarily indicate organic stenosis of the valve or functional stenosis of the infundibulum. The presence of a mitral diastolic murmur gives an indication that the shunt is fairly large.

At higher flow rates the right ventricular pressure increases due to functional infundibular narrowing or pulmonary hypertension. The elevated right ventricular pressure will diminish the flow through the defect, leading to disappearance of the mitral diastolic and lessening of the pulmonary systolic murmurs. As the right ventricular pressure rises further it exceeds the systemic pressure and venous blood from the right ventricle flows through the defect into the left ventricle causing central cyanosis (Eisenmenger's[29] syndrome).

Treatment.—Operation is generally indicated if the pulmonary to systemic flow rate is more than 3:1 especially if the right ventricular systolic pressure exceeds 50 mm Hg. Operation is contra-indicated when the Eisenmenger situation has developed. Polycythaemia commonly develops in congenital heart disease, it increases the viscosity of the blood and this offsets any advantage of increased oxygen capacity. If cyanotic congenital heart disease is associated with severe polycythaemia (Hb greater than 17 g per cent or PCV more than 65 per cent) venesection should be considered. The risk of thrombosis *in situ* is considerably increased in the presence of polycythaemia and if this is occurring anticoagulants may be indicated.

28. HENRI LOUIS ROGER (1811–1891). French physician.
29. VICTOR EISENMENGER. German physician.

Atrial Septal Defects

In the embryo the atria are at first separated by a crescentic septum which grows downwards to fuse with the atrioventricular rings, the gap between the two limbs of the crescent is the ostium primum. As the ostium primum closes a hole develops in the upper part of the septum—the ostium secundum. A second septum (the septum secundum) develops in the right atrium. In the fetus the lungs are not functioning and the right heart is responsible for pumping blood through the patent ductus arteriosus into the aorta, the blood entering the right heart comes from the umbilical vein of the placenta and is rich in oxygen and nutrients. At birth the lungs expand, the pressure in the right heart falls so that the pressure in the left atrium is higher than in the right. The septum primum is pressed against the septum secundum and the ostium secundum is obliterated and blood flow ceases. A small oval portion of the ostium secundum may remain patent and forms the foramen ovale. A secundum ASD is due to persistence of the whole of the ostium sedundum (i.e. the second hole in the septum primum is not blocked off by the septum secundum). A primum ASD is due to the persistence of the ostium primum. The septum primum is associated with the atrioventricular valve rings, hence primum defects are complicated by incompetence of the atrioventricular valves. The physical signs of a secundum ASD are an elevated *a* wave in the JVP (due to the stronger left atrial contraction being transmitted through the defect to the right atrium), a diastolic murmur at the tricuspid area and an ejection systolic murmur at the pulmonary area due to increased blood flow through the tricuspid and pulmonary valves. The pulmonary component of the second sound is widely split because the already overloaded right atrium and ventricle are unable to accommodate more blood during inspiration: splitting is already maximum in expiration (fixed splitting).

Right bundle-branch block usually occurs. The chest x-ray may show enlargement of the right atrium and large pulmonary arteries due to increased blood flow (pulmonary plethora). A primum ASD is also accompanied by a pansystolic murmur due to incompetence of the atrioventricular valves. The electrocardiogram may show right bundle-branch block with left axis deviation the explanation for which is not known. In contrast, the right bundle-branch block of a secundum defect is accompanied by right axis deviation.

Treatment.—Surgical correction is indicated if the pulmonary to systemic flow rate is 2–3 to 1 or there is evidence of increasing pulmonary hypertension. Patients in whom the diagnosis is made in adult life pose a special problem. They usually remain symptom-free until 30–40, the average age of death of unoperated cases being around 50. Operation is usually not performed in adults over the age of 45 or if the pulmonary vascular resistance is at systemic levels.

A patent ductus arteriosus results in a collapsing pulse and a murmur heard in systole and diastole since the systolic and diastolic pressures in the aorta exceed those in the pulmonary artery throughout the cardiac cycle.

Congenital heart defects which are unimportant haemodynamically are often the cause of subacute bacterial endocarditis. The defect itself need not be affected and associated lesions are frequently the only site infected, e.g. SBE develops in the right ventricle in a mild VSD where the stream of blood impinges on the wall of the ventricle or it develops on the bicuspid aortic valve associated with coarctation.

HYPERTENSION

The average blood pressure of most but not all *populations* of *healthy* people increases slowly with age (Miall and Oldham, 1963). However, the blood pressure of many individuals in the population remains the same throughout their lives. Rise in blood pressure with age seems to be proportional to the starting blood pressure (Miall and Lovell, 1967). The distribution curve of blood pressure in the general population probably does not show two peaks (one for normal people and one for people with hypertension) (Pickering, 1968). This is the crunch of the unsolved controversy whether essential hypertension is a distinct disease or whether blood pressure is a variable like height which means that no particular level of blood pressure can be said to be abnormal and therefore indicate the *disease* hypertension. Platt (1963) believes that essential hypertension is a distinct disease determined by a single pair of genes and that the distribution curve for blood pressure in the general population *does* show a bimodal distribution. He believes that other pieces of evidence suggest a dominant role for inheritance in the development of essential hypertension, namely the occurrence of hypertensive complications in pairs of identical twins, the fact that populations do exist in which blood pressure does *not* rise with age and the frequent strong family history of hypertension or hypertensive complications in patients with hypertension. Pickering believes that essential hypertension is not a distinct disease but that blood pressure, like height, is different in individuals, and that the complications of high blood pressure are not usually determined by inheritance but by environmental factors. Pickering does not discount inheritance completely, he believes that the inheritance of blood pressure is due to many genes. As in the case of dwarfs and giants in the height analogy occasionally high blood pressure is determined by single genes but it is usually determined by multiple genes as is the height of the vast majority of normal people.

The careful South Wales epidemiological surveys involving urban (Rhondda Valley) and rural (Vale of Glamorgan) populations support the polygenetic inheritance and environmental causes of raised blood pressure. The evidence favours "shared" genes, i.e. widespread occurrence of genes influencing blood pressure so that environmental factors are likely to be more important in causing the development of a high blood pressure. There is a close resemblance between the level of blood pressure and change of blood pressure in healthy individuals in the general population and their relatives (Miall and Oldham, 1963).

Two clear conclusions can be drawn from several surveys of life insurance blood pressure statistics: *mortality* from *most* hypertensive complications is related to the height of the diastolic pressure and the same level of raised diastolic pressure is more serious the younger the person. These figures only demonstrate a statistical association, they do not prove that an individual with a high diastolic pressure is at increased risk; none the less, for practical purposes we have to apply these group statistics to an individual case. Treatment of essential hypertension which reduces the blood pressure *reduces* the mortality and most of the complications. This applies particularly to malignant hypertension (Leishman, 1963). One of the largest series of mild and moderate hypertensives with Grade I or II retinopathy showed a significant improvement in mortality and complications, particularly cerebrovascular accidents and left ventricular failure (Smirk, 1966). There seems to be no reduction in the incidence of myocardial infarction (Smirk and Hodge, 1963). It is generally assumed that once antihypertensive treatment is started it must be continued for life; however, there is good evidence that up to a third of patients treated for *severe* hypertension may have their antihypertensive drugs withdrawn and the blood pressure remain within the normal range (Page and Dustan, 1962).

Treatment of hypertension is, therefore, based on these considerations:

1. There is no definite level at which the blood pressure becomes abnormal.

2. There is a slight increase in diastolic pressure with age.

3. The incidence of complications is related to the height of the diastolic pressure.

4. Complications may be reduced by the treatment of hypertension.

Causes of Hypertension

Unknown (essential).
Renal disease (glomerulonephritis, pyelonephritis).
Renal artery stenosis.
Coarctation of the aorta.
Cushing's syndrome.
Phaeochromocytoma.
Primary aldosteronism.

All the causes of secondary hypertension must be excluded before it is assumed that a patient has essential hypertension. Essential hypertension tends to be a familial disease, therefore, the presence of hypertension or its complications in a member of the patient's family is support (but not proof) for the diagnosis of essential hypertension.

Indications for Treatment of Hypertension

(1) **Malignant hypertension,** i.e. hypertension complicated by papilloedema or retinal haemorrhages and exudates: untreated, 90 per cent of patients with malignant hypertension will die within a year. (2) **Hypertensive encephalopathy.** (3) **Left ventricular failure** due to the hypertension. (4) **Evidence of other complications of hypertension,** i.e. cardiac enlargement, cardiographic evidence of left ventricular hypertrophy or hypertensive changes in the retinal arteries.

These factors in the presence of elevation of the diastolic pressure would be uncontroversial indications for the treatment of the raised diastolic pressure.

Other factors which may influence treatment are:

1. *Level of diastolic pressure.*—In view of the fact that no level can be said to be definitely abnormal, any figure given must be empirical. In practice a *sustained* diastolic pressure of 110 mm Hg is taken as indicating the presence of hypertension which warrants treatment.

2. *Sex.*—Males under the age of 45 have a poorer prognosis if untreated. Females at all ages are less likely to develop complications.

3. *Family history* of early death due to hypertension or its complications.

4. *Race.*—Negroes are more prone to complications.

5. *Obesity.*—Overweight is associated with elevation of the blood pressure which may fall with weight reduction.

6. *Age.*—Increasing age is normally accompanied by increasing diastolic pressure. A fall in systemic pressure may slow the flow through narrowed arteries precipitating thrombosis in heart or brain.

Special Considerations

1. **Hypertension under the age of 40.**—It is widely held that hypertension under the age of 40 is more likely to be secondary than essential. However, it is likely that only about a third of hypertensive patients under the age of 40 will have a possibly remediable cause and it is recommended that renal arteriography be limited to those patients in whom renal surgery is contemplated or to patients under 40 in whom control of blood pressure by drugs is difficult (Breckenbridge *et al.*, 1967).

2. **Hypertension due to unilateral renal disease.**—Nephrectomy may be

indicated if the hypertension is "significant" (i.e. causing cardio-vascular hypertrophy), overall renal function is good (blood urea less than 8 mmol/l and creatinine clearance more than 50 ml per minute) and when the damaged kidney is contributing less than 25 per cent of total renal function. This can usually be assessed by pyelography and isotope renograms, although occasionally divided renal function studies may be necessary. A renal arteriogram is essential before surgery (Luke *et al.*, 1968).

3. Hypertension in the presence of renal impairment.—Most of the antihypertensive drugs reduce renal blood flow and glomerular filtration and tend to make renal function worse in doses which control the blood pressure. The two drugs which do not usually reduce renal blood flow are α-methyldopa and hydralazine and both these may be used if it is believed that the hypertension is causing the renal failure or is increasing the cardiovascular damage (deteriorating ECG, fresh fundal exudates and haemorrhages or left ventricular failure which is difficult to control).

As a rule no attempt to lower the blood pressure is made if the blood urea is over 15 mmol/l. Renal function which is so impaired that the blood urea is more than 15 mmol is likely to be made worse by anti-hypertensive drugs. Occasional exceptions to this are made in malignant hypertension of recent onset or if the hypertension and not the renal failure is causing symptoms, e.g. severe headaches or left ventricular failure. Malignant hypertension is such a devastating disease that it is justified to grasp at every therapeutic straw; in respect to this it is important not to forget lumbar sympathectomy; although superseded in the treatment of benign essential hypertension sympathectomy should still be considered for the young patient with malignant hypertension who has failed to respond to all the standard drugs. Recently in the U.S. an aggressive antihypertensive regime in malignant hypertension with renal failure has been suggested using diazoxide and frusemide; limited personal experience of this regime has not been encouraging.

4. Hypertension with established cerebrovascular disease.—The length of survival and recovery following a cerebral thrombosis depends largely on the extent of the underlying atheroma. The value of anti-hypertensive drugs in a patient found to be moderately hypertensive after a stroke has been questioned on the grounds that in a large series prognosis was not improved by treating the raised blood pressure unless hypertension was severe (Adams, 1965). The question has been clarified by the finding that prognosis in hypertensive survivors of a stroke *is* improved if the diastolic hypertension is carefully treated in patients under the age of 65 (Carter, 1970).

5. Hypertension and the anaesthetist.—Antihypertensive drugs affect the vascular reflexes, particularly the compensatory reflexes to blood loss. Tilting the patient and induction of anaesthesia occasionally produce hypotension if antihypertensive drugs are not stopped. The response to vasoconstrictors is variably affected by previous antihypertensive drugs (Dingle, 1966). Antihypertensive drugs should be stopped for 7 days before a large elective operation provided the hypertension is not severe.

The most orthodox drug regimes are:

Mild hypertension (diastolic pressure below 110 mm Hg).—Sedation or sedation plus reserpine plus a thiazide diuretic.

Moderate hypertension (diastolic pressure above 110 mm).—Methyldopa plus a thiazide diuretic or methyldopa plus guanethidine plus a thiazide diuretic. Bethanidine or debrisoquine are often used instead of guanethidine. In resistant cases a β-blocking drug such as propranolol is used.

Reserpine (Serpasil) depletes stores of noradrenaline in sympathetic nerve endings and is a powerful mental depressant in some patients; other side-effects include nasal congestion, drowsiness, nightmares, salt retention and precipitation of heart failure. The usual dose is 0·25 mg twice daily.

Methyldopa (Aldomet) acts by depletion of noradrenaline stores and prevention of synthesis of noradrenaline. It does not alter cardiac output or decrease renal blood flow, therefore it is the best hypotensive drug to use in the presence of renal failure. Methyldopa does not cause much change of blood pressure with change to upright position or with exercise. Side-effects include sedation, depression, headaches, oedema and gastro-intestinal disturbances. The most serious toxic effects are leucopenia, liver damage and haemolytic anaemia; 10–20 per cent of patients on prolonged treatment develop a positive Coombs test. The positive Coombs test reverts to negative when the drug is stopped. The starting dose is 250 mg three times a day. The dose can be increased by 250 mg every two days.

Guanethidine (Ismelin).—This drug blocks transmission in the postganglionic nerve fibre of the sympathetic system and depletes the tissue stores of noradrenaline. In high doses it also blocks the ganglia of the parasympathetic system but this does not happen with therapeutic doses. Reduction of blood pressure is much greater in the upright position so that postural hypotension may occur; exercise may also cause hypotension. The main side-effects are diarrhoea, hypotension, fluid retention, gastro-intestinal disturbances and failure of ejaculation (but with normal erection).

The usual starting dose is 10 mg daily. The drug is cumulative over 5–7 days; if the blood pressure is not controlled the dose should be increased by 10 mg (as an out-patient) or 20 mg (as an in-patient) every week until the blood pressure is controlled. Absorption of guanethidine from the gastro-intestinal tract is variable from patient to patient but remains relatively constant in an individual patient. Bethanidine and debrisoquine are similar to guanethidine except that side-effects are less common and the drugs are not so cumulative, so that the dose can be increased every other day.

Combinations of drugs are used in order to reduce the incidence of side-effects due to large doses of one drug alone and to obtain better control of the blood pressure.

Guanethidine is used if the blood pressure is not reduced by methyldopa plus a thiazide diuretic. Guanethidine should not be used if the blood urea is raised or if there is severe cardiac failure. It should not be given with mono-amine oxidase inhibitors or in patients with a phaeochromocytoma.

Occasionally α-blocking drugs such as phenoxybenzamine are useful in cases of hypertension resistant to other drugs. Some physicians believe that α-blocking drugs are more effective in hypertension occurring during pregnancy.

Bethanidine, debrisoquine, phenoxybenzamine and β-blocking drugs cause less disturbance of sexual function than the other antihypertensive drugs.

MAIN ANTIHYPERTENSIVE DRUGS

	Dose increments (per day)	Interval
α-Methyldopa	250 mg	4–7 days
Guanethidine	10 mg	5–7 days
Bethanidine	5–10 mg	2–3 days
Debrisoquine	10 mg	2–3 days
Propranolol	60 mg	2–3 days

Malignant Hypertension and Hypertensive Encephalopathy

There is frequent quibbling about the exact definition of malignant hypertension. However, all are agreed that whatever the precise definition a blood pressure high enough to cause papilloedema needs urgent, prompt treatment in order to prevent irreversible renal damage, cerebral oedema and arterial damage.

In practice malignant hypertension is frequently accompanied by hypertensive encephalopathy in which severe headaches, convulsions, disturbances of consciousness and focal neurological signs accompany the hypertension; frequently there is also neck stiffness, papilloedema, left ventricular failure and deteriorating renal function.

Management.—The aims of treatment are to reduce the blood pressure and relieve cerebral oedema. Cerebral oedema, if severe, can be relieved with diuretics, mannitol, Ureaphil, by raising the head of the bed and occasionally with dexamethazone. The blood pressure can be quickly lowered with:

1. Hexamethonium intravenously, each dose is given at 5-minute intervals until the blood pressure is reduced. The starting dose is 2·5 mg and is repeated once; if necessary the dose is doubled and repeated and again doubled and repeated if the blood pressure is not reduced. Most patients have reduction of diastolic pressure on about 10 mg given at 5-minute intervals.

2. Pentolinium (Ansolysen) 1 mg every 5 minutes.

3. Reserpine (Serpasil) 2·5–5·0 mg i.m.

4. α-Methyldopa (Aldomet) 250–500 mg i.v. 6-hourly; this is given in 100 ml 5 per cent dextrose over 30 minutes and is effective in 3–4 hours.

5. Diazoxide and frusemide are occasionally used.

Longer-acting antihypertensives such as bethanidine or debrisoquine are given by mouth in large doses at the same time; when the blood pressure is reduced the parenteral therapy can be discontinued.

Renal Artery Stenosis

Renal ischaemia causes secretion of renin and hence aldosterone leading to the establishment of "vicious circle hypertension". Narrowing of one or both renal arteries may result in ischaemia. The bore of an artery must be reduced by 60–70 per cent before there is any reduction in blood flow. At postmortem, renal artery narrowing is common in normotensive people (Holley et al., 1964). and in life there may be arteriographic evidence of renal artery stenosis in normotensives (Eyler et al., 1962). Nevertheless, severe unilateral renal artery stenosis results in hypertension which is curable by repairing the stenosis. Unilateral renal artery stenosis is probably responsible for 2–5 per cent of cases of hypertension. Narrowing of the renal arteries may be due to an atheromatous plaque, fibromuscular hyperplasia, embolism or external compression. Fibromuscular hyperplasia is much commoner in women between the ages of 30–40, the stenoses are frequently multiple, tend to occur in the more distal parts of the arteries and to be accompanied by aneurysm formation (often multiple). Arteriosclerotic narrowing usually occurs in the proximal part of the artery, near its origin from the aorta. Clinical features which should lead to a "high index of suspicion" that renal artery stenosis may be present are sudden acceleration of previously mild hypertension, severe hypertension below the age of 35, the development of hypertension following an episode of renal pain suggesting embolism or infarction, and malignant hypertension. Careful auscultation may reveal a renal artery bruit.

Features in the IVP which are suggestive are a difference in size of more than 2 cm between the two kidneys and a delayed appearance time of the dye in one kidney with subsequent increased density of the dye on that side. The appearance time is delayed because of the decreased blood flow and the concentration increased because slower blood flow results in more time for more dye to be excreted. The next diagnostic step is usually a renal arteriogram to confirm the presence and location of the stenosis. The presence of the stenosis does not necessarily mean that the hypertension is due to the stenosis or that it is causing any alteration in the function of the kidney. In order to decide if the narrowing is likely to be responsible for hypertension it is usual to demonstrate a difference in function between the two kidneys. The easiest method of doing this is by noting the rate of uptake and excretion by the kidneys of a radioactive substance. A narrowed renal artery will delay uptake and excretion if the blood flow is significantly diminished. A gamma ray scintillation counter is used to count simultaneously over both kidneys. The two radioactive substances commonly used are I^{131}-labelled Hippuran and a diuretic, chlormerodrin, labelled with radioactive mercury (Hg^{203}). Occasionally "divided renal studies" (Stamey's[30] test) are performed to demonstrate the differences in function. Bilateral ureteric catheters are passed so that samples of urine can be collected from each kidney. The ischaemic kidney excretes urine more slowly than the normal and the urine contains less sodium because with slower urine flow through the renal tubules there is more time for more complete re-absorption of sodium from the tubules. For substances which are not re-absorbed by the tubules the concentration will be greater in the urine from the affected side (because the volume is smaller).

Hyperaldosteronism

The features of overproduction of aldosterone by an autonomous tumour of the adrenal cortex (Conn's[31] syndrome) are hypertension, hypokalaemia and an increased serum sodium. Alkalosis occurs because potassium lost from the cells is replaced by hydrogen ion which renders the extracellular fluid alkalotic. The alkalosis may lead to tetany by reducing the ionized calcium in the serum and the hypokalaemia may lead to muscle weakness and periodic muscular paralysis. There is polyuria and an increased urinary potassium, particularly in view of the low serum level. Oedema does not occur. The normal control of aldosterone production is probably by chemo- and volume-receptors in the juxtaglomerular apparatus of the kidney. An enzyme, renin, is released which acts on a protein called angiotensinogen circulating in the plasma forming angiotensin which causes the adrenal cortex to secrete aldosterone. Renal ischaemia caused by hypertension stimulates the production of renin and hence aldosterone. Secondary aldosteronism due to renal ischaemia secondary to hypertensive arterial narrowing will have many of the features of primary aldosteronism due to a tumour of the

30. T. A. STAMEY. Contemporary American surgeon.
31. W. J. CONN. Contemporary Michigan physician.

adrenal cortex. The best method of distinguishing between primary and secondary aldosteronism is to measure the plasma renin; in primary aldosteromism the plasma renin will be normal or low, whereas in secondary aldosteronism the plasma renin will be increased. Unfortunately the estimation of plasma renin is difficult to perform and not freely available. Renal biopsy may show hypertrophy of the juxtaglomerular apparatus indicating over-activity and excessive renin production in secondary but not primary aldosteronism.

It is possible to measure the 24-hour urine excretion of aldosterone or its metabolites; as a rule aldosterone secretion is much higher in primary than in secondary hyperaldosteronism, nevertheless, there is an overlap. The inability of a high sodium intake to suppress the rate of aldosterone secretion is further evidence of an autonomously functioning adrenal tumour.

The serum potassium may be reduced in patients on thiazide diuretics but in these patients the serum sodium is usually normal whereas in primary and secondary aldosteronism the serum sodium is usually elevated and the pH indicates an alkalosis (high bicarbonate and low chloride).

Suspicion of Aldosteronism

Hypokalaemia.
Inappropriately high urine potassium (more than 40 mEq/24 hours).
High or low plasma sodium.

Confirmation of Aldosteronism

Plasma and urine levels of aldosterone raised.
Reduction of *urine* potassium on a *low*-sodium diet.
Reversed ratio of sodium: potassium in sweat and saliva.

Diagnosing the Cause of Aldosteronism

Primary	*Secondary*
History: Tetany, paraesthesia, muscle weakness all commoner than in secondary aldosteronism.	Usually in diuretics.

Examination and Investigation:

Mild hypertension without retinopathy.	Severe hypertension often with retinopathy.
Plasma sodium increased or normal.	Plasma sodium decreased or normal.
Hypokalaemia despite potassium supplements.	Hypokalaemia often reversed by potassium supplements.

Plasma volume increased hence abnormal Valsalva manoeuvre.

Plasma volume normal or reduced hence normal Valsalva.

Spironolactone alone may reduce the blood pressure.

Spironolactone alone will not reduce the blood pressure.

Aldosterone level is high despite *high*-sodium diet.

Aldosterone level may be lowered by *high*-sodium diet.

Plasma renin low and remains *low* on a *low*-sodium diet and in the erect posture.

Plasma renin high.

Renal biopsy normal.

Renal biopsy may show hypertrophy of J-G apparatus.

Other conditions are associated with hypokalaemia but unlike primary aldosteronism and secondary aldosteronism due to hypertension they are not always accompanied by hypertension. The other main causes of hypokalaemia are:

1. Diarrhoea and vomiting.
2. Paralytic ileus in which potassium-rich fluid accumulates in the dilated small intestines.
3. Acidosis which promotes renal loss of potassium.
4. Other causes of hyperaldosteronism such as cirrhosis, heart failure and the nephrotic syndrome.
5. Cushing's syndrome.
6. Renal tubular defects.

Phaeochromocytoma

Tumours of the adrenal medulla produce catecholamines which result in hypertension which at first is paroxysmal but later becomes sustained. Hypertension causes damage to the arterioles of the kidney resulting in localised areas of renal ischaemia. These ischaemic areas cause further hypertension by stimulating renin formation and secondary hyperaldosteronism and a vicious circle is established ("vicious circle hypertension"). This is a feature of all forms of hypertension and is the mechanism by which episodic hypertension of phaeochromocytoma becomes sustained. There are usually other features of catecholamine release such as palpitations, pallor, severe headaches, perspiration and anxiety. There is often glycosuria and an increased BMR. The metabolites of the circulating catecholamines are excreted in the urine and the one most conveniently measured is vanillylmandelic acid (VMA). Certain drugs interfere with the estimation of VMA: these are barbiturates, salicylates and Aldomet. Drugs which block the effects of the circulating catecholamines may be used to confirm the diagnosis; phentolamine will block the alpha adrenergic activities of adrenaline and noradrenaline and cause a lowering of the blood pressure (a fall of

TABLE II

SHOWING THE MAIN ALPHA AND BETA EFFECTS OF ADRENALINE AND
NORADRENALINE (Lawrence, 1966)

Alpha Effects	Beta Effects
Excitatory except for intestinal relaxation	Inhibitory except for myocardial stimulation
Vasoconstriction (largely in the skin)	Vasodilatation (largely in the muscles)
Mydriasis	Myocardial stimulation (increased rate, force and excitability)
	Bronchial relaxation
Myometrial contraction	Myometrial relaxation
Intestinal relaxation	Intestinal relaxation

35 mm Hg in the systolic pressure is a positive response). The test must
not be performed if the patient has taken antihypertensive drugs in the
previous ten days. Surgical removal of the tumour is the treatment of
choice, both adrenals should be inspected because the tumours are
bilateral or multiple in 10 per cent of cases and may occur in extra-
adrenal sites, including thorax, bladder and sympathetic ganglia.
Medical treatment is used pre-operatively or if the tumours are malignant (10 per cent) and recur. The alpha effects of adrenaline and noradrenaline can be controlled with a long-acting alpha blocking drug
such as phenoxybenzamine (Dibenyline) and the beta effects by a beta
blocking drug such as propranolol. The main alpha and beta effects of
adrenaline and noradrenaline are shown in Table II. Adrenaline has
both alpha and beta effects, noradrenaline has predominantly alpha
effects while isoprenaline has mainly beta effects.

The advantages of α-blocking drugs in the management of phaeochromocytoma are (Ross *et al.*, 1967):

1. Pre-operative vasodilatation which permits re-expansion of con-
tracted blood volume.
2. Control of blood pressure.
3. Reduction of hypertension resulting from induction of anaesthesia.
4. No fall in blood pressure when the tumour is removed because
plasma volume is restored to normal.

The advantages of β-blocking drugs are:

1. To control tachycardia which may be aggravated by blocking drugs
2. To prevent dysrhythmias.
The aim is *partial* blockage of α and β adrenergic receptors. *Complete*

a and β blockage is accompanied by a number of disadvantages (Ross *et al.*, 1967):

1. The patient is more sensitive to the hypotensive effect of thiopentone.
2. Venous oozing is more pronounced in complete a blockage.
3. The patient is more susceptible to the hypotensive effect of haemorrhage.
4. Small amounts of blood loss produce a disproportionate tachycardia.

A suitable regime for the management of patients with a phaeochromocytoma is given in the paper by Ross and his colleagues (1967).

EFFORT SYNDROME

The patient has a large number of symptoms referable to the cardiovascular system. None of the symptoms are classical or characteristic of organic disease, although they may be sufficiently similar to cause diagnostic confusion—this is particularly so if the effort syndrome is superimposed on known organic heart disease. The hallmark of the syndrome is that physical exertion seems to require an excessive amount of effort and seems to produce exaggerated reactions. Physical examination usually reveals no abnormality. There are a number of simple tests which may be useful in diagnosing and assessing the condition. All these tests are based on demonstrating that autonomic reflexes are modified by higher centres of the brain. The autonomic reflex may be suppressed, e.g. when reflex apnoea is absent after hyperventilation; the reflex may be exaggerated, e.g. excessive tachycardia in response to hyperventilation. Four simple tests for evaluating the effort syndrome are:

1. Absence of reflex apnoea after 2 minutes' hyperventilation.
2. Inability to hold breath for 30 seconds.
3. Orthostatic and hyperventilation tachycardia of more than 100.
4. Slow return of pulse rate to normal after standard exercise.

CARDIOMYOPATHIES

The cardiomyopathies are a heterogeneous group of diseases in which the heart muscle is primarily involved. By convention, the group does not include heart muscle damage secondary to coronary artery disease, hypertension and valvular disease. In the American literature myocardiopathy, myocardosis and primary myocardial disease are synonymous. There are many classifications; one of the simplest (Goodwin *et al.*, 1961) is:

1. **Congestive:** with features of congestive heart failure.
2. **Constrictive:** with features of constrictive pericarditis.

3. **Obstructive:** with features of functional obstruction of the ventricular outflow tracts.

A more recent classification (Table III) is into two main groups: "primary" and "secondary"—those in which the main disorder is of the heart itself and those in which the heart disorder is secondary to some more generalised disease (Goodwin, 1966).

The accepted definition of cardiomyopathy (Goodwin, 1970) is: "A subacute or chronic disorder of heart muscle of unknown or unusual cause, often with associated endocardial and sometimes pericardial involvement." The functional classification into congestive, constrictive and obstructive has been modified. Constrictive (restrictive)

TABLE III

CLASSIFICATION OF CARDIOMYOPATHIES

Primary		Secondary	
Infective	Viral Bacterial Parasitic	Nutritional	Starvation Kwashiorkor
		Toxic	Alcohol
Obstructive			Drugs
Endomyocardial fibrosis		Infiltrations	Amyloidosis Haemochromatosis Glycogen storage disease
Fibroelastosis			Sarcoidosis
Puerperal			Fat
Idiopathic	Familial Non-familial	Collagen disease	Rheumatoid arthritis SLE Scleroderma Polyarteritis nodosa
		Endocrine	Myxoedema Acromegaly Myasthenia gravis
		Congenital	Friedreich's ataxia Muscular dystrophies Gargoylism

cardiomyopathy is rare, the most usual cause being amyloid infiltration. Hypertrophic cardiomyopathy may occur without obstruction to the outflow tract but the main haemodynamic disturbance may be difficulty in ventricular filling due to decreased compliance of the hypertrophied ventricle. Obliterative cardiomyopathy refers to those cases in which there is encroachment on the cavity of the ventricles and usually endocardial thickening.

The diagnosis of cardiomyopathy should only be made when the commonest cause of myocardial damage (i.e. ischaemia due to coronary artery disease) has been excluded. Exclusion of coronary artery disease can be extremely difficult.

Occasionally patients with a congestive cardiomyopathy have hypertension or develop angina. Rarely hypertrophic obstructive cardiomyopathy can follow left ventricular hypertrophy due to some other cause such as hypertension. In obstructive cardiomyopathy the β-blocking drugs successfully lower the end-diastolic pressure. Anticoagulants are indicated if a dysrhythmia (usually atrial fibrillation) is present. Bacterial endocarditis in association with obstructive cardiomyopathy has been described.

PRIMARY CARDIOMYOPATHIES

Infective

Viral.—The commonest cause of viral myocarditis is the Coxsackie B virus. The illness is often biphasic—initial malaise is followed about ten days later by fever, tachycardia, cardiac dilatation and arrhythmias. Virus may be isolated from throat swab and stool; however Coxsackie virus is often found in the stools of healthy children so that virus isolated from the stools after the third week of the illness may have been acquired coincidentally. Neutralising antibodies to the virus are found in the serum, a fourfold rise in titre between acute and convalescent sera is confirmatory.

Myocarditis is occasionally seen in other viral infections such as poliomyelitis, influenza, mumps and glandular fever.

Bacterial.—The best known bacterial myocarditis is diphtheria in which the myocarditis usually presents in the third week of the illness with cardiac enlargement, ECG changes and circulatory collapse. Complete recovery in non-fatal cases is the rule. True myocarditis may occur with tuberculosis and probably occurs with miliary spread of the disease. Active carditis occurs in rheumatic fever, streptococcal infections and meningococcal septicaemia. Other bacterial infections which may be complicated by a myocarditis are Weil's[32] disease, toxoplasmosis and trypanosomiasis (particularly in South America where the organism is *Trypanosoma cruzi* and the disease is known as Chagas'[33] disease).

32. ADOLF WEIL (1848–1916). Wiesbaden physician.
33. CARLOS CHAGAS (1879–1934). Brazilian physician.

Hypertrophic Obstructive Cardiomyopathy (HOCM)

During systole, the ventricle contracts progressively from apex to infundibulum. If this sequence is abnormal, and the infundibulum contracts before the end of systole it will obstruct the flow of the blood from the ventricle. Abnormal infundibular contraction may occur in either ventricle, it may be congenital or acquired.

There is a day-to-day variability of the symptoms which include angina, syncope and dyspnoea. The pulse is characteristically jerky— with a rapid upstroke unlike the anacrotic pulse of aortic stenosis. There is an ejection murmur which is late in onset and best heard at the apex and left sternal edge. The rapid upstroke of the pulse is due to early rapid emptying of the ventricle; the functional narrowing of the outflow tract occurs late in systole, which corresponds with the late onset of the ejection murmur. Abnormal contraction of the ventricular muscle may interfere with the function of the papillary muscles, tending to distort the cusps of the mitral valve and so cause mitral regurgitation. There is often a double impulse at the apex during systole which may be due to a palpable atrial impulse or to forward displacement of the apex when the hypertrophied muscle of the outflow tract contracts. Drugs which improve the efficiency of myocardial contraction, such as isoprenaline and digitalis, tend to make the obstruction worse, beta adrenergic drugs such as propranolol decrease the obstruction.

Endomyocardial Fibrosis (EMF)

As its name implies both the endocardium and myocardium are involved. The endocardium becomes thickened and stiff leading to constriction of the ventricular cavity and distortion of the papillary muscles which causes incompetence of the atrioventricular valves. The myocardium becomes thickened and fibrotic. The disease occurs only in the tropics but expatriates as well as the indigenous population may be affected. The onset is sometimes a febrile illness accompanied by malaise, dyspnoea and tachycardia. Occasionally there is an accompanying eosinophilia but no other evidence of an infecting organism. The disease is usually complicated by intractable heart failure, pulmonary hypertension or emboli—both pulmonary and systemic.

Fibroelastosis

The endocardium may become thickened at the site of excessive turbulence as in the McCallum patch seen in the left atrium in mitral incompetence, where the blood impinges on the atrial wall. Endocardial thickening also occurs secondary to myocardial disease, for example EMF and myocardial infarction and in congenital heart disease, especially in the presence of desaturated blood. Nevertheless, excessive fibrosis of the endocardium occurs in the absence of any known causes. Primary fibroelastosis usually presents in the first few months of life as intractable heart failure; rarely the disease presents in adult life. The majority of children with fibroelastosis have a positive skin test to mumps antigen at an age when a positive reaction is unusual (Noren *et al.*, 1963).

SECONDARY CARDIOMYOPATHIES

Nutritional

Congestive cardiac failure is frequently seen in severe malnutrition and is probably related to dietary deficiency of B_1 (thiamin), electrolyte imbalance if associated pellagra causes severe diarrhoea or protein deficiency as in kwashiorkor (kwashiorkor—red boy—a reference to the characteristic brown hair and skin pigmentation; another interpretation is "disease of the jealous child"—referring to the occurrence of the disease in children who have been prematurely weaned because the mother is again pregnant).

Toxic

Alcoholic cardiomyopathy.—Excessive consumption of alcohol to the exclusion of adequate vitamin intake, may result in beri beri and high output heart failure because of widespread peripheral vasodilatation. However, a congestive type of cardiomyopathy may occur in alcoholics in the absence of the signs of beri beri. Alcoholic cardiomyopathy should be considered in anyone who has drunk continuously, for ten years or more, a bottle of spirits or ten to fifteen pints of beer a day (Brigden and Robinson, 1964). The ECG findings are variable but specific abnormalities have been described (Evans, 1959). These are the "spinous" T waves, in which left ventricular T waves become heightened and pointed; "cloven" T waves in which the upright T wave has a small depression near its summit, and the "dimple" T wave in which the normal T wave is absent and is replaced by a small dimple in an otherwise isoelectric S–U period. Treatment of the heart failure, prolonged bed rest and total abstinence from alcohol may result in a complete cure in the early stages.

Drugs.—Emetine hydrochloride, used to treat amoebiasis, and sodium or potassium antimony tartrate, used to treat bilharzia, both cause a myocarditis. The myocardium may be involved in sensitivity reaction to drugs.

Infiltration of the Myocardium

Amyloidosis.—The heart is a common site for deposition in primary amyloidosis other common sites being muscle, skin and gums. The heart usually is small and restricted by the amyloid tissue (an example of a "constructive" type of cardiomyopathy). The heart is rarely involved in secondary amyloidosis, the main sites of deposition in which are kidney, liver and spleen. Curiously, the distribution of the amyloid deposits secondary to myelomatosis resembles that of primary amyloid.

Haemochromatosis.—Excessive absorption of iron due to lack of the normal "mucosal block" or a congenital deficiency of the iron-carrying beta globulin (transferrin) results in excessive storing of iron in the tissues. The stored iron acts as an irritant, causing fibrosis, which in the heart leads to congestive failure, usually both sides of the heart are involved and conduction defects are common.

Fat.—Extreme obesity may be associated with infiltration of fat into the myocardium, hampering ventricular contraction. Rarely, the heart may be the site of deposition of the lipoid material in histiocytosis X.

Sarcoidosis.—The heart is frequently involved in cases of sarcoidosis severe enough to come to autopsy. This may lead to cardiomegaly, arrhythmias and congestive cardiac failure.

Glycogen storage disease.—In this disease there is excessive deposition of glycogen in different tissues especially the heart, liver and skeletal muscles. There may be increased glycogen in the blood and urine. The affected infant usually presents with cardiomegaly or hypoglycaemia.

Collagen Diseases

Rheumatoid arthritis.—Cardiac involvement in rheumatoid arthritis usually causes a pericardial effusion. Rarely a rheumatoid nodule may cause fibrosis of the myocardium and congestive heart failure.

Systemic lupus erythematosus.—The most usual cardiac manifestations of SLE are sterile pericarditis and effusion and the verrucous non-embolising endocarditis of Libman[34]-Sacks.[35] SLE may also cause widespread fibrosis of the myocardium and congestive cardiac failure without valvular or pericardial involvement.

Scleroderma.—The commonest organs involved are the gastro-intestinal tract, skin, lungs and peripheral nerves; involvement of the arteries results in Raynaud's phenomenon and ischaemia. Myocardial fibrosis is fairly common, and causes congestive failure or conduction defects if the bundle of His is involved. Cor pulmonale may occur secondary to pulmonary hypertension, due to lung fibrosis.

Polyarteritis nodosa.—Polyarteritis nodosa may cause heart failure secondary to associated hypertension or myocardial infarction due to involvement of the coronary arteries. In addition there is frequently pericardial involvement and focal myocardial fibrosis, which may result in heart failure out of proportion to the severity of the hypertension or the degree of coronary artery involvement.

34. EMANUEL LIBMAN (1872–1946). New York physician.
35. BENJAMIN SACKS (b. 1896). New York physician.

Endocrine Diseases

Myxoedema.—Cardiac enlargement in myxoedema is usually due to the presence of a pericardial effusion and angina to co-existing coronary artery disease. However myxoedema may cause heart failure due to infiltration with mucoprotein. The ECG changes of myxoedema usually revert to normal promptly with thyroxine, suggesting that they are due to a rapidly reversible cause such as electrolyte disturbance of the myocardial cells.

Acromegaly.—The heart is usually large in acromegaly as part of the general splanchnomegaly or as a result of associated hypertension. However, there is also an increase in myocardial fibrosis which leads to heart failure more readily than would be expected from the associated hypertension alone.

Myasthenia gravis.—Identical changes may occur in heart muscle to those which occur in voluntary muscles, i.e. lymphorrhages, atrophy of muscle fibres and necrosis.

Congenital

Friedreich's ataxia.—This hereditary disease, appearing before adolescence and characterised by degeneration of the spinocerebellar tracts, posterior columns, and pyramidal tracts and by skeletal deformity (kyphoscoliosis and pes cavus) also affects the heart. There may be cardiac enlargement, arrhythmias and conduction defects.

Muscular dystrophies.—All the muscular dystrophies may be accompanied by myocardial involvement but it is most frequently seen in the pseudohypertrophic type and dystrophia myotonica. ECG abnormalities are common.

Gargoylism.—The myocardium may be involved in the widespread deposition of mucopolysaccharide characteristic of this condition.

REFERENCES

ADAMS, G. F. (1965). *Brit. med. J.*, **2**, 253.
ALTSCHULE, M. D. (1966). In *Controversy in Internal Medicine*. Ed. Ingelfinger, F. J., Relman, A. S., and Finland, M. Philadelphia: W. B. Saunders.
American Heart Association (1956). *Circulation*, **13**, 617.
BAILEY, R. R., ABERNETHY, M. H., and BEAVEN, D. W. (1967). *Lancet*, **1**, 970.
BEARD, O. W., HIPP, H. R., ROBINS, M., TAYLOR, J. S., EBERT, R. V., and BERAN, L. G. (1960). *Amer. J. Med.*, **28**, 871.
BORDLEY, J., CHARLES, A. R., CONNOR, M. D., HAMILTON, W. F., KERR, W. J., and WIGGERS, A. R. (1951). *Circulation*, **4**, 503.
BRECKENRIDGE, A., PREGER, L., DOLLERY, C. T., and LAWS, J. W. (1967). *Quart. J. Med.*, **36**, 549.
BRIGDEN, W., and ROBINSON, J. (1964). *Brit. med. J.*, **2**, 1283.
BROWSE, N. L., (1969a). *Fifth Symposium on Advanced Medicine*, Royal College of Physicians, London.

BROWSE, N. L. (1969b). *Brit. med. J*, **4**, 676.

BROWSE, N. L., LEA THOMAS, M., and PIM, H. P. (1968). *Brit. med. J.*, **3**, 717.

BURNS COX, C. J. (1967). *Lancet*, **1**, 1194.

BYWATERS, E. G., and THOMAS, G. T. (1962). *Brit. med. J.*, **8**, 221.

CARTER, A. B. (1970). *Lancet*, **1**, 485.

CLEAVE, T. L., and CAMPBELL, G. D. (1969). *Diabetes, Coronary Thrombosis and the Saccharine Disease*. Bristol: John Wright.

Combined Rheumatic Fever Study Group (1965). *New Engl. J. Med*, **272**, 63.

DAVIES, J., and DAVIES, I. J. T. (1968). *Hosp. Med.*, **2**, 686.

DINGLE, H. R. (1966). *Anaesthesia*, **21**, 151.

DORFMAN, A., GROSS, J. I., and LORINCZ, A. E. (1961). *Pediatrics*, **27**, 692.

DUGUID, J. B. (1948). *J. Path. Bact.*, **60**, 57.

EVANS, W. (1959). *Brit. Heart J.*, **21**, 445.

EYLER, W. R., CLARK, M. D., GARMAN, J. E., RIAN, R. L., and MEININGER, D. E. (1962). *Radiology*, **78**, 879.

FLANC, C., KAKKAR, V. V., and CLARKE, M. B. (1969). *Brit. med. J.*, **1**, 806.

FLEMMING, H. A., and BAILEY, S. M. (1966). *Brit. med. J.*, **1**, 1322.

FRIEDBERG, C. K. (1966). *Diseases of the Heart*, p. 898. Philadelphia: W. B. Saunders Co.

FULMER, H. S., and ROBERTS, R. W. (1963). *Ann. intern. Med.*, **59**, 740.

GOODWIN, J. F. (1966). In *Symposium on Disorders of the Heart and Circulation*, Publication No. 31, Royal College of Physicians of Edinburgh.

GOODWIN, J. F. (1970). *Lancet*, **1**, 731.

GOODWIN, J. F., GORDON, H., HOLLMAN, A., and BISHOP, M. B. (1961). *Brit. med. J.*, **1**, 69.

GROEN, J. J., TIJONG, K. B., KOSTER, M., WILLEBRANDS, A. F., VERDONEK, G., and PIERLOOT, M. (1962). *Amer. J. clin. Nutr.*, **10**, 456.

GROSS, R. E. (1950). *Circulation*, **1**, 41.

GSELL, D., and MAYER, J. (1962). *Amer. J. clin. Nutr.*, **10**, 471.

HILDEN, T., IVERSON, K., RAASCHOU, F., and SCHWARTZ, M. (1961). *Lancet*, **2**, 327.

HOCKEN, A. G. (1967). *Lancet*, **1**, 466.

HOLLEY, K. E., HUNT, J. C., BROWN, A. L., KINCAID, O. W., and SHEPS, S. G. (1964). *Amer. J. Med.*, **37**, 14.

HONEY, G. E. and TRUELOVE, S. C. (1957a). *Lancet*, **1**, 1155.

HONEY, G. E. and TRUELOVE, S. C. (1957b). *Lancet*, **1**, 1209.

International Anticoagulant Review Group (1970). *Lancet*, **1**, 203.

JACOBS, A. L. (1963). *Amer. Heart. J.*, **65**, 716.

KAGAN, A., LIVSIC, A. M., STERNBY, N., and VIHERT, A. M. (1968). *Lancet*, **2**, 1199.

KAMATH, V. R., and THORNE, M. G. (1969). *Lancet*, **1**, 1025.

KANNEL, W. B., DAWBER, T. R., FRIEDMAN, G. D., GLENNON, W. E., and MCNAMARA, P. M. (1964). *Ann. intern. Med.*, **61**, 888.

KEYS, A., ANDERSON, J. T., and GRANDE, F. (1963). *Metabolism*, **14**, 766.

KIRBY, B. J., and MCNICOL, M. W. (1966). *Lancet*, **2**, 1054.

LAWRENCE, D. R. (1966). In *Second Symposium on Advanced Medicine* at the Royal College of Physicians of London (Ed. Trounce, J. R.), p. 360. London: Pitman Med. Pub. Co.

LEISHMAN, A. W. (1963). *Lancet*, **1**, 1284.
LILLEHEI, R. C., LONGERBEAM, J. K., BLOCH, J. H., and MANAX, W. G. (1964). *Clin. Pharmacol. Ther.*, **5**, 63.
LOWTHER, C. P., and TURNER, R. W. (1962). *Brit. med. J.*, **1**, 1027 and 1102.
LUKE, R. G., KENNEDY, A. C., BRIGGS, J. D., STRUTHERS, N. W., and STIRLING, W. B. (1968). *Brit. med. J.*, **3**, 764.
MCANDREW, G. M., and OGSTON, G. (1965). *Brit. med. J.*, **1**, 425.
MCMICHAEL, J., and PARRY, E. H. (1960). *Lancet*, **2**, 991.
MCNICOL, M. W., KIRBY, B. J., BHOOLA, K. D., EVEREST, M. E., PRICE, H. V., and FREEDMAN, S. F. (1965). *Brit. med. J.*, **2**, 1270.
MANN, G. V., SHAFFER, R. D., ANDERSON, R. S. and SANDSTEAD, H. H. (1964). *J. Atheroscler. Res.*, **4**, 289.
MATTINGLY, T. W. (1962). *Amer. J. Cardiol.*, **9**, 395.
MAVOR, G. E., and GALLOWAY, J. M. (1967). *Lancet*, **1**, 871.
MAVOR, G. E., and GALLOWAY, J. M. (1969). *Brit. J. Surg.*, **56**, 45.
MAVOR, G. E., GALLOWAY, J. M., and KARMODY, A. M. (1970). *Proc. roy. Soc. Med.*, **63**, 126.
Medical Research Council (1964). *Brit. med. J.*, **2**, 837.
Medical Research Council, (1969). *Brit. med. J.*, **1**, 335.
MIALL, W. E., and LOVELL, H. G. (1967). *Brit. med. J.*, **2**, 660.
MIALL, W. E., and OLDHAM, P. D. (1963). *Brit. med. J.*, **1**, 75.
NOREN, G. R., ADAMS, P., and ANDERSON, R. C. (1963). *J. Pediat.*, **62**, 604.
NORRIS, R. M., BRANDT, P. W., CAUGHEY, D. E., LEE, A. J., and SCOTT, P. J. (1969). *Lancet*, **1**, 274.
NORRIS, R. M., CAUGHEY, D. E., DEEMING, L. W., MERCER, C. J., and SCOTT, P. J. (1971). *Lancet*, **2**, 485.
OLIVER, M. F. (1962). *Lancet*, **1**, 653.
OLIVER, M. F., KURIEN, V. A., and GREENWOOD, T. W. (1968). *Lancet*, **1**, 710.
PAGE, I. H., and DUSTAN, H. P. (1962). *Circulation*, **25**, 433.
PATERSON, J. C., ARMSTRONG, R., and ARMSTRONG, E. C. (1963). *Circulation*, **27**, 229.
PAUL, O., LEPPER, M. H., PHELAN, W. H., DEPERTINS, W., MACMILLAN, A., MCKEAN, H., and PARK, H. (1963). *Circulation*, **28**, 20.
PELL, S., and D'ALONZO, C. A. (1964). *New Engl. J. Med.*, **270**, 915.
PICKERING, G. W. (1968). *High Blood Pressure*. London: J. & A. Churchill.
PLATT, R. (1963). *Lancet*, **1**, 899.
POLLER, L., and THOMSON, J. M. (1965). *Lancet*, **1**, 1475.
POMERANTZ, H. Z. (1962). *Canad. med. Ass. J.*, **86**, 57.
RIFKIND, B. M., and DICKSON, C. (1965). *Lancet*, **1**, 312.
RITLAND, S., and LYGREN, T. (1969). *Lancet*, **1**, 122.
ROSENBAUM, F. F., and LEVINE, S. A. (1941). *Arch. intern. Med.*, **68**, 913.
ROSS, E. J., PRICHARD, B. N., KAUFMAN, L., ROBERTSON, A. I., and HARRIES, B. J. (1967). *Brit. med. J.*, **1**, 191.
RUSSEK, H. I., ZOHMAN, B. L., DOERNER, A. A., RUSSEK, A. S., and WHITE, La V. G. (1952). *Circulation*, **5**, 707.
SEVITT, S. (1968). *Proc. roy. Soc. Med.*, **61**, 143.
SEVITT, S., and GALLAGHER, N. (1961). *Brit. J. Surg.*, **48**, 475.
SLEIGHT, P. (1964). *J. Physiol. (Lond.)*, **173**, 321.

SMIRK, F. H. (1966). In *Antihypertensive Therapy: Principles and Practice*. Ed. Gross, F. Berlin: Springer.

SMIRK, F. H., and HODGE, J. V. (1963). *Brit. med. J.*, **2**, 1221.

STAMLER, J. (1969). In *Modern Trends in Cardiology*, p. 88. Ed. Jones, A. M. London: Butterworth.

TURNER, R. W. (1968). *Brit. med. J.*, **2**, 383.

VALENTINE, P. A., FLUCK, D. C., MOUNSEY, J. P., REID, D., SHILLINGFORD, J. P., and STEINER, R. E. (1966). *Lancet*, **2**, 837.

WAHLBERG, F. (1962). *Acta med. scand.*, **171**, 1.

WILLIAMS, R. C., and KUNKEL, H. G. (1962). *J. clin. Invest.*, **41**, 666.

WILSON, M. G. (1960). *Advanc. Pediat.*, **11**, 243.

WRIGHT, I. S., MARPLE, C. D., and BECK, D. F. (1954). *Myocardial Infarction*. New York: Grune and Stratton.

2

RESPIRATORY SYSTEM

RESPIRATORY ADVENTITIOUS SOUNDS

There are two separate conventions for naming the main varieties of adventitious sounds arising from the lungs and airways. Laennec, in his *Treatise on Mediate Auscultation* published in 1819, used "râle" (death-rattle) to describe the sound made by patients dying of advanced tuberculosis—for humanitarian reasons he used the Latin translation, "rhonchus", in front of patients. Thus he used râle and rhonchus interchangeably to describe *all* adventitious sounds. His treatise was quickly and poorly translated into English and "râle and "rhonchus" came to signify different types of sound.

The two main types of adventitious sound either continue more or less throughout one or both phases of the respiratory cycle or are an interrupted series of short sounds. The two nomenclatures are:

Adventitious sounds (râles)   ⎰ crepitations (interrupted sounds)
                                               ⎱ rhonchi (continuous sounds)
Adventitious sounds   ⎰ râles (interrupted sounds)
                                               ⎱ rhonchi (continuous sounds)

Thus, interrupted sounds are either called "râles" or "crepitations". Synonyms sometimes used are:

crepitations (râles)	*rhonchi*
moist sounds	dry sounds
crackling	musical sounds
explosive sounds	wheezes
discontinuous sounds	continuous sounds

Crepitations (râles) were believed to be caused by air bubbling through fluid in the alveoli and/or airways. It is possible to distinguish fine and coarse crepitations (râles) depending on the size of the airways through which the air was thought to be bubbling through the fluid. High-pitched and low-pitched rhonchi (wheezes) were believed to correspond to the size of the airways which are narrowed—high-pitched rhonchi (wheezes) being produced by the smaller airways. Recently these widely held views of the origins of the adventitious sounds have been disputed and plausible alternative explanations produced (Forgacs, 1969). The reasons why the traditional explanations for adventitious sounds are unlikely to be correct are:

1. The viscosity and surface tension of secretions in the small airways cannot be overcome by physiological pressure gradients.

2. Crepitations (râles) are common during inspiration alone—sounds caused by air bubbling through fluid should be heard in both phases of breathing.

3. Recordings of crepitations show that individual crackles recur constantly in each respiratory cycle—this would not be the case if air was bubbling through fluid.

4. Crepitations occur constantly in localised and diffuse fibrosis of the lungs when no excess fluid is present.

5. Crepitations heard over dependent parts of the lungs sometimes disappear in the *next* breath following a change of posture long before fluid could have had a chance to move to the new dependent part.

Crepitations are probably a sign of abnormal deflation and are due to an alteration in the elastic properties of the lungs. Air bubbling through fluid only occurs in the larger airways and then randomly in both phases of breathing.

6. Rhonchi (wheezes) do not vary in pitch when a low-density gas (such as helium) is breathed whereas the pitch of wind instruments depends on the density of the vibrating gas; however, the pitch of instruments containing a vibrating reed is independent of the density of the vibrating gas. This suggests that a closer analogy to explain the generation of wheeze is a vibrating reed rather than a vibrating column of air. Furthermore, attempts to recreate wheeze by blowing through postmortem airways have failed.

The vibrating reed analogy probably explains why some patients with severe airway obstruction do not have rhonchi (wheezes). The velocity of gas necessary to vibrate a reed is fairly high if ventilation is reduced or hyperinflation is severe; exhaled air will not reach a sufficient velocity to cause the obstructed airways to vibrate. Wheeze is also sometimes absent due to collapse of the large airways or poor sound conduction through hyperinflated lungs. It follows that the pitch of the wheeze is not an indication of the size of the airway obstructed—this is supported by the fact that a high-pitched wheeze is sometimes heard when a tumour or foreign body obstructs a large airway.

RADIOLOGY OF THE LUNGS

X-ray films are the records of shadows cast by structures between the film and the source of x-rays. The shadows may be distorted by variations in technique. An exact diagnosis is usually not possible on a single x-ray, the shadow thrown by a radio-opaque mass will not disclose the composition of the mass. Past experience and training will suggest the probability of a shadow being due to a known cause. Sometimes there is virtual certainty, as in the case of Kerley's "B" lines being due to engorgement of septal lymphatics; at other times diagnosis involves discussion of possibilities and probabilities.

The following routine of examining a chest film is essential in order to avoid missing obvious abnormalities:

1. **Degree of penetration.**—Normally it should be just possible to see individual intervertebral discs behind the heart shadow and the division of trachea into the main bronchi.

2. **Centering of the film** and whether it has been taken in full inspiration.

3. **Name of the patient.**—This avoids mistakes like diagnosing coalminers' pneumoconiosis in a woman. Check the nationality of the name—in a Greek patient a solid round opacity is likely to be hydatid cyst, in a Welshman fine nodular opacities may be due to pneumoconiosis. If the patient is a female check that both breast shadows are present. If one breast has been removed check for secondary deposits in the bones. An absent breast shadow will cause increased translucency in the lower zone. Check also for shadowing suggesting past irradiation, viz. lung fibrosis and associated periostial calcification.

4. **Check the right and left side of the film.**—The heart shadow is a poor guide as dextrocardia may be present. Right and left markers should be seen on the film.

5. **Bone abnormalities** such as rib fractures, rib notching, periostitis, rib erosions or congenital fusion of the ribs. Note whether there is any kyphosis, scoliosis or calcification of the ligaments of the spine.

6. **Soft tissues** for abnormal swellings or calcification.

7. **Size and silhouette of the heart shadow,** paying particular attention to shadows behind the heart. A double shadow behind the heart may be due to hiatus hernia, collapsed left lower lobe, paravertebral abscess or mediastinal tumour.

8. **Diaphragm.**—The right diaphragm in full inspiration is normally at the posterior end of the tenth rib and the anterior end of the sixth rib. The left diaphragm is about $\frac{1}{2}$ inch lower. Costophrenic angles should be acute in the absence of pleural effusion.

9. **Gastric gas bubble.**—If not under the left diaphragm check whether it is on the other side or in the mediastinum (hiatus hernia). It may be absent if there is a large abdominal mass, splenomegaly or a full stomach.

10. **Trachea** should be central and not indented (by an external mass). It is usually possible to see its division into the main bronchi at the anterior end of the second rib.

11. **Mediastinum.**—Note widening or displacement. Any shadow continuous with the mediastinum may arise from it even though it extends well out into the lung fields.

13. **Lung fields.**—The "lung markings" of normal lungs are vascular

shadows. Note whether the markings are normal and regularly distributed or if they are crowded together anywhere suggesting collapse of a lobe. The radiotranslucency of both sides should be the same. The lung markings should extend to the edge of the chest wall. If a pneumothorax is anticipated a chest film should be taken in expiration—the volume of the lung will decrease but the volume of air in the pleura will stay the same so that the lung is pushed further away from the chest wall during expiration.

Each lung field is conventionally divided into zones:

Upper zone: above the anterior end of the second rib.

Middle zone: from the level of the anterior end of the second rib to the level of the anterior end of the fourth rib.

Lower zone: below the anterior end of the fourth rib.

The horizontal fissure of the right lung may be seen in a normal film, it runs from the middle of the hilar shadow to meet the sixth rib in the axilla. Occasionally an azygos lobe is present in the right upper zone, a fold of pleura may be seen extending to a small protrusion at the upper right hilum, the azygos vein. An azygos lobe occurs in approximately 1 in 1000 chest x-rays.

The size, number, homogeneity, density and distribution of abnormal shadows in the lung fields should be noted.

Terms Used to Describe Shadows (Simon, 1962):

Homogeneous opacity.—Uniformly radio-opaque opacity.

Patchy shadow.—Non-homogeneous opacity. Each of these may be well- or ill-defined; the size and location should be stated.

Bullous area.—An area of hypertranslucency.

Ring shadow.—An area of hypertranslucency surrounded by an opaque wall.

Honeycomb shadowing.—Numerous small ring shadows.

Oval or circular shadows.—1. *Fine or miliary mottling:* shadows less than 2 mm in size. 2. *Coarse mottling:* shadows 2 mm to 2 cm in size. 3. *Large circular shadow:* measuring 2 cm or more.

The presence of cavitation or calcification of all shadows should be noted. Lung shadows may be associated with other abnormalities in the chest x-ray, for example an ill-defined area of patchy shadowing in the right middle and lower zones may be due to aspiration pneumonia which may have occurred as a result of a dilated oesophagus. This may be seen as a well-defined opacity parallel to the right upper mediastinum in which there may be a fluid level or food residue.

Causes of Miliary Mottling

Miliary tuberculosis.

Sarcoidosis.

Pneumoconiosis.
Secondary deposits.
Previous bronchogram.
Haemosiderin.
Histoplasmosis.
Pulmonary oedema.

To locate a shadow anatomically it is essential to have a lateral film; it is most unwise to attempt an anatomical diagnosis unless two views are available. In the lateral film the main fissure may be seen separating lower from middle and upper lobes on the right, and lower from upper lobe on the left. On the left side there is no middle lobe, it is represented by the lingula whose bronchus comes off anteriorly from the upper lobe bronchus. The fissures may be the sites of accumulation of fluid which may remain in the fissures after it has cleared elsewhere, particularly following left ventricular failure. The main fissure runs roughly in the line of the sixth rib; on the right side it is met by the horizontal fissure.

Aspiration or inhalation pneumonias are associated with shadowing in particular lobes depending on the position of the patient during aspiration:

1. Apical segment of right lower lobe or less commonly the apical segment of the left lower lobe if the patient was on his back.

2. Axillary subsegments of anterior or posterior segments of right upper lobe with the patient lying on his right side, depending on whether the patient was lying more on his back or on his face.

3. Axillary subsegments of anterior and apico-posterior segments of the left upper lobe if the patient was lying on his left side.

4. Right middle lobe and lingula if the patient was prone (as in swimming breast stroke, seen particularly in shipwrecked sailors who have swum in oil-covered water).

5. Posterior or lateral basal segment of either lower lobe if aspiration occurs while the patient is sitting upright as in the dentist's chair.

The sites from which material may be aspirated are:

1. Upper respiratory tract and mouth, fauces, sinuses and septic teeth.

2. Lower respiratory tract: blood and pus can be aspirated into healthy bronchi from areas of bronchiectasis or bleeding.

3. Oesophagus: pharyngeal diverticula, achalasia of the cardia, hiatus hernia and neuromuscular inco-ordination as in bulbar palsy.

Level of a Pleural Effusion

The true upper level of a pleural effusion is a straight line at or above the top of the level that the effusion appears to have reached in the axilla

on a P.A. x-ray film of the chest. The apparent rise of the fluid in the
axilla as seen on the P.A. film of the chest is an artefact due to the x-rays
penetrating an increased thickness of fluid at the periphery. This has
been convincingly shown by x-raying plaster casts of pleural effusions
and by x-rays of a model which consisted simply of a balloon in a
bucket of water (Davis *et al.*, 1963).

The rising line of dullness in the axilla (Ellis' or Damoiseau's S-
shaped line) can be explained in a similar way. It is a common experience
that aspiration of a large volume of a pleural effusion can be successfully performed at the upper level of dullness to percussion. That a thin
layer of pleural fluid causes no shadowing on x-ray can be shown by
x-raying in the supine position a patient known to have a pleural
effusion. The fluid then occupies the most dependent position and is
a uniform thickness. This explains why a large pleural effusion is often
completely missed in a very ill patient who has a chest x-ray performed
in the supine or near supine position.

TESTS OF RESPIRATORY FUNCTION

The function of the respiratory system is to provide an adequate
supply of oxygen and to remove carbon dioxide from the blood. Air is
moved in and out of the chest by a bellows-like action—expansion of
the rib cage by intercostal muscles and active descent of the diaphragm.
During normal breathing (tidal breathing) about 500 cc of air is inhaled and exhaled at each breath (tidal volume). The maximum amount
of air which can be blown out after maximum inspiration is about 5
litres (vital capacity). Air enters the chest through the trachea and is
distributed to all parts of the lungs through the bronchi and bronchioles.
Thus, without considering the lungs themselves we have three functions
of respiration which can be measured:

1. Ability to cause air to move in and out of the chest or bellows
function (ventilation).

2. The ability to allow this volume of air through the airways
(obstruction).

3. The equality of distribution of this air to different parts of the
lungs (distribution).

The ability to move air in and out of the chest is measured by recording the volume of air which can be blown out after a maximum inhalation (vital capacity or VC). This does not take into account the speed of
breathing; this is measured by recording the volume of air blown out
in one minute when breathing as fast as possible (maximum breathing
capacity or MBC) normally 120 litres per minute.

The ability to allow air through the airways depends on their bore.

It takes a longer time for a given volume of air to flow through a narrow tube than a wide one. Similarly, there is less air flow in a given time. These two facts form the basis of the tests for narrowing or obstruction of the airways. The FEV_1 is the volume of air flowing in the first second of a forced expiration. In diseases causing obstruction to the airways, the forced expiratory volume in the first second (FEV_1) is reduced. Furthermore, the ratio of FEV_1 to VC is also reduced; normal people can usually exhale 75 per cent of their vital capacity in the first second. In obstruction to the airways, the FEV_1 to VC ratio is less than 75 per cent. Another method of measuring volume of air flow in a given time is to record the maximum rate of flow (volume per minute) which is known as the peak expiratory flow rate (PEFR). It is measured with a Wright peakflow meter. The units of measurement are litres per minute and the normal is 400–600 litres per minute—note that this is a maximum *rate* of flow and does not indicate the actual volume flowing in one minute. The FEV_1 and PEFR measure volume flowing in a given time. It is also possible to measure the time taken to displace a given volume of air. The tidal volume is about 500 ml and by listening over the trachea the length of time taken to exhale this volume of air during quiet respiration can be noted. Obstruction to the airways will prolong expiration time.

The equality of distribution can be measured by adding a small amount of radioactive gas to the inspired air and counting the radioactivity over each part of the lung, the part of the lung receiving less radioactive gas will emit less radioactivity. The radioactive gas used is an isotope of xenon (^{133}Xe). An older method of measuring equality of distribution is known as the "nitrogen wash-out method". The patient breathes 100 per cent oxygen, the concentration of nitrogen in the expired air is measured, the amount of nitrogen in the expired air falls as pure oxygen replaces nitrogen in the recesses of the lung. In a normal person it takes about 7 minutes for the volume of nitrogen in the expired air to reach a constant. In a patient with maldistribution of air it takes longer to wash out the nitrogen from the underventilated parts of the lung. Another method of measuring equality of distribution is the "helium wash-out time" which is based on the same principle as the nitrogen wash-out time except that only a single breath of helium is taken whereas in the nitrogen wash-out time 100 per cent oxygen is inspired continuously. These are the most widespread clinical tests of ventilation, obstruction and distribution.

From the alveoli, oxygen has to diffuse across the alveolar epithelium, across the interstitial "space" and the endothelium of the alveolar capillaries before coming into contact with haemoglobin, contained within the red cells. This transfer of alveolar air to haemoglobin, which takes about 0·8 seconds, can be deranged in several ways:

1. Decrease in the number of alveoli.
2. Increase in the interstitial "space".
3. Inadequate supply of haemoglobin (heart failure).

Decrease in the number of alveoli results in failure to supply enough oxygen to the blood, causing a reduction of the partial pressure of oxygen in arterial blood (Po_2). Carbon dioxide diffuses much more readily than oxygen and reduction of the number of alveoli never occurs to the extent that transfer of carbon dioxide is interfered with. If the number of alveoli were reduced so that carbon dioxide transfer was affected the amount of oxygen able to pass into the blood would be insufficient to maintain life.

The diffusion of carbon dioxide and oxygen across the alveolar wall depends on a difference in the partial pressure of the two gases on either side of the alveolar wall. If the partial pressure of carbon dioxide in the alveoli increases, then CO_2 will not be able to diffuse from the blood and the partial pressure of CO_2 in the blood will rise. In widespread narrowing of the airways there is reduction in ventilation of the alveoli and failure to "wash away" carbon dioxide which accumulates in the alveoli and prevents CO_2 diffusing from the blood. This explains why in chronic bronchitis and emphysema the Po_2 is reduced (in emphysema there is loss of alveoli) and the Pco_2 is raised (bronchitis causes widespread narrowing of the bronchi).

Increase in the interstitial space interferes with the diffusion of oxygen much more than carbon dioxide. Disease sufficient to hamper CO_2 diffusion would so impede oxygen transfer that the patient would not survive. Disorders which affect the interstitial space will cause a reduction of the partial pressure of oxygen in the blood. Patients compensate for anoxia by increasing the rate of respiration, this hyperventilation usually results in a reduction of the amount of carbon dioxide in the blood. Diffusion defects are, therefore, characterised by an increased respiratory rate, a low Po_2 and a low Pco_2—other tests of respiratory function are usually normal. Lesser degrees of impairment of oxygen transfer can be found by measuring the rate of transfer of an easily detected gas which has much the same diffusing capacity as oxygen, such a gas is carbon monoxide. The rate at which carbon monoxide is removed from the inspired air is measured; CO is so rapidly taken up by the haemoglobin that the limiting factor is assumed to be the interstitial space. This assumption is only justified if other respiratory function tests have not been severely abnormal, for example, inequalities of ventilation or distribution of blood will invalidate carbon monoxide diffusion tests. The rate of uptake of carbon monoxide depends on its partial pressure in the inspired air. The normal uptake is about 15 ml/min/mm Hg at rest; this should approximately double after exercise, due to an increase in ventilation and an increase in the blood supply to the lungs.

Abnormal distribution of blood to the lungs may result in failure of gas transfer. Blood flowing through an unventilated part of the lung will not come into contact with air-containing alveoli and is thus "short-circuited" from pulmonary artery to pulmonary vein. Systemic arterial blood will be undersaturated with oxygen because of the "shunt effect". Similarly parts of the lungs may be well ventilated but not perfused with blood (dead space effect). As with diffusion defects, "shunt" and "dead space" effects are never severe enough to cause an elevated Pco_2 in the blood; in order to reduce arterial Po_2 below 60 mm (90 per cent saturation) at least a third of the venous blood must bypass the lungs. The simplest method of deciding whether peripheral desaturation is due to a "shunt" effect is to have the patient breathe 100 per cent oxygen. This will increase the oxygen saturation of arterial blood, because even the poorly ventilated alveoli will now be receiving enough oxygen; in contrast, if there is an anatomical shunt there is almost no rise in arterial Po_2. The same thing occurs when ventilation of normally under-ventilated lung is increased by exercise. A rise in oxygen saturation after breathing 100 per cent oxygen occurs in diffusion defects, ventilation/perfusion inequality, and hypoventilation. The rise in oxygen saturation breathing 100 per cent oxygen is much less when an anatomical shunt is present. 30 per cent oxygen improves oxygen saturation in diffusion defects but does not raise oxygen saturation due to shunts at all. 100 per cent oxygen does cause a small rise in oxygen saturation when a shunt is present because some oxygen becomes dissolved in the plasma. Under-saturation of arterial blood due to a diffusion disorder will become rapidly worse after exercise due to increased tissue utilisation of oxygen which cannot be offset by increasing diffusion of oxygen from alveoli to alveolar capillaries.

CHANGES IN ARTERIAL Po_2 WITH OXYGEN AND EXERCISE
IN PULMONARY CONDITIONS CAUSING HYPOXIA

	100% oxygen	30% oxygen	Exercise
Ventilation/Perfusion inequality	improved	unchanged	improved
Shunt	unchanged	unchanged	worse
Diffusion defect	improved	improved	worse
Underventilation	improved	improved	improved

Abnormalities of blood flow to different parts of the lungs can be detected by injecting intravenously a radioactive substance and counting the radioactivity over the different zones of the lungs. The radio-active substances given are xenon (^{133}Xe) and I^{131}-labelled macro-aggregated albumin which is transiently bound to the pulmonary arteriolar walls.

The last respiratory function measurement which may be of clinical value is the elastic property (compliance) of the lungs. The elasticity of the lungs will be reduced by pulmonary fibrosis, pulmonary venous congestion, and left-to-right shunts in which increased pulmonary artery blood flow causes the arteries to be turgid and stiff and to hold the lungs outwards like the spokes of an umbrella. Diseases which cause stiffening and deformity of the chest wall such as ankylosing spondylitis and kyphoscoliosis will also diminish the effective elasticity of the lungs. The compliance of the lungs and chest wall are usually measured by intra-oesophageal pressure balloons and "whole body plethysmograph" in which the external pressure on the chest can be varied and the changes in tidal volume and rate of respiration noted.

Occasionally bronchitis damages the cartilaginous rings of bronchi and trachea: during attempted expiration the intrathoracic pressure rises and may cause collapse of the damaged intrathoracic airways. In an effort to maintain a high intratracheal pressure such patients will exhale slowly against a resistance—they will purse their lips and allow air to escape slowly. On the spirograph record of the vital capacity such airways collapse is seen as a sudden temporary cessation of airflow.

Formal tests of respiratory function do not obviate the need for a careful clinical history, accurate examination and consideration of the chest x-ray. Respiratory function tests enable lung function to be assessed at a single moment in time but the history is the best way of assessing retrospective progression of the disease.

The chest x-ray may be useful in anticipating which lung function tests are going to be helpful. A large radiotranslucent area surrounded by a thin wall will suggest an underventilated lung cyst, local attenuation of pulmonary arteries will suggest abnormal distribution of blood and bilateral lower zone patchy shadowing will suggest interstitial pulmonary fibrosis as a cause of a diffusion defect.

ACID-BASE BALANCE

The pH of blood is one of the most constant physiological para-meters. Tissue metabolism continuously produces acid metabolites which constantly tend to increase the hydrogen ion concentration of the blood. The pH is maintained around 7·4 by the action of "buffers" which are the salts of a strong base and a weak acid. The salt is neutral, i.e. has a pH of 7, if more acid is added to a buffer then either more neutral salt is formed or the base is so much stronger than the added acid that no appreciable change of pH occurs until vast unphysiological amounts of acid are added. There are many buffer systems in the body but the most important clinically is the bicarbonate-carbonic acid system. Bicarbonate is the strong base and carbonic acid the weak acid; the concentration of the bicarbonate in the blood is about twenty times that of carbonic acid. The pH of the blood depends on the proportion of base to acid. This is expressed in the infamous Henderson[36]-Hasselbalch[37] equation: $pH = pK + \log \frac{Base}{Acid}$. From a clinical point of view the only thing we have to note is that in order for the pH to remain constant, $\frac{Base}{Acid}$ must also remain constant, so that any increase in base should be accompanied by an increase in acid, otherwise, $\frac{Base}{Acid}$ would increase. The weak acid, carbonic acid, readily dissociates into carbon dioxide and water ($H_2CO_3 \rightleftharpoons CO_2 + H_2O$) so that the CO_2 concentration of the blood is an indirect way of measuring the acid component of the most important buffer system in the body.

The CO_2 release from the body is controlled by the lungs, any tendency to alter the CO_2 content of the blood is *respiratory*. Any *primary* increase in CO_2 is a *respiratory* acidosis (as CO_2 is a measure of the carbonic acid) and any primary decrease in CO_2 is a *respiratory* alkalosis.

Any change in one component of the $\frac{Base}{Acid}$ ratio will be compensated for by a similar change in the other component. Thus a respiratory acidosis (elevation of CO_2) will be accompanied by a rise in bicarbonate.

Any *primary* change in bicarbonate is called a *metabolic* change and is accompanied by a similar change in the CO_2 content. Thus, a metabolic acidosis is accompanied by a fall in bicarbonate and then a fall in CO_2. Measurement of the P_{CO_2} and bicarbonate concentration will usually indicate whether an acidosis or alkalosis is present. The compensatory alteration of either bicarbonate or CO_2 is usually less than the primary abnormality. If the pH is also known it is even simpler to determine whether a patient is suffering from a compensated metabolic or respiratory acidosis or alkalosis. The normal P_{CO_2} of arterial blood is 40 mm Hg and of venous blood 46 mm Hg. The normal plasma bicarbonate is 23 mmol/l. Example: $P_{CO_2} = 50$ mm, HCO_3 25 mmol/l—could theoretically be either a respiratory acidosis (raised P_{CO_2} or a metabolic alkalosis (raised HCO_3). However, the largest change is the elevation of the P_{CO_2} from the normal of 40 mm to 50 mm so a respira-

36. LAWRENCE JOSEPH HENDERSON (1878–1942). Boston biochemist.
37. KARL HASSELBALCH (b. 1874). Copenhagen biochemist.

tory acidosis is probably present. When you know that the accompanying pH was 7·32 it will unequivocally be a respiratory acidosis. Similarly a Pco_2 of 20 mm and a bicarbonate of 10 mmol/l (both reduced) could theoretically be a metabolic acidosis or respiratory alkalosis. However, the bicarbonate is very low at 10 mmol/l and as this is probably the primary abnormality a metabolic acidosis is probably present; the accompanying pH of 7·3 makes it a metabolic acidosis for certain. Figure 9 shows the relationship between pH, bicarbonate and Pco_2. At a given pH a rise in Pco_2 will be accompanied by a rise in bicarbonate and vice versa.

The medullary respiratory centre is normally sensitive to changes in arterial Pco_2. An elevated Pco_2 stimulates hyperventilation of the lungs via the respiratory centre and the excess carbon dioxide is rapidly blown off.

Excretion of bicarbonate and hydrogen ion via the renal tubules is a much slower process. There are three mechanisms by which hydrogen ion is secreted into the urine:

1. Plasma bicarbonate excreted as carbonic acid

$$HCO_3 + H^+ \rightarrow H_2CO_3$$

2. Excretion of ammonium salts from ammonia manufactured in renal tubules

$$NH_3 + H^+ \rightarrow NH_4^+$$

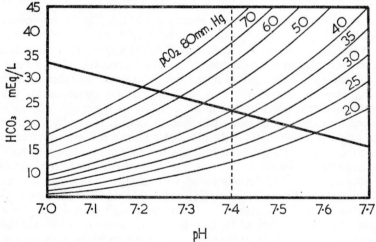

FIG. 9.—The interrelationship between pH, Pco_2 and bicarbonate in the plasma. (By courtesy of Dr. E. W. O'Brien.)

3. Excretion of sodium hydrogen phosphate manufactured from disodium phosphate

$$Na_2HPO_4 + H^+ \rightarrow NaH_2PO_4$$

The bicarbonate-carbonic acid buffer system is the most important clinically but there are several other buffer systems involved in keeping the blood pH constant. Proteins including haemoglobin and the plasma proteins act as weak acids and form buffer systems with strong bases such as bicarbonate and phosphate. Oxyhaemoglobin is more acid than reduced haemoglobin, hence in the tissues, where oxyhaemoglobin is reduced to more basic reduced haemoglobin, the acid metabolites are buffered by the reduced haemoglobin. Haemoglobin combines loosely with carbon dioxide, forming "carbamino compounds", when oxyhaemoglobin reaches the tissues where acid metabolites and CO_2 have accumulated it rapidly loses its oxygen at the same time, becoming more avid for carbon dioxide. The process is reversed in the lungs. Reduced haemoglobin, therefore, is important as a buffer against acid metabolites and as a transporter of CO_2.

When blood is collected for estimation of bicarbonate, CO_2 will immediately start to come out of solution unless the blood is collected anaerobically. Because the buffering properties of blood still remain intact (even though it is in a bottle) the bicarbonate level will also fall. In order to allow for this *in vitro* change in bicarbonate and CO_2 content the bicarbonate is estimated when the blood has been in contact with a PCO_2 of 40 mm Hg (the PCO_2 of arterial blood)—this value is the plasma "standard bicarbonate" concentration.

Causes of Disturbed Acid-Base Balance

Respiratory acidosis (CO_2 retention).

1. Airways obstruction (asthma and bronchitis).
2. Failure of bellows function:
   obesity
   ankylosing spondylitis
   poliomyelitis
   chest injuries
   relaxant drugs.
3. Depression of respiratory centre:
   drugs (morphia, barbiturates)
   cerebrovascular accident
   encephalitis
   coma.

Respiratory alkalosis (reduced PCO_2).

Overbreathing:
hysteria
diffusion defects
salicylates (cause stimulation of respiratory centre).

Metabolic acidosis (decrease in bicarbonate).

Ketosis due to diabetes or starvation.
Renal failure.
Cyclical vomiting in children (causes ketosis).
Severe dehydration.
Ingestion of ammonium chloride.
Uretero-colic anastomosis.
Severe anoxia (lactic acid accumulates).

Metabolic alkalosis (increase in bicarbonate).

Repeated vomiting (pyloric stenosis).
Intestinal fistulae.
Milk-alkali syndrome (excessive ingestion of alkalis).
Aldosteronism.
Cushing's syndrome.
Diuretic therapy.

Treatment

Respiratory acidosis.—The elevated Pco_2 of respiratory failure may be lowered by reversing airways obstruction, stimulating the respiratory centre or mechanical ventilation.

Respiratory alkalosis.—Rebreathing in a closed circuit will raise the Pco_2 (e.g. hysterics should be made to breathe in and out of a paper bag).

Metabolic alkalosis.—Usually no specific treatment is necessary apart from removal of the cause. Severe alkalosis whether metabolic or respiratory is accompanied by tetany which is due to a reduction in the ionised calcium in the serum. It can be stopped by intravenous calcium chloride (10 ml of 10 per cent solution). Metabolic alkalosis may be caused by hypokalaemia; the cells become depleted of potassium which is replaced by hydrogen which is withdrawn from the extracellular fluid causing an excess of bicarbonate.

Metabolic acidosis.—Diabetic coma should usually be treated with intravenous infusion of bicarbonate (or lactate) as well as rehydration and insulin. Insulin is thought to be less easily utilised in an acid medium (see p. 357 for treatment of diabetic coma).

Standard bicarbonate (BP) is a 1·4 per cent solution and contains 167 mmol/l of bicarbonate and sodium ions. Sixth molar lactate also contains 167 mmol/l of bicarbonate. The 8·4 per cent bicarbonate solution used in the correction of acidosis following cardiac arrest and in the forced alkaline diuresis treatment of salicylate and barbiturate overdose contains 1 mEq/ml. of bicarbonate (see p. 408 for treatment of drug overdosage).

Replacement of electrolytes which are found mainly in the extracellular fluid is based on the fact that the extracellular fluid is about one-fifth of the body weight (usually about 15 litres). In the case of bicarbonate this regime has to be modified since bicarbonate is also an intracellular ion; it has been found empirically that an assumption that bicarbonate is distributed through fluid equivalent to one-third of the body weight results in adequate replacement of the ion. The plasma is a representative sample of the extracellular fluid, the normal plasma bicarbonate is approximately 25 mmol/l hence the amount of bicarbonate replacement needed is the plasma deficit per litre multiplied by the number of litres involved, i.e. one-third of the body weight in kilograms (1 litre weighs 1 kilogram).

Example: A 60 kilogram diabetic in diabetic coma has a plasma bicarbonate of 20 mmol/l. He is 5 mmol/l short of bicarbonate, he therefore requires $5 \times 20 \text{ mEq} = 100 \text{ mmol}$.

This is 100 ml. of 8·4 per cent bicarbonate (1 mmol per ml.) or about $\frac{1}{2}$ litre of 1·4 per cent bicarbonate (167 mmol/l).

CHRONIC BRONCHITIS AND EMPHYSEMA

Chronic bronchitis is a condition characterised by excessive mucus secretion from the bronchial tree and recurrent cough productive of sputum every day, for three months of the year for at least two successive years. Infection of the bronchi is usually, but not invariably present, the commonest infecting organisms being *Haemophilus influenzae* and the pneumococcus; the part played by respiratory viruses in initiating and perpetuating infection is probably much underestimated. Factors which predispose to and aggravate, but probably do not cause, chronic bronchitis are general atmospheric pollution (dust and sulphur dioxide), inhalation of cigarette smoke, damp climate and occupational exposure to harmful dusts and irritant fumes.

The excessive mucus production characteristic of chronic bronchitis is produced by hypertrophied and more numerous mucus-producing goblet cells in the bronchial epithelium and by dilated mucous glands within the bronchial wall. The severity of the bronchitis can be correlated with the increase in size of the mucous glands. Infection results in thickening of the mucous membrane, micro-abscess formation and viscous infected sputum. The bronchi are narrowed by the thickened oedematous mucous membrane and viscous infected mucus which is difficult to expectorate. These changes may be confined to the larger bronchi but more usually the bronchioles are also involved—for this reason the term "obstructive airways disease" is preferable to "chronic bronchitis".

Emphysema is defined as enlargement of the air spaces distal to the respiratory (the most distal) bronchioles due to dilatation or destruction of the alveolar walls. Emphysema is a frequent accompaniment of chronic bronchitis. It is suggested that if the bronchioles as well as bronchi are chronically infected, infection can spread to and destroy alveolar walls leading to loss of functioning lung tissue, fusion of many alveoli and hence to a dilated air space. If the infection is more or less confined to the larger airways the dominant features will be widespread narrowing and obstruction to air flow. Emphysema does not always follow chronic bronchitis and chronic bronchitis is not always followed by emphysema.

The late clinical features of chronic bronchitis tend to be different depending on whether the dominant effect is widespread airways obstruction or destruction of lung tissue (emphysema). In their pure forms these two effects are seen clinically as the "blue bloater" and the "pink puffer". Loss of alveolar wall as in emphysema diminishes the area over which diffusion of O_2 and CO_2 can take place; the effect of this is to diminish the Po_2 in the blood. The diffusing surface is never reduced to the extent that diffusion of CO_2 is affected because CO_2 is much more easily diffusible than O_2 and a reduction of diffusing surfaces which would interfere with CO_2 diffusion would so impede O_2 diffusion that the blood would contain virtually no oxygen. The medullary respiratory centre normally responds only to alteration of the blood CO_2; however, there are chemoreceptors in the carotid and aortic bodies which are sensitive to anoxia. Stimulation of these chemoreceptors by the anoxia results in an increase in the depth and rate of breathing which will increase the diffusing surface available to oxygen, and the blood oxygen will rise. The oxygen saturation of the blood is only kept normal by rapid and deeper breathing; in its extreme form this becomes "dyspnoea". The respiratory centre of "pink puffers" remains sensitive to a small rise in Pco_2 and their chemoreceptors remain sensitive to a small fall in Po_2, whereas the respiratory centre of "blue bloaters" becomes "set" for a higher level of Pco_2 and their chemoreceptors do not respond to anoxia. The patients who have severe emphysema but no airways obstruction, therefore, are not cyanosed (i.e. "pink") but are usually dyspnoeic (i.e. "puffing"). The patients with widespread airways obstruction have a normal ability to allow gases to diffuse from alveoli to blood but a diminished ability to move air in and out of the alveoli through the airways. This does not affect the content of oxgen in the blood very much because the partial pressure of oxygen in the alveoli has to be reduced considerably before there is a fall in oxygen content of the blood. This is because haemoglobin has a very high affinity for oxygen and will absorb any oxygen available no matter how small the amount. However, for CO_2 the situation is different, the CO_2 content of the blood is proportional to the concentration of the CO_2 in the alveoli. Hence, any condition which causes underventilation of the alveoli and therefore increases the alveolar concentration of the CO_2 will result in the blood leaving the alveoli containing normal amounts of oxygen but increased amounts of CO_2. The high CO_2 content of the blood causes narrowing of the pulmonary arteries leading to pulmonary hypertension. Obstruction to the airways results in collapse of small areas of the lung which are then not ventilated but may be perfused with blood, which is, therefore, effectively shunted from pulmonary artery to pulmonary veins. This right-to-left shunting leads to oxygen desaturation of the arterial blood and cyanosis ("blue"). The pulmonary hypertension results in cor pulmonale, right heart failure and peripheral oedema ("bloater").

The pulmonary hypertension is due to a combination of several factors; there is a reduction in the number of capillaries with a consequent reduction in the cross-sectional area of the blood vessels; anoxia causes: (i) pulmonary arteriolar vasoconstriction, (ii) increased pulmonary blood flow, (iii) increased blood viscosity. Air trapping within the alveoli increases the intra-alveolar pressure causing compression of capillaries.

"Blue bloaters" tend to be obese and the mechanical work of moving the heavy chest wall outstrips the oxygen which can be supplied by the inadequate lungs; there is probably some central mechanism which reduces the ventilating capacity in obesity.

Normal people respond to a raised P_{CO_2} by hyperventilating; however, chronic CO_2 retention does not cause hyperventilation—the respiratory centre becomes "set" for a higher level of P_{CO_2}. Thus "blue bloaters" with chronic CO_2 retention lose their compensatory over-ventilating mechanism. Should this failure of adaptation of the respiratory centre to a chronically raised P_{CO_2} not occur the patient may be dyspnoeic the whole time in an attempt to blow off CO_2 and keep the blood P_{CO_2} normal. There are, therefore, several mechanisms for the clinical differences between "blue bloaters" and "pink puffers":

1. Airways obstruction results in an increased P_{CO_2} whereas emphysema results in a reduced P_{O_2} and anoxic stimulation of the carotid and aortic chemoreceptors.

2. In "blue bloaters" the work of breathing causes a compensatory reduction of respiratory effort.

3. "Blue bloaters" have lost the ability to respond normally to a raised P_{CO_2} whereas the respiratory centre of "pink puffers" still responds in the normal way to small rises in the P_{CO_2}.

In practice, airways obstruction and emphysema so frequently co-exist that differentiation into distinct clinical groups is only rarely possible. Patients with dominant airways obstruction frequently develop secondary polycythaemia, the dominant emphysema patients very rarely do so; there is no satisfactory explanation for this difference.

The only physical signs of uncomplicated chronic bronchitis are those of narrowing of the airways leading to prolongation of expiration more than inspiration since the bronchi usually dilate on inspiration and the effect of narrowing will therefore be more marked on expiration. Rhonchi may be heard due to localised areas of bronchial narrowing. When bronchial narrowing becomes widespread "wheeze" is heard. Crepitations are not a feature of bronchitis; if they occur, they are due to associated left ventricular failure, bronchopneumonia or bronchiectasis. Bronchiectasis is commonly associated with chronic bronchitis. On the plain chest x-ray there are no diagnostic features of bronchitis; the thickened bronchial walls are rarely visible. In fibrocystic disease in children bronchial thickening and bronchiectasis may be seen as parallel line shadows ("tram-lines"). In the bronchogram the narrowed bronchi of chronic bronchitis are visible and the dilated mucous glands fill with lipiodol and are easily seen, the bronchi also end sooner and more abruptly than in normals ("sawn-off tree" appearance).

Antibiotics in Chronic Bronchitis

The two organisms most frequently present in acute attacks of bronchitis are *Strept. pneumoniae* and *H. influenzae*. In the majority of cases *H. influenzae* is the real pathogen. Acute infections are always associated with infection and inflammation within the walls of the bronchi and bronchioles; however, the mucus acts as a reservoir of organisms between acute attacks. Unfortunately antibiotics can only enter the mucus in *bacteriocidal* concentration when there is exudation present, i.e. when the sputum is purulent. Pathogenic organisms are recoverable from the sputum even when it is mucoid *between* acute attacks. Factors other than infection are likely to be responsible for acute exacerbations of bronchitis. This is supported by the fact that serum precipitins to *H. influenzae* are found only in a quarter of patients with simple bronchitis (Burns and May, 1967). For these reasons it is sometimes recommended that antibiotics should only be used in acute exacerbations if the sputum is purulent, i.e. contains pus (May, 1968). *H. influenzae* is always sensitive to ampicillin and tetracycline; it is, therefore, suggested that it is unnecessary to culture the sputum in acute exacerbations of bronchitis unless:

1. There is a failure to respond to treatment.
2. Pneumonia is suspected.
3. Bronchiectasis is known to be present.

The quantity of antibiotic in purulent sputum cannot be increased above a certain concentration. In acute exacerbations with purulent sputum ampicillin or tetracycline 1 g. 6-hourly should be given for 5 days or longer if the sputum remains purulent; in this dose bacteriocidal concentrations should be reached in the sputum; when the sputum ceases to be purulent ideally the dose should be reduced to 250–500 mg 6-hourly at which dose bacteriocidal levels still occur in the tissues. The lowest effective dose of antibiotic should be given because of the danger of superinfection with staphylococci and fungi and the danger of producing antibiotic-resistant organisms which are possibly a source of danger to the patient and the community. For recurrent attacks of acute bronchitis there are two logical courses: one is to give continuous antibiotics and the other is to give antibiotics immediately an acute exacerbation starts. The orthodox management is to give continuous antibiotics if the sputum remains purulent between attacks. If the sputum is mucoid between acute attacks antibiotics should not be given continuously but the patient should have his own supply so that he can start a course as soon as he notices symptoms of an acute exacerbation.

The evidence with regard to prophylactic antibiotics reducing the frequency and/or severity of acute attacks is conflicting. Prophylactic antibiotics probably reduce the duration of acute attacks but not their frequency. There is little evidence that lung damage can be prevented by suppression of bronchial infection (M.R.C. Report, 1966).

Physical Signs

The physical signs of "hyperinflation" of the chest are:

1. Reduced expansion of lower ribs.
2. Diminished breath sounds.
3. Increased resonance on percussion.
4. Reduced cardiac and liver dullness.
5. Use of accessory muscles of respiration.
6. The presence of rhonchi (wheezes).
7. Filling of the *external* jugular veins during expiration.

Less familiar signs of airways obstruction and hyperinflation have been emphasised by Campbell (1969):

1. Length of the trachea palpable above the sternal notch in expiration. The length of trachea becomes less in hyperinflation because of elevation of the sternum relative to the hilum.
2. Tracheal descent with inspiration. When there is hyperinflation of the chest the trachea moves downwards during inspiration probably because the diaphragm is lower than in the normal.
3. Palpable hardening of the sternomastoid and scalene muscles

during inspiration indicating excessive use of the accessory muscles of respiration.

4. Indrawing of the suprasternal and supraclavicular fossae during inspiration indicating an excessive fall in intrathoracic pressure during inspiration (in order to try to "suck" more air through the narrowed airways).

5. Forced expiration time. During forced expiration with the mouth open *following* maximum inspiration, the time should normally be less than 4 seconds.

The x-ray features of hyperinflation are:

1. Hypertranslucency of the lung fields.
2. Low and flat diaphragms which, on screening, show diminished excursion.
3. Increase in A-P diameter of the chest.
4. Increase in normal retrosternal translucent area.
5. Splaying out of the pulmonary vessels whose angles of bifurcation are thereby increased.
6. Rarely, bronchial "tram-lines" may be seen because of the increased "contrast" due to the hyperinflated chest.

Respiratory Failure

The function of the respiratory system is to supply oxygen to the blood and to eliminate carbon dioxide. Failure of the respiratory system will therefore mean a rise in PCO_2 (above 50 mm) and a fall in PO_2 (below 60 mm),

Hypercapnoea.—Elevation of the PCO_2 gives rise to a number of clinical features. The most important are (Gross and Hamilton, 1963):

1. Peripheral vasodilatation
2. Rapid, bounding pulse
3. Small pupils
4. Engorged fundal veins
5. Confusion or drowsiness
6. Depressed tendon reflexes
7. Extensor plantar responses
8. Headache
9. Papilloedema
10. Coma.

Elevation of the PCO_2, if compensated, results in a rise in serum bicarbonate. The kidneys compensate by reabsorbing bicarbonate (with sodium) from the tubules—this results in sodium (and water) retention, and peripheral oedema. Peripheral oedema in the absence of heart failure, peripheral vasodilatation and a high cardiac output have given rise to the suggestion that heart failure occurs much less commonly than it is diagnosed in the presence of hypercapnoea. It is important to be aware of this possibility because digoxin dosage may be unnecessarily increased to try and control "heart failure" which is not present. Patients with respiratory acidosis often develop hypokalaemia and may not respond to diuretics until potassium supplements have been given.

EMPHYSEMA

Emphysema has already been defined as an increase in the size of the air spaces distal to the respiratory bronchiole due to dilatation or destruction of the alveolar walls. Recently the detailed pathology of various types of emphysema has been elucidated (Reid, 1967). The lung consists of discrete lobules or acini each supplied by several respiratory bronchioles; leaving the respiratory bronchiole are alveolar ducts which lead into individual alveoli. In all types of emphysema (compensatory, focal, bullous, senile or atrophic) there is either dilatation or destruction of the alveolar walls or destruction of the walls of the respiratory bronchioles. Destruction of the walls of the respiratory bronchioles whether due to bronchitis or deposition of dusts will lead to several respiratory bronchioles fusing together and forming a large air space in the middle of the lobule, the periphery of the lobule still being composed of normal alveoli. This centrilobular emphysema is the type of focal emphysema seen particularly in dust disease and sometimes in the early stages of bullous emphysema. If all the alveoli in the lobule (or acinus) are involved in the emphysema it is said to be panacinar. Panacinar emphysema occurs with dilatation of the air spaces as in compensatory emphysema when part of the lung enlarges to replace damaged lung or it occurs if there is destruction of alveolar walls as in bullous emphysema. The mechanisms of alveolar wall destruction in panacinar (bullous) emphysema are extension of infection from bronchioles, rupture through constant coughing, damage by irritants (cigarette smoke and air pollution) and possibly "avascular necrosis" due to interference with blood supply.

The radiological features of emphysema are those of hyperinflation of the chest with the addition of dilated proximal pulmonary arteries and attenuated peripheral arteries if there is accompanying pulmonary hypertension.

It should not be forgotten that α_1 antitrypsin deficiency in both the heterozygotes and homozygotes may cause primary emphysema particularly involving the lower zones. The homozygotes almost always have cirrhosis as well but the heterozygotes may have α_1 antitrypsin levels about 50 per cent of normal. They tend to develop primary emphysema but there is evidence that its onset can be delayed if the patient abstains from smoking.

Cadmium inhalation also causes emphysema and cigarette smoke contains appreciable and measurable amounts of cadmium.

ASTHMA

Asthma is defined as "a disease characterised by variable dyspnoea due to widespread narrowing of intrapulmonary airways which varies over short periods of time either spontaneously or as a result of treatment" (Scadding, 1963).

Note that this definition does not mention allergy, hypersensitivity, or bronchospasm; it emphasises that asthma is dyspnoea due to narrowing of the airways and is to be distinguished sharply from those conditions which cause variable dyspnoea (usually by inhaled allergens) which is due to sudden impairment of diffusion of gases across the alveolar walls (transfer defects). This group of conditions is described on page 102. Their superficial similarity to asthma can lead to unnecessary over-investigation.

The main causes of asthma are:

1. Allergy to known or unknown allergens. The allergens are usually inhaled but may be ingested or injected as in the case of an anaphylactic reaction. Asthma of this type is commonly called "extrinsic asthma".

2. Intrinsic asthma, in which there may be some evidence of an allergic origin (e.g. eosinophilia and occasional hypersensitivity to salicylates). However, the natural history of intrinsic asthma differs from extrinsic asthma in which the evidence for external allergy is more definite although the exact allergen may not have been identified.

3. Asthma secondary to bronchitis or oedema of the bronchial walls as in cardiac or renal failure.

In chronic bronchitis there is no dispute that the major airways are narrowed due to thickening of the mucous membrane while the remainder of the bronchial wall is of a normal thickness; this thickening results from squamous metaplasia and increase in the number of goblet cells. It is such a constant finding in chronic bronchitis that it is one of the ways of assessing chronic bronchitis postmortem; the changes are irreversible. Superimposed on this irreversible airway narrowing there is usually a reversible component.

The reversible component is due to:

1. Inflammatory or allergic oedema.
2. Plugging of bronchi by exudate and eosinophils.
3. Spasm of bronchial wall smooth muscle.

In simple asthma only the reversible component of airways narrowing is present. There is controversy about the importance of muscle spasm in asthma and the reversible component of airways narrowing in bronchitis.

The main arguments in favour of bronchial mucosal oedema as the most important factor in reversible airways narrowing are:

1. In some cases the airways narrowing is only slowly reversible when corticosteroids are used.

2. Mucosal oedema and airways narrowing are present postmortem. If the narrowing is mainly due to muscle spasm this should relax after death.

3. Airways narrowing is a feature of pulmonary oedema.

4. The agents which induce asthma, e.g. histamine, are known to produce a sudden allergic oedema in other sites, e.g. the skin and larynx (as in angioneurotic oedema).

5. The same drugs which can rapidly reverse angioneurotic oedema (e.g. adrenaline, aminophylline and hydrocortisone) can also rapidly relieve asthma.

The main arguments in favour of spasm of the bronchiolar muscles as the most important factor in reversible airways narrowing are:

1. Hypertrophy of the bronchiolar smooth muscle may be seen at autopsy.

2. The speed of the changes which can occur in asthma are more suggestive of active muscle spasm than oedema analogous to angioneurotic oedema which is a relatively rare manifestation of an allergic state.

3. Isolated fragments of bronchiolar muscle have been seen to contract actively when they come into contact with allergens to which the patient is sensitive.

4. The pressure generated by bronchial muscle contraction can be measured by balloons in a segmental bronchus.

Extrinsic Asthma

This usually starts in infancy and occurs in "atopic" subjects. Atopy refers to a type of hypersensitivity unique to man. There is a predisposition to asthma, hay-fever, eczema, migraine, rhinitis, urticaria and food allergies. These people become sensitive to many ubiquitous foreign proteins which are not usually antigenic. Antibodies produced by these antigens in atopic subjects circulate in the blood sensitising the cells of the skin, bronchi and gastro-intestinal tract. They are known as "reaginic" antibodies and induce an immediate (Type I) hypersensitivity reaction. The "reaginic" antibodies are usually in the IgE component of the immunoglobulins.

An important factor in the management of a patient with extrinsic asthma is a careful and detailed history. It is important to know if the asthma is equally severe throughout the year—if it is, then it suggests that the patient is in constant contact with the offending allergen and makes house dust, bedding, occupational factors or pets the most likely causes. The most likely allergen in house dust is probably the mite *Dermatophagoides pteronyssinus*. Asthma which is seasonal is more likely to be caused by fundal spores, pollen or food (strawberries, rhubarb, etc.). Despite the general disillusionment about the usefulness of skin testing, in most cases of asthma the occasional patient can be considerably helped when only a few offending allergens can be demonstrated. As a working rule any patient with seasonal or occasional asthma should have skin testing performed with a limited number of probable allergens. All asthmatic patients should probably have skin tests with extracts of the fungus *Aspergillus fumigatus* which is an important cause of extrinsic asthma in adults. Skin testing is much safer and more reliable if performed by pricking or scratching the skin through the allergen being tested. The reaction produced by skin tests is suppressed if the patient is receiving antihistamines or bronchodilators but not affected by corticosteroids or disodium cromoglycate (Intal). Testing for hypersensitivity to allergens by inhalation tests is occasionally necessary but is usually carried out by special departments. Asthmatic attacks induced by inhaled allergens may not develop for several hours after inhalation.

If exposure to known allergens induces asthmatic attacks then these allergens should be removed if possible (e.g. using foam mattresses instead of hair; vacuum cleaning beds and bed linen) to see whether such manoeuvres reduce the asthmatic attacks. They may occasionally do so in individual patients, although a controlled trial of rigorous precautions in the home has not shown that these precautions help the majority of asthmatics.

Seasonal asthma in which there is demonstrable allergy to the prevalent pollen is often treated with hyposensitisation in which increasing doses of the offending allergen are given subcutaneously. Slow release ("depot") preparations of allergens are available but they occasionally give rise to severe attacks of asthma.

Steroid inhalation aerosols are now available (beclomethasone). They should be used when the dose of oral steroids is more than 10 mg of prednisone per day so that the systemic effects of steroid therapy may be lessened.

Management

The severe acute attack is treated with bronchodilators by injection. Status asthmaticus is present if bronchodilators are ineffective in relieving the attack after 24 hours or if the attack is so severe that the patient is unable to speak in sentences. A suitable regime for managing most adult cases of status asthmaticus is:

1. Aminophylline 250–500 mg i.v.
2. Isoprenaline by i.v. infusion.
3. Hydrocortisone 100 mg i.v. 6-hourly if the patient has not previously received long-term corticosteroids. If the patient has been receiving corticosteroids, 500–1000 mg hydrocortisone i.v. 6-hourly should be given. There is evidence that patients on long-term steroids metabolise them much more quickly than normal.
4. Take arterial blood for Pco_2, Po_2 and pH, Hb, PCV electrolytes, ECG, chest x-ray (to exclude pneumothorax).
5. Oxygen 28–35 per cent by Ventimask.
6. Fluid replacement. Dehydration encourages bronchial plugging; the patient may have been too breathless to drink fluid. If renal function is normal Dextrose 5 per cent 500 ml 6-hourly should be given to severe cases.
7. Antibiotics. Many attacks of status asthmaticus are precipitated by infection hence ampicillin or tetracycline 500–1000 mg 6-hourly should be given.

Artificial ventilation and bronchial lavage.—The main guide to the need for artificial ventilation is the level of the Pco_2. The main indication for artificial ventilation is if the Pco_2 is more than 50–60 mm on admission and does not fall after eight hours' treatment (Rees *et al.*, 1968).

Bronchial lavage with warm dilute saline is indicated in desperate cases. Occasionally this results in removal of surprisingly large bronchial plugs and clinical improvement.

Other Facets of Severe Asthma (Rees *et al.*, 1968)

Hypoxia occurs because of disturbed ventilation/perfusion relation-ships in the lungs; the Po_2 may not return to normal despite an improvement in FEV_1. Furthermore the Po_2 may remain at dangerously low levels despite marked symptomatic improvement; before dis-charging a patient with severe asthma from hospital it is wise to check that the Po_2 has returned to normal. Practical experience suggests that patients admitted with status asthmaticus who are discharged early from hospital are often readmitted with another attack of status asthma-ticus within a few days of returning home. In the early stages of status asthmaticus there is an inverse relationship between the arterial oxygen pressure and the pulse rate. If other causes of tachycardia can be excluded a pulse rate above 130/min is suggestive of an arterial oxygen pressure below 50 mm. Hypoxaemia, when severe, may lead to a meta-bolic acidosis superimposed on a respiratory acidosis if the Pco_2 is raised; treatment with bicarbonate is sometimes indicated. The level of the Pco_2 is not always a reliable guide because severe asthma may result in hyperventilation and a low Pco_2; an elevated Pco_2 always indicates a severe attack.

The FEV_1, and PFR are not always reliable guides—sometimes the patient improves symptomatically and the Po_2 rises despite the fact that the FEV_1 remains unchanged. The vital capacity may be a more useful monitor of progress. The reason for this is that airways narrowing results in trapping air within the lungs increasing the functional residual capacity (FRC) causing stretching of the lungs. The work needed to move the tidal volume in and out of these stretched lungs is much more than the work needed to move the same tidal volume out of lungs which are not stretched. The FEV_1 measures airways narrowing; the airways may remain the same size but the work needed to move the tidal volume in and out is less if the lungs are not stretched. Clinical improvement in asthma may occur because the FRC is reduced and not because the FEV_1 has improved.

Other physiological disturbances may occur:

1. Transient right ventricular hypertrophy on ECG.
2. Transient hypokalaemia possibly caused by steroids and over-ventilation.
3. Transient elevation of blood urea.

When the acute attack of allergic asthma is over the FEV_1 usually returns to normal or near normal until the next attack. Corticosteroids used to treat the acute attack can be stopped as soon as the attack is over. Some airways obstruction occasionally persists between acute attacks, particularly in intrinsic asthma. It may then be reasonable to give long-term corticosteroids. These should be given if they can be shown to improve significantly the FEV_1. When being considered for long-term steroid treatment the patient should be admitted to hospital and daily FEV_1 measurements recorded for 4–5 days *before* starting on steroids and then for 5–7 days afterwards. It sometimes takes seven days for steroids to produce an improvement, however; if, after this, the mean FEV_1 readings are the same as before steroids they should not be given continuously in extrinsic asthma. The situation is not quite so clear-cut in intrinsic asthma; the poor prognosis of this condition may justify continuous steroids on the grounds that they *may* reduce the frequency of acute attacks even if they do not improve airways obstruction between attacks. There is some evidence that prednisone taken on alternate days gives rise to fewer steroid adverse reactions.

Disodium cromoglycate (*Intal*).—This prevents the release of histamine following an antigen-antibody reaction and has been shown to reduce the frequency and severity of attacks of allergic asthma. The effects in intrinsic asthma are much poorer. The drug is administered as a powder by inhalation from a "Spinhaler".

Intrinsic Asthma

Most chronic asthmatics are in this group. The disease is much commoner in women over the age of 40; there is no previous history of allergy or evidence of atopy. There is often higher blood eosinophilia than in extrinsic asthma. The prognosis is poor and early, continuous corticosteroids may be justified. It is particularly in this group of asthmatics that the asthma may lead to chronic bronchitis, exacerbations of which in turn aggravate the asthma.

Asthma and Bronchitis

Chronic bronchitis causes permanent airways narrowing; in some patients this is accompanied by additional narrowing of the airways which may vary over short periods of time either spontaneously or as a result of treatment; therefore, by definition, these patients have asthma as well. In some patients with chronic bronchitis acute exacerbations are dominated by this asthmatic component, in others further infection and inflammatory oedema are dominant in the acute exacerbation. Chronic bronchitics in whom the asthmatic component is predominant may have eosinophils in blood and sputum in the same way as other asthmatics; similarly the acute exacerbation may respond to treatment of the asthmatic component more than treatment of the infection. In these patients the question always arises whether the asthmatic component is due to the infecting organisms acting as allergens. This is a difficult thing to prove; attempts to do so have not been entirely successful— however, such a reasonable hypothesis should not be lightly discarded.

Allergic Lung Disease other than Asthma

Extrinsic allergic asthma is associated with narrowing of the airways which is a response of Type I (immediate) hypersensitivity reactions. Another type of hypersensitivity reaction is the Type III (Arthus) reaction. Following repeated exposure to antigen, circulating antibodies develop. On re-exposure to the antigen an antibody antigen reaction takes place which differs from the immediate one of Type I allergy: it takes 3–6 hours to develop and is associated with vascular damage and local oedema. This reaction occurs at the site of exposure to the antigen which in the respiratory system is the alveoli. Unlike Type I reactions the severity of this reaction is related to the dose of antigens. Extrinsic allergic alveolitis describes the conditions caused by these Type III hypersensitivity reactions. All the conditions have a number of features in common as a result of their common type of hypersensitivity:
1. Symptoms begin suddenly 3–6 hours *after* exposure.
2. Repeated exposure at short intervals will result in a chronic disease.
3. The acute symptoms are caused by alveolar wall oedema which

causes sudden dyspnoea and cough. There is also a systemic reaction which generally consists of pyrexia, shivering and malaise. There is *no* evidence of airways obstruction.

4. The chronic disease is caused by organising fibrosis of the alveolar oedema and results in restrictive lung function tests (impaired ventilation tests) as well as diffusion abnormalities.

5. Circulating, precipitating antibiotics may be present in the serum.

The known diseases causing extrinsic allergic alveolitis are:

Farmers' lung
Bird breeders' lung
Bagassosis
Weavers' cough
Pituitary snuff-takers' lung
Smallpox handlers' lung
Mushroom pickers' lung
Maple bark disease
Wheat weevil (flour) disease
Suberosis
Malt weevil lung
Thatchers' lung
Cheese washers' lung
Paprika splitters' lung.

Long-standing cases of allergic (extrinsic) alveolitis often develop fibrosis of the interstitial tissues of the lung. Similar fibrosis may develop in the absence of any of the known predisposing causes; this idiopathic type of pulmonary fibrosis used to be called "diffuse interstitial pulmonary fibrosis" but is now called "cryptogenic (idiopathic) fibrosing alveolitis".

Diffuse fibrosing alveolitis is a disease characterised by an inflammatory process in the lungs beyond the terminal bronchioles having as its essential features:

1. Cellular thickening of the alveolar walls.

2. The presence of large mononuclear cells presumably of alveolar origin within the alveolar spaces (Scadding and Hinson, 1967).

Clincally fibrosing alveolitis is characterised by dyspnoea, dry cough, crepitations particularly over the lower zones and finger clubbing. In extrinsic allergic alveolitis clubbing is less common and the disease tends to affect the upper lobes. Corticosteroids are more useful when there are a large number of mononuclear cells present. They are unlikely to be of value if there is thickening of the alveolar walls. There is no constant relationship between the biopsy appearances and length of survival. Spontaneous remissions occur (Scadding and Hinson, 1967).

The pathology of the two conditions, extrinsic allergic alveolitis and cryptogenic fibrosing alveolitis, is compared in the Table below (Turner-Warwick, 1973).

Pathology	Extrinsic Allergic Alveolitis	Cryptogenic Fibrosing Alveolitis
Acute		
Granuloma	Yes	No
Giant cells	Yes	No
Inclusions	Yes	No
Alveolar wall infiltration	Patchy	Diffuse
Chronic		
Wall fibrosis	Yes-patchy	Yes
Honeycombing	Yes	Yes
Plasma cells	+++	+
Lymphoid follicles	+++	+

PNEUMONIAS

Pneumonia usually implies infection of alveoli although there are exceptions to this such as lipoid and aspiration pneumonias.

Classical lobar pneumonia is due to *Streptococcus pneumoniae*. Complications are minimal with prompt antibiotic treatment with the drug of choice which is penicillin. Among the complications which may occur are sterile pleural effusion, empyema (infection in the pleural space), lung abscess, pericardial involvement and septicaemia leading to meningitis and endocarditis.

Staphylococcal pneumonia frequently complicates other pneumonias such as influenza and aspiration pneumonias as well as complicting staphylococcal septicaemia. In children staphylococcal pneumonia may occur as a primary infection and is common in cystic fibrosis. Characteristically it causes multiple, cavitated, ill-defined round opacities on the chest x-ray. Hospital acquired infection will be due to a coagulase-positive (virulent), penicillinase, producing organism. Frequent blood cultures should be taken as staphylococcal septicaemia is a frequent complication. Pyopneumothorax is a common complication in children.

Recurrent Pneumonia

In a patient who has had several attacks of pneumonia always consider if one of the following are present:

1. Lowered resistance to infection (leucopenia or hypogammaglob-ulinaemia).
2. Diabetes mellitus.
3. Aspiration.
4. Bronchial obstruction (adenoma, carcinoma, foreign body, external compression of the bronchus).
5. Bronchiectasis of the bronchus of the infected lobe.

Note: bronchiectasis may be secondary to fibrosis caused by old tuberculosis; in these cases the recurrent pneumonia is often in the upper lobes.

6. Recurrent pulmonary infarcts.

Aspiration Pneumonia

A second attack of pneumonia within six months or a second attack in the same lobe as a previous attack at any time should alert to the probability that aspiration is occurring. There may be a clear history of dysphagia or possible inhalation of a foreign body (e.g. the party trick of throwing up nuts and catching them in the open mouth or a bout of coughing following a dental extraction). However aspiration pneumonia may occur when sinusitis is present; pus is aspirated at night while the patient is asleep. Liquid paraffin taken for constipation is sometimes aspirated during sleep and nose drops with an oil base may be accidentally aspirated. Microscopic globules of oil may be coughed up in the sputum if aspiration of any oil has occurred. In cases of recurrent pneumonia it is always worth having the sputum examined for oil droplets. Pneumonia may recur in lobes with normal bronchi if pus is aspirated from bronchi which are bronchiectatic.

Friedländer's[38] Pneumonia

This is usually a severe pneumonia in which the patient coughs up odourless thick, gelatinous reddish-green sputum (due to blood staining of the green pus characteristic of Friedländer's bacillus). The upper lobes are more frequently affected than the lower and abscess formation is very common. The pneumonia may be followed by fibrosis or bronchiectasis.

Virus Pneumonias

Strictly speaking "virus pneumonia" or primary atypical pneumonia is not due to a virus—it is due to the Eaton agent or *Mycoplasma pneumoniae*. Mycoplasmas are not viruses as they can be cultured on non-living media and divide by binary fission. Primary atypical pneumonia is associated with a sudden onset of cough and fever accompanied by headache and myalgia. Dyspnoea may be marked in the absence of

38. CARL FRIEDLÄNDER (1847–1887). Berlin pathologist.

physical signs in the lungs. The chest x-ray may show extensive bilateral patchy or modular shadows which are sometimes of lobar distribution. About 60 per cent of patients develop a rising titre of "cold agglutinins" (antibodies which will agglutinate group O red cells at 4°C.) They appear in the blood one to four weeks after infection and may remain for several months. Confirmatory evidence of primary atypical pneumonia is the demonstration of complement-fixing antibody in the serum to *M. pneumoniae* and isolation of *M. pneumoniae* from the sputum or throat swab. The organism is slow growing and the sputum cultures may take several weeks to become positive. The organism is sensitive to tetracycline. The complications of primary atypical pneumonia are central nervous system involvement (headaches, photophobia and meningism), haemolysis and peripheral venous thrombosis due to a high titre of circulating cold agglutinins. Rarely, arthralgia, pleural effusions and skin lesions resembling erythema multiforme occur. A useful diagnostic feature is the high ESR and normal white cell count. A normal white cell count makes bacterial pneumonia unlikely.

In epidemics of influenza the B virus may cause a fulminating rapidly fatal viral pneumonia; between epidemics the pneumonia is much milder. Psittacosis (ornithosis) is an acute respiratory illness due to a virus acquired from the excreta of birds which are usually ill. The birds are not necessarily psittacine birds such as parrots and budgerigars; chickens and pigeons may also be responsible. Systemic features such as splenomegaly and meningo-encephalitis occur. The disease is modified by tetracycline and chloramphenicol. Other virus illnesses such as chickenpox, measles and cytomegalic inclusion disease may cause a specific pneumonia.

PULMONARY EMBOLISM AND INFARCTION

Recent experimental and clinical work has suggested that the mechanical obstruction effects of a clot lodging in the pulmonary circulation are the most important factors leading to death from pulmonary embolism. Small pulmonary emboli can be lysed and disappear. In a patient with no previous heart or respiratory disease over half the pulmonary circulation must be occluded before death occurs, although patients with emphysema, mitral stenosis or previous left ventricular failure are unable to tolerate emboli of this size. The purely mechanical effects of a pulmonary embolus have been under-emphasised; however, it is also probable that other factors are involved. Following pulmonary embolism there is tachypnoea; this does not occur when the pulmonary artery is experimentally occluded, suggesting a *reflex* nervous mechanism; hypoxia frequently occurs: theoretically this should not happen if the circulation to one lung alone is obstructed, suggesting that *reflex* bronchial constriction also occurs.

Clinically tachypnoea and slight cyanosis may be the earliest or only signs of pulmonary embolism. Emboli which occlude so much of the pulmonary arteries that the circulation through the lungs virtually ceases cause hypotension, hypoxia, shock and cardiac arrest. Pulmonary embolism occasionally causes chest pain which is indistinguishable from the pain of myocardial ischaemia. In fact the chest pain of a large embolus is probably due to a sudden reduction of blood flow to the coronary arteries.

Pulmonary emboli which do not cause sudden death or are not soon dispersed usually produce signs of right ventricular strain. A rare physical sign is a transient murmur over the affected pulmonary artery due to blood passing the obstruction. In the plain chest x-ray there are only three signs of pulmonary embolism:

1. Enlarged pulmonary arteries.
2. Abrupt ending of a pulmonary artery.
3. Hypertranslucency of part of the lung fields due to absent blood flow.

Pulmonary Infarction

If the thrombo-emboli are small enough to block the small pulmonary arteries then infarction of part of the lung may occur. Infarction caused by small pulmonary artery occlusion occurs much more readily if pulmonary vein function is also disturbed. Infarction of the part of the lung generally occurs in a cone, with the base of the cone on one of the pleural surfaces—it may, therefore, be on one of the *interlobar fissures*. In effect this means that the shape of the resulting shadow on x-ray can be anything from triangular or round to linear. Sometimes the only x-ray sign is the resulting pleural effusion which is usually bloodstained but can be serious; elevation of the diaphragm is occasionally the only x-ray sign. The intrapulmonary shadowing following a pulmonary infarct may not appear for up to 24 hours after pleuritic chest pain; haemoptysis or pyrexia suggest that infarction has occurred. The electrocardiogram in both pulmonary infarction and pulmonary embolism may be normal or may show a dysrhythmia, right ventricular hypertrophy pattern, or features of posterior myocardial infarction due either to unidentified pulmonary-coronary reflexes or reduced blood flow.

A normal lung scan and chest x-ray virtually excludes significant pulmonary embolism. However, the reverse is not necessarily true, namely filling defects in the lung scan may be due to pathologies other than pulmonary embolism; for example asthma or bronchitis may result in small areas of collapse which are not perfused. This can be overcome by combining perfusion lung scanning, using labelled macro-aggregated albumin with a labelled xenon ventilation scan. This requires a gamma camera which is not widely available. It is disconcerting that 25–30 per cent of all patients undergoing surgery develop evidence of deep vein thrombosis as judged by the labelled fibrinogen uptake test and that about 20 per cent of patients have evidence of pulmonary embolism as judged by combined ventilation and perfusion scanning. The figures correspond to those obtained from autopsy material.

Management.—In a case of suspected pulmonary embolism two additional investigations may be mandatory, viz. lung scanning and pulmonary arteriograms. The pulmonary arteriograms can be performed after some practice in any x-ray department; the catheter should be placed if possible in the pulmonary artery so that contrast in the right ventricle does not obscure the view of the lower pulmonary arteries. It is not essential to make pressure recordings in the cardiac chambers.

Emergency pulmonary arteriography is a comparatively safe procedure.

Treatment of Pulmonary Embolism and Infarction

1. Prevention of further thrombosis: heparin.
2. Lysis or removal of established pulmonary emboli.
3. Attention to the source of the emboli (see page 70).
4. Prevention of thrombo-embolic pulmonary hypertension.

As a general rule, pulmonary infarcts which are judged to be small, in that the embolus which caused them has not produced any haemodynamic disturbance, should not be over-investigated or treated by thrombolysis. If on clinical, electrocardiographic and radiological evidence a pulmonary embolus is judged to be large then pulmonary angiography should be performed and the embolus located or the extent of occlusion of pulmonary arteries demonstrated. If it is then decided to institute thrombolytic treatment the catheter is left in the appropriate pulmonary artery and streptokinase and hydrocortisone infused for 24 hours in the same dose as for deep vein thrombosis. Further pulmonary arteriograms should then be obtained.

It has been shown that thrombolytic therapy can dissolve large pulmonary emboli. It should be considered in the relatively uncommon occurrence of pulmonary embolism in which death is not immediate and in which there is evidence of persisting haemodynamic disturbances due to the embolus or when x-rays reveal resisting obstruction of one or more of the major pulmonary arteries.

Pulmonary embolectomy is considered if the patient is unlikely to survive long enough for thrombolytic therapy to have time to work or if there is no evidence of clot lysis or improvement after 24 hours.

The evidence of the Urokinase Pulmonary Embolism Trial Study Group indicates that the patients who will benefit most from thrombolytic therapy are those who are critically ill from massive pulmonary embolism. There is no evidence that thrombolytic therapy in the early stage of embolism will reduce the incidence of late complications. Further deterioration with heparin or thrombolytic therapy would be an indication for pulmonary embolectomy.

There are numerous references to the long-term dangers following either pulmonary embolism or deep vein thrombosis (Phear, 1960; Goodwin et al., 1963). As a general rule all cases of deep vein thrombosis and pulmonary embolism or infarction should receive oral anticoagulants for at least 6 months. The risks and importance of repeated thrombo-embolism are so great that anticoagulants for this length of time are essential. The common practice of discontinuing oral anticoagulants when a patient is mobile or after an empirical period of 6 weeks after a deep vein thrombosis is difficult to justify.

There are particular dangers of thrombo-embolism in women on oestrogen-containing oral contraceptives. It is wise to consider giving prophylactic anticoagulants to any woman who is to have an operation and who is taking or who has taken them within the previous two months.

TUBERCULOSIS

Pulmonary tuberculosis is acquired by droplet infection with human *Mycobacterium tuberculosis*. The first infection of the lung produces an acute inflammatory response at alveolar level which soon forms a typical tubercle consisting of fibrous tissue, lymphocytes and Langhans[39] giant cells. The lung is very rich in lymphatics and living tubercle bacilli disseminate by lymph spread to the hilar lymph glands, here the disease may be contained. The combination of initial tuberculous infection of the lung together with lymphatic spread to the hilar lymph glands is known as the "primary" complex. Lymphatic spread of the bacilli in the primary infection may be responsible for infection of pleura and vertebrae. Live tubercle bacilli may be disseminated from the original infected alveoli to other parts of the lung by the airways or an infected lymph gland may rupture into a blood vessel causing haematogenous spread. By far the commonest occurrence is complete healing of the primary focus and its associated primary complex.

About 4–6 weeks after the first tuberculous infection all the cells in the body become sensitised to the presence of tubercle bacilli or protein

39. THEODOR LANGHANS (1839–1915). Berne pathologist.

products derived from them. As a result of this hypersensitivity further contact with tubercle bacilli produces an extremely vigorous inflammatory response. This inflammation is accompanied by caseation and fibrosis. Within such a fibrocaseous mass tubercle bacilli may either become walled off and harmless or, less commonly, liquefaction may occur and tubercle bacilli multiply and spread (fibrocaseous or post-primary tuberculosis).

Primary Tuberculosis

For the first four weeks after infection there are no abnormal signs; after this the patient develops signs of tuberculin sensitivity: erythema nodosum, phlyctenular conjunctivitis and a positive tuberculin skin test. After eight to twelve weeks the primary lung focus may be seen in the chest x-ray. It may be accompanied by hilar lymphadenopathy which, if severe, causes bronchial obstruction leading to consolidation and collapse. At this stage haematogenous (miliary) and lymphatic spread to pleura and bone may occur.

Primary tuberculosis may occur at any age; the frequency of complications depends upon the age group:

Ages 0–7 years: High incidence of miliary spread particularly 3–6 months after infection. Pleural effusions and cavitation are unusual.

Age 7–12 years: Relatively few complications.

Age 13–20 years: Pleural effusions 3–6 months after infection are common. Progress of the intrapulmonary primary focus to cavitated fibrocaseous tuberculosis is common.

Meningitis tends to occur about a year after primary infection, bone and kidney involvement later. Pleural effusion tends to occur after about 5 months and erosion of bronchial walls at about 9 months (Miller *et al.*, 1963).

Management.—Clinical evidence of tuberculous infection at any age is always treated whether it be pleural effusions of change of tuberculin skin test from negative to positive. Treatment is continued for at least two years with at least two anti-tuberculous drugs to which the bacilli are fully sensitive. Pleural effusions are treated with repeated aspirations as well as anti-tuberculous chemotherapy. If the effusion persistently recurs intrapleural hydrocortisone is used. Tuberculin testing is done with old tuberculin (OT), which is a heat-sterilised protein derivative of human *Mycobacterium tuberculosis*. The Mantoux test involves the intradermal injection of 0·1 ml of 1 in 10,000 (1 unit) of old tuberculin, the test is read in 2–4 days and the size of both the erythema and the accompanying induration should be recorded. Induration with a diameter of more than 0·5 cm is a positive reaction. If the reaction is negative the test should be repeated, using 0·1 ml of 1 in 1000 OT (10 **units**).

The Heaf[40] test involves intradermal injection to a depth of 1 mm. of a concentrated solution of Purified Protein Derivative (PPD) by means of a mechanical gun with 6 pointed prongs which project for 1 mm when the gun is fired. A positive Heaf test corresponds to a positive Mantoux test at a dilution of OT of approximately 1 in 1000. PPD is a purer form of the antigen from tubercle bacilli than old tuberculin. Certain factors may depress the skin reaction in a patient who should have a positive tuberculin test:

Inactive old tuberculin.
Old age.
Healed childhood tuberculosis.
Sarcoidosis.
Miliary tuberculosis.
Corticosteroid administration.
Malignant lymphomas.
Exanthemata.
Severe febrile illness.

Following a primary tuberculous infection the patient becomes tuberculin positive and this gives some natural immunity if the patient is again infected. Artificial immunity can be given by vaccination with BCG vaccine (Bacille Calmette[41]-Guérin[42]) which is an attenuated strain of bovine tubercle bacilli. It is given intradermally to people who are known to be tuberculin negative. Usually a small primary lesion develops at the site of injection six weeks later and the patient becomes tuberculin positive. Occasionally BCG vaccination is accompanied by ulceration, induration and regional lymphadenopathy, particularly if given accidentally to a tuberculin positive patient. This may require anti-tuberculous chemotherapy. In this country it is usual to offer BCG to:

1. All school children at the age of 13–14 who are not already tuberculin positive.
2. All tuberculin negative contacts of cases of tuberculosis.
3. People at special risk such as doctors and nurses.
4. The newborn children of tuberculous mothers.

Post-primary (Adult) Tuberculosis

Following primary tuberculosis living tubercle bacilli may remain dormant in the healed primary complex. Post-primary tuberculosis arising from infection by these organisms is "endogenous reinfection"— this is probably unusual. The common method of reinfection is by

40. FREDERICK ROWLAND GEORGE HEAF. Contemporary British physician.
41. LÉON CHARLES ALBERT CALMETTE (1863–1933). Paris bacteriologist.
42. CAMILLE GUÉRIN (1872–1961). Paris bacteriologist.

inhalation of a fresh dose of tubercle bacilli from outside—"exogenous reinfection". These external bacilli may be immediately involved in an intense inflammatory reaction which prevents their multiplying further. However, the inflammatory reaction may be insufficient to contain them and the organisms and inflammatory reaction continue to "fight it out". The inflammation heals by caseation and fibrosis; if caseation occurs into a bronchiole the patient will cough up live tubercle bacilli and cavitation is said to have occurred. The evidence of exogenous reinfection is:

1. Coinciding with a fall in open cases of tuberculosis in the population there has been a parallel decrease in notifications of new cases of tuberculosis.

2. People who had primary tuberculosis before the advent of anti-tuberculous chemotherapy occasionally develop post-primary (adult) tuberculosis due to *drug-resistant* organisms.

3. Post-primary tuberculosis due to ordinary *M. tuberculosis* occasionally develops in people who have previously had BCG; if endogenous reinfection occurred then their tuberculosis should be due to the organisms given in the BCG.

4. Occasionally cluster cases of tuberculosis occur in close contacts, suggesting case-to-case transmission of organisms.

The patient who coughs up live tubercle bacilli is said to be "sputum positive" or an "open case". Haemoptysis will occur if cavitation involves a blood vessel. Fibrosis may lead to contraction of the part of the lung involved (together with distortion of neighbouring structures such as trachea, pleura, chest wall and interlobar fissures) it may also lead to dilatation of neighbouring bronchi, bronchiectasis and secondary infection. Common methods of presentation of adult tuberculosis are weight loss, night sweats, haemoptysis, cough and sputum. The chest x-ray may show evidence of old primary tuberculosis, ill-defined patchy shadowing usually in one upper zone, which may be cavitated or calcified and accompanied by evidence of fibrosis. Post-primary tuberculosis generally involves the apical segment of the upper lobes and the primary focus the peripheral part of the middle or lower zones—the reason for the difference in distribution is not known. Tomography is often necessary to confirm cavitation or calcification.

The annual number of deaths from tuberculosis in England and Wales is still over 1300. This number far exceeds the death rate from any other notifiable infectious disease. It is salutary to note that 20 per cent of cases dying from tuberculosis were diagnosed only after death. In other words every District General Hospital in the country should expect to have at least one patient a year dying of unsuspected tuberculosis. Asian immigrants are more than 20 times as liable to have tuberculosis as the indigenous population. They are also more likely to have a non-respiratory manifestation of the disease. The most common forms of presentation of pulmonary tuberculosis are (Citron, 1973):

1. Middle-aged smoker with persistent cough.
2. Unresolved pneumonia.
3. Discovered by Mass Miniature Radiography. This has now been abandoned routinely because the yield was less than one active case per 1000. However, the equipment remains available for certain categories in which the yield remains high, e.g. contacts, immigrants, prisons and mental hospitals.
4. Deterioration in general health and weight loss.
5. Ill health in immigrants.
6. Haemoptysis.
7. Patients on steroids, diabetics and post-gastrectomy patients.

Non-respiratory Tuberculosis

It is important to note that, in the elderly, tuberculosis may present as a wasting illness with fever and without pulmonary manifestations. Ante-mortem diagnosis may depend on marrow, lymph node or liver biopsy. In cases of doubt a therapeutic trial with PAS and ioniazid is justified.

In immigrants non-respiratory tuberculosis is the rule and the features may include fever, generalised cervical or hilar lymphadenopathy, hepato-splenomegaly, as well as bone or genito-urinary involvement.

Treatment of Tuberculosis (Citron, 1974)

Primary chemotherapy refers to treatment for patients who have never previously had any anti-tuberculous chemotherapy. In Britain about 4 per cent of newly diagnosed patients have infection with organisms which are resistant to at least one of the main primary drugs and in order to prevent the emergence of resistant strains of organisms at least two of the drugs must be given. In practice this means starting initial intensive therapy with three drugs in case the patient happens to be one of the 4 per cent whose organisms are resistant to one drug. The result of tubercle bacillus sensitivity to chemotherapy will not be known for at least 6 weeks after treatment.

In Britain streptomycin and isoniazid are always included in the initial stage of primary therapy and the third drug in primary therapy may be PAS, ethambutol or rifampicin. In developing countries thio-cetazone may be used because of its cheapness. Initial therapy is continued for at least 6 weeks but the exact duration depends on the site and extent of the disease.

Continuation therapy is with two drugs to which the organism is known to be sensitive. Continuation therapy is continued for at least 1 year for non-cavitated disease and for $1\frac{1}{2}$–2 years for cavitated disease. All combinations of drugs used in continuation therapy contain isoniazid. The second drugs in the various regimes are PAS, ethambutol, rifampicin and thiocetazone.

Retreatment of relapsed tuberculosis and drug resistant organisms.— If the organisms are still sensitive to the primary drugs then these drugs may again be used. If the organisms have developed resistance, rifampicin and ethambutol are the most useful drugs provided they have not been used previously because the incidence of side-effects is lower with these than with the other reserve anti-tuberculous drugs. Abroad (particularly India and East Africa), successful treatment of tuberculosis has been obtained both with carefully controlled intermittent chemotherapy and short course regimes but these are not used in this country.

Examination of contacts.—Adult contacts who are tuberculin negative six weeks after the patient has been in hospital should be given BCG and regular chest x-rays (BCG is given if the contact is tuberculin negative after a delay of six weeks after the patient's admission as the contact may already be in the process of developing a positive tuberculin test as a result of his last contact with the patient). Adult contacts who are tuberculin positive should receive regular chest x-rays and tuberculin tests. All the children who are tuberculin negative six weeks after the patient has been admitted should be given BCG. Children who have not previously had BCG and are tuberculin positive should receive two years anti-tuberculous chemotherapy if they are between the ages of 0 and 7, and 12 and 20. Opinion is divided about tuberculin positive children between the ages of 7 and 12. Some would advocate regular check-ups and no anti-tuberculous chemotherapy unless further evidence of tuberculosis develops, others would give anti-tuberculous chemotherapy on the grounds that most children at this age are tuberculin negative and that a child who is tuberculin positive has evidence of tuberculous infection which has probably recently been acquired from the newly discovered hospital case. The reason why 7 to 12 years is a special age group is that the complications of primary tuberculosis at this age are less than in infants and adolescents.

The principal side-effects of the anti-tuberculous drugs in *reverse* order of frequency of incidence are:

Isoniazid: Peripheral neuropathy. This is commoner in patients who inactivate isoniazid slowly ("slow inactivators"). It can be prevented by giving pyridoxine at the same time. There is no evidence that the rate of healing of tuberculosis is different in slow and fast inactivators of isoniazid on the same dose of the drug. Psychosis, intellectual impairment, insomnia and epilepsy occur rarely with isoniazid. There have been reports of a possible carcinogenic effect of isoniazid.

Streptomycin: Vestibular disturbances (nystagmus, ataxia, vertigo), fever, skin rash and very rarely deafness. It is a wise precaution for everyone having steptomycin to have caloric and audiometry tests before starting on the drug. When the drug is stopped the vestibular disturbances are usually reversible. Deafness is usually not reversible.

PAS: Gastro-intestinal disturbances, goitres, hypothyroidism, hypokalaemia, liver damage and a glandular-fever-like syndrome.

Ethambutol: The only major toxic effect so far is a reversible form of optic neuritis which presents as blurring of vision. A unique form of red-green colour blindness and an arcuate central scotoma may be associated. Visual function should be tested before the drug is given. The drug is mainly excreted via the kidneys, hence renal failure may cause accumulation.

Rifampicin: No serious toxic effects have yet been reported. Mild gastro-intestinal disturbance, and liver impairment have occurred. The drug causes a red colour of urine and sputum. It also interferes with colour reaction for bilirubin in the serum giving false high bilirubin readings.

Capreomycin: The side-effects are similar to although less frequent than those of kanamycin; the most important are nephrotoxicity and ototoxicity.

Pyrazinamide: Liver damage (therefore fortnightly transaminase estimations for the duration of treatment), gout, fever and photosensitivity.

Cycloserine: Severe depression, epilepsy and confusion.

Prothionamide: Gastro-intestinal disturbances, liver damage, peripheral neuropathy, gynaecomastia and possibly teratogenic (hence to be avoided in pregnancy).

Other Mycobacteria

Mycobacteria are acid- and alcohol-fast bacilli of which *M. tuberculosis* and *M. leprae* are two types. Most of the others occur as opportunists in man and rarely can cause disease. *Histologically* the disease they cause is identical to that caused by *M. tuberculosis* but *clinically* the diseases are very different. These opportunist mycobacteria were called "atypical" or "anonymous". For practical clinical purposes there are three important opportunist mycobacteria in this country:

1. *M. kansasii.*
2. *M. avium—Battey bacillus.*
3. *M. marinum (M. balnei).*

The opportunist mycobacteria are classified into groups according to certain biochemical, cultural and morphologic differences. The opportunist mycobacteria grow rather more rapidly than *M. tuberculosis,* therefore a culture report back in four weeks instead of the usual six should alert one to the possibility that opportunist mycobacteria are present.

Some of the opportunist mycobacteria are saprophytes and are normally found in soil and water; they are occasionally found in association with M. tuberculosis. They should only be assumed to be causing the disease if they are repeatedly isolated. Infection by individual opportunist mycobacteria can be tested for by Mantoux testing using antigen prepared from the organism. The incidence of infection with opportunist mycobacteria varies in different parts of the world from 10 per cent of all tuberculosis in some parts of the United States to about 1·5 per cent in this country. Some of the opportunist mycobacteria are partially sensitive to the first line anti-tuberculous drugs.

1. *M. kansasii* can cause a pulmonary disease virtually identical to that caused by *M. tuberculosis*. Certain differentiating chest x-ray appearances have been claimed, namely more cavitation and less fibrosis (Chapman and Guy, 1959). Infection with *M. kansasii* is much commoner among urban dwellers and coal miners with pneumoconiosis. It is virtually confined to adult men, some of whom have had previous tuberculosis due to *M. tuberculosis*; there is no evidence of spread of the disease in close contacts; *M. kansasii* does *not* exist in the soil or water (Marks, 1969).

2. *M. avium* (*Battey bacillus*). This causes cervical adenitis particularly in children and is now the commonest cause of "tuberculous" adenitis (Keay, 1969).

3. *M. marinum* (*M. balnei*). This rarely causes outbreaks of skin granulomas (swimming-bath granulomas).

SARCOIDOSIS

Sarcoidosis is characterised by involvement of various organs with non-caseating granulomas. Similar granulomas occur in foreign-body reactions, tuberculosis, fungus infections and in lymph glands draining a carcinoma. The relationship of sarcoidosis to tuberculosis is still not clear, most cases have a negative tuberculin test but the incidence of tuberculosis in patients with sarcoidosis is 10 per cent. The clinical course of the disease is variable; an acute form with a duration of three to four weeks is more common in young women under the age of 30. They develop erythema nodosum and hilar lymphadenopathy and only occasionally involvement of other organs. The chronic form develops insidiously and often begins with fever, cough and dyspnoea, the pulmonary manifestations being hilar lymphadenopathy and infiltration by fibrous tissue. On the chest x-ray this is seen as soft irregular nodular shadows and linear streaks often radiating from the hilum. The acute form commonly has a good prognosis and the chronic form a poor prognosis. In the chronic form pulmonary function tests usually show a diffusion defect but the impairment of diffusion bears no relationship to the severity of the x-ray shadowing. A diffusion defect is sometimes found when the chest x-ray is normal. Other organs which are frequently involved are lymph nodes, eyes (uveitis and kerato-conjunctivitis sicca), skin (erythema nodosum), spleen, liver, bone, salivary glands and nervous system. Bone cysts occur in the terminal phalanges of the hands, they do not occur unless there is skin involvement. Nervous system involvement has been recorded in the absence of any other signs. Neurosarcoid is more common with the acute variety; response to corticosteroids is usually poor. Hypercalcaemia, which may cause nephrocalcinosis, is probably due to hypersensitivity to vitamin D resulting in excessive gastro-intestinal absorption of calcium; hypercalcuria may occur in the absence of hypercalcaemia. Increased gamma globulins also occur.

The diagnosis is confirmed by a negative tuberculin test, a positive Kveim[43] test and histological evidence. The most usual sites for biopsy are liver, scalene node and conjunctiva. Rarely it may be necessary to obtain a paratracheal gland by mediastinoscopy or a bronchial biopsy by bronchoscopy. The Kveim test is almost always positive in acute sarcoid although it may be negative in chronic sarcoid. Occasional false positive Kveim tests occur—their frequency depends on the antigen used.

Corticosteroids are used for the treatment of the hypercalcaemia, involvement of eyes and nervous system, disfiguring skin lesions, diffusion defects and intrapulmonary shadowing which remains unchanged for three months. Progressive dyspnoea, particularly in the early stages, is an indication for high doses of steroids which should be reduced when there is clinical improvement but should probably be continued in smaller doses for at least three months. In younger patients enlarged hilar lymph glands usually disappear within a year. They are more likely to remain in older patients when they may calcify. Pleural effusions do not occur in sarcoidosis.

DRUG-INDUCED LUNG DISEASE

A large number of drugs have adverse reactions involving the respiratory system. The lungs and airways may be involved in a generalised reaction caused by the drug (e.g. drugs causing a syndrome resembling systemic lupus erythematosus or asthma as part of an anaphylactic reaction). Involvement of the lungs may be the only adverse reaction produced (e.g. pulmonary eosinophilia). The drug-induced

43. MORTEN ANSGAR KVEIM. Contemporary Oslo physician.

lung diseases have been comprehensively reviewed by Dr. P. D. B. Davies from whose paper the following lists are taken (Davies, 1969).

Asthma

Penicillin
Tetracycline
Erythromycin
Streptomycin
Griseofulvin
Cephaloridine
Ethionamide
Monoamine oxidase inhibitors
Organic iodides
Local anaesthetics

Mercurials
Vitamin K
Bromsulphthalein
Iron dextran
Suxamethonium
Antisera
Vaccines
Aspirin
Indomethacin
Pituitary snuff

Pulmonary eosinophilia

Nitrofurantoin
Para-amino salicylic acid
Penicillin

Sulphonamides
Imipramine

Systemic lupus erythematosus

Penicillin
Tetracycline
Gold
Sulphonamides
Phenylbutazone
Griseofulvin
Hydrallazine
Isoniazid

Phenytoin
Streptomycin
Procainamide
PAS
Thiouracil
Tridione
Methyldopa
Carbamazepine

Polyarteritis

Iodides
Mercurials
Hydantoins
Penicillin

Gold salts
Thiouracils
Phenothiazines
Sulphonamides

Lipoid pneumonia

Liquid paraffin
Ephedrine nose drops

Cod liver oil

Intra-alveolar oedema and fibrosis

Busulphan

Hexamethonium and other
ganglion-blocking drugs

Local atelectasis and alveolar oedema
Oxygen—when administration of high concentrations is prolonged.

Local pleural fibrosis
Methysergide

Mediastinal and generalised lymphadenopathy

Phenylbutazone ⎫   Histology of glands in these conditions may
PAS   ⎬   resemble sarcoidosis, glandular fever and
Hydantoins   ⎭   lymphoma respectively

Pulmonary infarcts
Oral contraceptives

BRONCHIAL CARCINOMA

The evidence implicating cigarette smoking as a cause of bronchial carcinoma is now overwhelming. The carcinogen in cigarette smoke thought to be responsible is 3-4-benzpyrene. Atmospheric pollution probably plays a minor role in causation but the evidence is conflicting; the incidence of bronchial carcinoma is lower in coal miners even though their smoking habits are the same. It is suggested that pneumoconiosis results in obstruction of lung lymphatics limiting lymphatic spread of carcinoma. Certain mining and industrial processes are associated with a high incidence of bronchial carcinoma in exposed workers, e.g. asbestos, nickel, chromate, arsenic workers and pitchblende and uranium miners.

Carcinoma of the bronchus is responsible for over one-third of cancers in men and is responsible for nearly 10 per cent of all deaths in men. Despite widespread publicity of its dangers the amount of tobacco consumed in this country has not declined, nor has the incidence of bronchial carcinoma. It is interesting that the incidence of death from bronchial carcinoma is now constant in men below the age of 60 but the incidence in younger women, and in men over this age, is still increasing. This corresponds to the two periods when cigarette smoking became widespread in this country—among men during the First World War and among women during the Second World War.

The main pathological types are:

Squamous cell (or epidermoid—because the cells resemble the epithelium of the bronchi).—These tend to occur in the main bronchi.

Anaplastic, a common variety of which is the oat-cell carcinoma. This is the most common type associated with non-metastatic endocrine abnormalities. This type is highly malignant and is often associated with massive involvement of the mediastinum.

Adenocarcinoma.—This tends to occur in the periphery of the lung, it is the commonest bronchial carcinoma in women and is not associated with smoking. It accounts for less than 5 per cent of bronchial carcinoma in men and is mainly responsible for the uncommon occurrence of bronchial carcinoma in non-smokers. It is the commonest histological type associated with asbestosis.

Alveolar cell carcinoma.—These are uncommon and are usually widespread throughout the lung, they may arise from several foci or spread by aspiration metastasis. Histologically they resemble adenocarcinoma. Rarely they may be responsible for defects of diffusion; on x-ray alveolar cell carcinoma is seen as diffuse small ill-defined nodules.

Histological proof of the diagnosis of carcinoma is desirable and is obtained by bronchoscopy sputum cytology, pleural biopsy, pleural aspiration or lymph node biopsy. For ten days following bronchoscopy cells may appear in the sputum which are indistinguishable from carcinoma cells when no carcinoma is present; if the patient is suffering from tuberculosis or chronic bronchitis the sputum may contain cells which are similar to neoplastic cells. Cells derived from a pleural effusion due to pulmonary infarction may resemble adenocarcinoma cells. Approximately 10 per cent of bronchial carcinomas present with evidence of central nervous system involvement.

Treatment

The two main forms of treatment are surgery or radiotherapy. Apart from differences in the tumour histology there are a number of factors which exclude surgery:

1. Severe coincidental lung disease; chronic bronchitis severe enough to cause an FEV_1 less than 60 per cent of the predicted normal for age and weight is a contra-indication to surgery.

2. Severe coincidental disease in other systems.

3. Old age. The operative mortality of most series increases over the age of 65.

4. Mediastinal involvement with evidence of widening of the carina on bronchoscopy or paratracheal gland involvement.

5. Pleural effusion which recurs after aspiration, provided infection distal to bronchial obstruction is not responsible for the persisting effusion.

6. Paralysed diaphragm, recurrent laryngeal palsy or Horner's syndrome.

7. Extension to the chest wall.

8. Metastases—very occasionally exceptions are made when there is a solitary cerebral metastasis.

The current orthodox policy is to advise surgery for cases of squamous and adenocarcinoma deemed operable and radiotherapy for anaplastic and oat-cell carcinomas. There has now been a 5-year M.R.C. follow-up of cases of anaplastic carcinmoa treated by surgery and radiotherapy; results indicate that radiotherapy is marginally better than surgery for oat-cell and small-cell anaplastic tumours (Medical Research Council, 1969).

The question of earlier diagnosis of lung cancer in people at risk (smokers over the age of 40) is important. It seems that earlier detection of cases by regular six-monthly chest x-rays does improve the 5-year survival in operable cases (Brett, 1969).

If a tumour is found to be inoperable at thoracotomy implants of radioactive gold, if available, are inserted around the tumour. Inoperable and anaplastic tumours are treated with radiotherapy; sometimes this is combined with cyclophosphamide or nitrogen mustard. Recurrent pleural effusions are treated with radioactive gold, nitrogen mustard or pleurodesis.

Bronchial carcinoma of whatever type in women carries a worse prognosis than in men (Bignall and Martin, 1972).

NON-METASTATIC EXTRAPULMONARY COMPLICATIONS OF BRONCHIAL CARCINOMA

Endocrine

1. Cushing's syndrome. This is due to formation by the tumour of a peptide resembling ACTH. Often the first manifestation of Cushing's syndrome is a severe hypokalaemic alkalosis which is extremely resistant to treatment with potassium infusion and spironolactone. Most cases of Cushing's syndrome arise in young women. The occurrence of the disease in a middle-aged man should arouse the suspicion that a bronchial neoplasm is responsible. This is the commonest endocrine manifestation of carcinoma of the bronchus. Severe muscle weakness and pigmentation are usually present.

2. Hypercalcaemia. This is caused by a parathormone-like substance elaborated by the tumour. The hypercalcaemia may cause thirst, polyuria, fits and mental confusion, muscle weakness and constipation. The level of serum calcium can be brought down with steroids and the syndrome usually improves when the tumour is treated either surgically or with radiotherapy.

3. Inappropriate secretion of ADH. This results in a dilutional hyponatraemia; symptoms do not occur unless the serum sodium drops below 120 mmol/l. Paradoxically there may be sodium in the urine. There may also be a renal tubular defect resulting in glycosuria,

aminoaciduria and potassium loss. The condition can be improved with fludrocortisone.

4. Carcinoid syndrome. This syndrome can occur with bronchial carcinomas as well as adenomas.

5. Hypo- and hyperglycaemia.

6. Thyrotoxicosis.

7. Acromegaly.

8. Gynaecomastia.

9. Red cell aplasia.

10. Polycythaemia.

Other tumours associated with polycythaemia are:

1. Renal carcinoma.

2. Benign renal tumours.

3. Cerebellar haemangiomas.

4. Fibroids.

5. Adrenal carcinoma or hyperplasia.

6. Ovarian tumours.

7. Hepatomas.

8. Phaeochromocytoma.

Neurological Complications

All parts of the nervous system may be affected.

1. Encephalopathy with dementia, cerebral degeneration or leuco-dystrophy.

2. Cerebellar degeneration.

3. Extrapyramidal syndromes.

4. Myelopathy.

5. Neuropathy (motor and sensory).

6. Myasthenia.

7. Motor neurone disease.

Other Non-metastatic Manifestations:

1. Dermatomyositis.

2. Pulmonary osteoarthropathy.

3. Enteropathy resulting in malabsorption.

4. Thrombophlebitis.

5. Haemolytic anaemia, bleeding diatheses due to excess fibrinolysins, megaloblastic anaemia due to the tumour utilising all available folic acid.

6. Skin disorders (see page 330).

The course of these syndromes is very variable; in some patients they remit if the primary tumour is treated, in others they progress despite "adequate" treatment of the primary. Some, particularly the neuropathies, fluctuate regardless of treatment of the primary. The syndromes may antedate the appearance of the bronchial carcinoma by several years. In the neuromyopathies the CSF may show a rise of cells and protein and a Lange curve which is paretic (hence resembling multiple sclerosis or GPI).

PULMONARY FIBROSIS

Some diseases are associated with the involvement of the interstitial tissue of the lungs as opposed to primary involvement of the bronchi or pulmonary blood vessels. In general these diseases produce extensive fibrosis which manifests itself by interference with diffusion of gases before severely affecting ventilation. Characteristically, this results in dyspnoea and cyanosis without carbon dioxide retention. Diffuse interstitial pulmonary fibrosis (fibrosing alveolitis) is a disease of insidious onset and unknown aetiology characterised clinically by cough but no sputum, exertional dyspnoea, hyperventilation, clubbing and bilateral basal crepitations. The disease is slowly progressive and the downward progress is not prevented by corticosteroids although these may give some symptomatic relief. In the U.S. this condition is usually called the Hamman[44]-Rich[45] syndrome. However, Hamman and Rich originally described an acute illness which was rapidly progressive and sometimes associated with areas of consolidation and eosinophilic infiltration (Hamman and Rich, 1944). Another cause of interstitial fibrosis is pulmonary congestion.

Other Causes of Pulmonary Fibrosis

Chronic infections
  Bronchiectasis
  Fibrocystic disease

Collagen diseases
  Rheumatoid arthritis
  Scleroderma
  Systemic lupus erythematosus
  Polyarteritis nodosa

Dust and physical agents
  Silicosis
  Asbestosis

44. LOUIS VIRGIL HAMMAN (1877–1946). Baltimore physician.
45. A. R. RICH. Contemporary American physician.

Berylliosis
Fumes
Irradiation (deep x-ray therapy)

Granulomatous diseases
Sarcoidosis
Tuberculosis
Wegener's granuloma

Neoplasms
Alveolar-cell carcinoma
Lymphangitis carcinomatosa
Leukaemias

Histiocytosis
Letterer[46]-Siwe's[47] disease
Hand[48]-Schüller[49]-Christian[50] disease
Eosinophilic granuloma

Miscellaneous
Goodpasture's[51] syndrome
Alveolar proteinosis
Alveolar microlithiasis
Pulmonary haemosiderosis

Goodpasture's syndrome consists of multiple haemorrhages into the
lungs in association with glomerulonephritis and is a variant of polyarteritis nodosa. In pulmonary haemosiderosis there are also multiple
haemorrhages into the lungs but this disease is much more chronic and is
not associated with nephritis; it may be idiopathic or secondary to
chronic pulmonary venous congestion as in mitral valve disease.
Alveolar proteinosis and microlithiasis are very rare diseases in which
a protein substance and numerous minute calcified particles respectively
are deposited in the alveoli.

INDUSTRIAL DUST DISEASE

Silicosis

Silicosis is due to inhalation of particles of silica in exposed workers.

46. ERICH LETTERER. Contemporary Tübingen pathologist.
47. STURE AUGUST SIWE. Contemporary Lund physician.
48. ALFRED HAND (1868–1949). Philadelphia paediatrician.
49. ARTHUR SCHÜLLER (b. 1874). Vienna neurologist.
50. HENRY ASBURY CHRISTIAN (1876–1951). Boston physician.
51. ERNEST WILLIAM GOODPASTURE (1866–1960). Nashville pathologist.

Small amounts of silica dust can be disposed of by the ordinary processes of phagocytosis; inhalation of larger amounts result in silica particles remaining in the substance of the lung, and this provokes an intense inflammatory reaction—the silicotic nodule. With continued exposure these nodules will appear throughout both lungs and in the lymphatics and lymph glands. The silicotic nodules enlarge and coalesce; this may be avoided if the patient is removed from exposure. The conglomeration is greatest in the upper zones and is possibly associated with tuberculosis; distortion of the lung by fibrosis results in bullous emphysema. Cor pulmonale and pneumothorax are frequent complications.

On x-ray the first appearance is of well-defined, dense nodules throughout both lung fields, later the nodules enlarge and become ill-defined. Conglomeration of nodules is seen particularly in the upper zones; the hilar lymph glands are enlarged and frequently calcified. Later when emphysema supervenes the masses are even easier to see and they tend to move medially and finally may become continuous with the enlarged lymph glands of the mediastinum.

Coal-miners' Pneumoconiosis

This may develop in workers exposed to pure coal dust (e.g. stokers and trimmers aboard coal-burning ships) as well as coal-miners. In miners pneumoconiosis is often accompanied by silicosis. The x-ray appearances in the first instance are similar to those of silicosis with progression to coarse nodules. Unlike silicosis, these nodules are less well-defined and are not associated with bullous emphysema or lymph gland enlargement. Clearing of the dust particles is slower from alveoli which are relatively fixed, i.e. those in the centre of the lung lobules and those immediately underlying pleura and lung septa. This results in emphysema which is characteristically "focal"—this is the stage of simple pneumoconiosis. Complicated pneumoconiosis is said to have occurred when the nodules in the upper zone coalesce, a process called progressive massive fibrosis (PMF); tubercle bacilli are frequently isolated at postmortem from the fibrotic areas but clinical tuberculosis is uncommon in coal-miners' pneumoconiosis. Treatment prophylactically with anti-tuberculous drugs has no effect on the development of PMF. The lesions of PMF frequently cavitate and calcify; they result in compression and distortion of neighbouring lung tissue and frequently cause bronchiectasis and thrombosis of arteries and veins. Obstruction of lymphatics in the dust diseases result in inefficient clearing of any fluid; hence, pulmonary oedema tends to occur more readily than when lymph drainage from the lungs is normal. Patients with coal-miners' pneumoconiosis are more breathless than those with pure silicosis who have a similar amount of shadowing. Cor pulmonale is more common in coal-miners' pneumoconiosis, clinical tuberculosis more common in silicosis.

There is an international classification of radiological opacities in the lung fields provoked by inhalation of mineral dusts. Categories numbered 1 to 3 indicate the "profusion" of the opacities (extent and density of distribution). Category 1 indicates that the opacities occupy an area of one-third of both lung fields, Category 2 that most of both lung fields are involved and Category 3 that the opacities are very numerous. The size of the opacities is indicated by letters: p (punctiform) indicates nodules up to 1·5 mm, m (micronodular) indicates nodules 1·5–3 mm and n (nodular) nodules 3–10 mm in size. The letters A, B and C indicate the extent of massive fibrosis; the letter D denotes distortion of any thoracic structure (mediastinum, lung fissures, diaphragms, trachea or pleura) by the fibrosis of complicated pneumoconiosis (Pneumoconiosis and Allied Occupational Chest Diseases, 1967). Compensation for pneumoconiosis is possible from Category 2 onwards; at this stage PMF may develop even if the miner is removed from exposure. The presence of pneumoconiosis does not always mean that a miner has to leave mining; further compensation is not affected by the fact that he continues to work in the mines and later develops more severe pneumoconiosis. In men who have or are destined to have rheumatoid disease the radiological appearances of pneumoconiosis are atypical (Caplan's syndrome). Usually on a background of Category 1 or 2 pneumoconiosis, well-defined round opacities may appear suddenly in the periphery of any part of the lungs. They may come and go in crops, they may calcify or they may disappear leaving thin-walled cavities. The opacities can be very large and result in surprisingly little functional impairment.

Asbestosis

Is due to inhalation of dust containing the silicates of magnesium and iron in workers and miners who handle asbestos and mica. Characteristically there is fine mottling and streaky diffuse shadows particularly in the lower zones. The pleura and pericardium are thickened and shaggy in outline. Clubbing is common and there is probably no predisposition to tuberculosis. Minimum exposure is necessary to develop the disease; people exposed to asbestos dust cough up "asbestos bodies" in the sputum but these do not necessarily mean that the person has lung fibrosis due to asbestos; they merely indicate previous exposure to asbestos.

Exposure to asbestos dust leads to a predisposition to develop mesotheliomata which are malignant tumours of serous membranes such as pleura, pericardium and peritoneum. Mesotheliomata are much commoner in exposure to blue or Cape asbestos (Crocidolite); they appear to be commoner in people exposed to asbestos dust but who have not worked with asbestos, e.g. the wives of asbestos workers and local populations near asbestos mines. The relationship between pleural plaques and mesothelioma has not yet been established. There is also a predisposition to develop bronchial carcinoma, particularly peripheral adenocarcinoma.

FUNGUS INFECTIONS

Aspergillus Fumigatus

Aspergillus fungus may infect a lung previously damaged by a tuberculous cavity, unresolved pneumonia, pulmonary infarct or bronchiectasis. If a mycetoma or fungus ball forms the serum contains precipitins against the fungus; there is no immediate-type skin hypersensitivity but delayed-type skin hypersensitivity may be present. Mycetomas can cause haemoptysis but do not usually cause any other symptoms. In an old tuberculous cavity a mycetoma is seen as a solid round shadow lying on the floor of the cavity; above the mycetoma is a layer of air which appears as a crescentic translucency. The fungus ball may be seen to have moved if x-rays are taken in different positions.

Allergic aspergillosis.—Atopic subjects whose bronchi become infected with *Aspergillus fumigatus* usually develop wheezing accompanied by transient intrapulmonary shadowing. The aspergillus affects the more *proximal* bronchi causing localised proximal bronchiectasis—in contrast to *distal* bronchiectasis when pyogenic organisms are the cause. Allergic type of aspergillosis causes serum precipitins and both immediate and delayed types of skin tests. On rare occasions the allergic type of aspergillosis can produce localised proximal bronchiectasis and transient lung shadows without the patient having a wheeze or objective evidence of airways obstruction.

REFERENCES

BIGNALL, J. R., and MARTIN, M. (1972). *Lancet*, 2. 60.

BRETT, G. Z. (1969). *Brit. med. J.*, 4, 260.

BURNS, M. W., and MAY, J. R. (1967). *Lancet*, 1, 354.

CAMPBELL, E. J. M. (1969). *Thorax*, 24, 1.

CHAPMAN, J. S., and GUY, L. R. (1959). *Pediatrics*, 23, 323.

CITRON, K. M. (1973). *Brit. med. J.*, 2, 296.

CITRON, K. M. (1974). *Brit. J. hosp. Med.*, 12, 731.

DAVIES, P. B. (1969). *Brit. J. Dis. Chest*, 63, 57.

DAVIS, S., GARDNER, F., and QVIST, G. (1963). *Brit. med. J.*, 1, 436.

FORGACS, P. (1969). *Brit. J. Dis. Chest*, 63, 1.

GOODWIN, J. F., HARRISON, C. V., and WICKEN, D. E. (1963). *Brit. med. J.*, 1, 701 and 777.

GROSS, N. J., and HAMILTON, J. D. (1963). *Brit. med. J.*, **2**, 1096.

HAMMAN, L. V., and RICH, A. R. (1944). *Bull. Johns Hopk. Hosp.*, **74**, 177.

KEAY, A. (1969). *J. Tuberc.*, **50**, 85.

MARKS, J. (1969). *J. Tuberc.*, **50**, 78.

MAY, J. R. (1968). *The Chemotherapy of Chronic Bronchitis*. London: English Universities Press.

MEDICAL RESEARCH COUNCIL REPORT (1966). *Brit. med. J.*, **1**, 1317.

MEDICAL RESEARCH COUNCIL REPORT (1969). *Lancet*, **2**, 501.

MILLER, F. J., SEAL, R. M., and TAYLOR, M. D. (1963). *Tuberculosis in Children*. London: J. & A. Churchill.

PHEAR, D. (1960). *Lancet*, **2**, 832.

PNEUMOCONIOSIS and ALLIED OCCUPATIONAL CHEST DISEASES (1967). London: H. M. Stationery Office.

REES, H. A., MILLAR, J. S., and DONALD, K. W. (1968). *Quart. J. Med.*, **37**, 541.

REID, L. (1967). *Pathology of Emphysema*. London: Lloyd-Luke (Medical Books).

SCADDING, J. G. (1963). *Brit. med. J.*, **2**, 1428.

SCADDING, J. G., and HINSON, K. W. (1967). *Thorax*, **22**, 291.

SIMON, G. (1962). *Principles of Chest X-ray Diagnosis*, p. 4. London: Butterworth & Co.

TURNER-WARWICK, M. (1973). In *Recent Advances in Medicine*, 16th edit. Eds. Baron, D. N., Compston, N., and Dawson, A. M. Edinburgh: Churchill-Livingstone.

3

GASTRO-ENTEROLOGY

EXAMINATION OF THE ALIMENTARY SYSTEM

The external and remote clues of disorders of the alimentary tract are often as informative as the detailed examination of the abdomen itself. It is, therefore, mandatory to look carefully for circumstantial evidence of alimentary disease. One of the most frequently overlooked pointers to alimentary disease is an abnormality at the beginning of the alimentary tract, namely in the mucosa of the mouth and tongue.

The examination of the alimentary system should begin at the finger tips. Clubbing of the nails occurs in cirrhosis, Crohn's[52] disease and chronic diarrhoeas, whereas koilonychia occurs in severe iron deficiency anaemia and it is a feature of the Kelly[53]-Paterson[54] or Plummer[55]-Vinson[56] syndrome (dysphagia, iron deficiency anaemia and koilonychia). White crescents in the nails or leukonychia are said to be a feature of alcoholic cirrhosis; pigmentation of the nails occurs with excessive use of phenolphthalein as a purgative.

The hands may show palmar erythema involving the finger tips, thenar and hypothenar eminences; the condition occurs in cirrhosis but is also seen in pregnancy, following oestrogen ingestion and in patients with rheumatoid arthritis. Tylosis palmaris or hyperkeratosis of the palms occurs in carcinoma of the oesophagus. The skin creases should be inspected for pallor and pigmentation; pigmentation of the skin creases is highly suggestive of Addison's disease.

The hair should be observed—there may be changes due to pernicious anaemia (premature greying) or kwashiorkor (reddening of the hair). The hair and skin may be involved in vitamin deficiencies such as scurvy and pellagra. The skin should be carefully inspected for spider naevi as evidence of liver disease; they are often diagnostic but may occur in pregnancy, weather-beaten facies and following oestrogen ingestion. The skin may also show jaundice with scratch marks and bruising as evidence of liver disease.

Careful inspection of the mouth is essential before proceeding to the abdomen. Carious teeth and abnormally shaped teeth should be noted.

52. BURRIL BERNARD CROHN (b. 1884). New York physician.
53. ADAM BROWN KELLY (1865–1941). Scottish laryngologist.
54. DONALD ROSS PATERSON (1863–1939). Cardiff laryngologist.
55. HENRY STANLEY PLUMMER (1874–1937). Rochester, Minnesota, physician.
56. PORTER PAISLEY VINSON (b. 1890). Rochester, Minnesota, physician.

Hutchinson's[57] teeth occur in congenital syphilis and only the permanent teeth are affected: they are abnormally widely spaced and the incisors are notched and pointed. The gums are swollen and often bleed if there is gingivitis, scurvy, primary amyloid or hypertrophy due to anticonvulsant drugs. The gums may be stained in fluorosis or with tetracycline administration at an early age. The gums may become swollen and necrotic with chronic mercury poisoning (e.g. excessive mersalyl).

The mucous membranes of the mouth may be involved in systemic skin disorders such as scleroderma, pemphigus and lichen planus. They are also involved as part of the Stevens[58]-Johnson[59] syndrome, Behçet's[60] disease, generalised allergic reactions and vitamin deficiencies.

Loss of the filiform papillae of the tongue occurs in iron deficiency and pernicious anaemia as well as riboflavin deficiency which may cause angular stomatitis in addition. The mucosae may be involved in any bleeding diathesis; the ones most relevant to the alimentary system are Henoch-Schönlein purpura, liver disease and hereditary telangiectasia. The mucosae may be pigmented in Addison's disease; circumoral pigmentation occurs in the Peutz[61]-Jeghers[62] syndrome (circumoral pigmentation and small intestinal polyposis). Circumoral purpura are a feature of scleroderma associated with acrosclerosis and calcification of the soft tissues of the fingers (Thibierge[63]-Weissenbach syndrome). The lymph drainage of the stomach is ultimately into the left supraclavicular glands; these glands frequently become the seat of metastases from carcinoma of the stomach. A large number of eponyms have been given to these glands when they are enlarged; the most macabre is that of Troisier[64] who noted the ill-fated physical sign in himself.

The abdomen itself is then inspected: its general shape, movement with respiration and distension are observed. The presence of operation scars, abnormal peristalsis, dilated veins and hernias should be noted. The abdomen should be palpated with the patient lying flat. Before starting to palpate, it is essential to ask the patient if there is any local tenderness. After inspecting the abdomen carefully palpation should only be performed while looking at the patient's face in order to catch the first sign that palpation is causing pain. The abdomen is

57. SIR JOHNATHAN HUTCHINSON (1823–1913). London hospital surgeon.
58. ALBERT MASON STEVENS (b. 1884). New York paediatrician.
59. F. C. JOHNSON. Contemporary American physician.
60. HULUSI BEHÇET (1889–1948). Turkish dermatologist.
61. J. L. A. PEUTZ. Contemporary Dutch physician.
62. HAROLD JOSEPH JEGHERS (b. 1904). New Jersey physician.
63. GEORGES THIBIERGE (1856–1926). French dermatologist.
64. CHARLES ÉMILE TROISIER (1844–1919). Paris physician.

conventionally divided into nine segments: right and left hypochondrium, right and left lumbar region, right and left iliac fossae, epigasttrium, umbilical region and hypogastrium. Each segment should be palpated twice—the first time lightly and the second time more firmly.

The liver may be enlarged, tender or shrunken. Regeneration nodules may be palpable; the presence of umbilicated nodules is pathognomonic of secondary carcinoma. In amyloidosis the liver is often very large but there is seldom any evidence of hepatocellular failure or portal hypertension. The liver may be smaller than normal due to fibrosis; the small liver can only be detected by percussing the upper border which should lie at the level of the fifth rib in the mid-clavicular line in the normal. A Riedel's[65] lobe may extend down into the right lumbar region; this is a normal variant and is more often seen in women.

The characteristics of a splenic enlargement are:

1. Well-defined medial border which is notched.
2. It is impossible to get above the swelling.
3. A groove is felt between the swelling posteriorly and the erector spinae whereas no such groove occurs with renal swellings.
4. The swelling is dull to percussion.

The normal spleen can be percussed; percussion should begin posteriorly and extend along the 10th rib towards the mid-line. The limit of dullness of the normal spleen is the mid-axillary line.

The gall bladder, if palpable, is generally felt as a smooth rounded swelling projected below the edge of the liver. Enlargement of the liver displaces it downwards. If the liver is not enlarged the surface markings of the gall bladder are either the intersection of the right costal margin and a line drawn from left superior iliac spine through the umbilicus or the angle between the costal margin and the lateral border of the right rectus abdominis muscle.

Renal swelling is characterised by being felt in the loin, by being able to get above the swelling, by movement with respiration and by a band of resonance extending over it anteriorly due to gas in the colon.

ABDOMINAL PAIN

There is a very useful and sometimes life-saving dictum—"Any abdominal pain lasting more than six hours is likely to be surgical".

These are some tips which may be useful:

1. Digoxin causes vomiting and diarrhoea *but do not assume* that in a patient who is on digoxin vomiting is due to digoxin *until* you have *examined* the abdomen.

65. BERNHARD MORITZ CARL LUDWIG RIEDEL (1846–1916). Jena surgeon.

2. In all cases of abdominal pain always *examine carefully all* the hernial orifices.

3. Strangulation of part of the gut wall can occur in a hernia which *later* reduces itself (Richter's hernia).

4. Intestinal obstruction may *not* cause vomiting until very late.

5. Localised perforation and peritonitis going on later to generalised peritonitis can occur when the bowel sounds and abdominal x-rays remain *absolutely* normal.

6. Any cause of severe abdominal pain, e.g. acute cholecystitis or pyelitis, may cause a reflex paralytic ileus—the abdominal x-ray may show multiple fluid levels *but* the gut is *not* usually distended.

7. Ileus may be caused by drugs and electrolyte disturbances.

8. Feel the femoral pulses and listen for bruits—abdominal aortic aneurysms can cause abdominal pain.

9. So can a mesenteric embolus.

10. In a coloured patient, remember sickle-cell anaemia—the abdominal pain is usually due to infarcts in the mesentery or anterior abdominal wall—the gut sounds are often normal in the presence of quite severe pain.

11. Diabetic ketosis and porphyria may cause severe abdominal pain.

12. Always do the serum amylase—pancreatitis is surprisingly common *but* as a rule any cause of local or general peritonitis can cause a rise in the serum amylase to levels which are claimed to be diagnostic of pancreatitis. Pancreatitis does not always cause pain in the back.

13. Don't forget the rectal examination. Tenderness PR is *not* normal. If the patient is tender PR peritonitis either localised or generalised is probably present.

14. Ask for a second opinion sooner rather than later.

RADIOLOGY OF THE ALIMENTARY SYSTEM

Chest X-ray

A dilated oesophagus is seen as a well-demarcated opacity continuous with the right upper mediastinum; in the lower chest it may cause a double outline to the right border of the heart. Within the dilated oesophagus there may be particles of food and fluid levels. Associated with a dilated oesophagus there may be evidence of aspiration pneumonia or consolidation in aspiration segments. Scleroderma may cause oesophageal narrowing with dilatation above as well as abnormal lung shadowing which is usually bilateral and which may progress to "honey-comb" lung.

A "rolling" hiatus hernia may cause an abnormal shadow with fluid levels behind the heart, a lateral film shows that the shadow is situated posteriorly. Rare types of diaphragmatic hernia may be seen in the chest x-ray; one is herniation through the foramen of Morgagni[66] which is situated anteriorly and is an area of weakness at the attachment of the diaphragm to the sternum, it occurs much more commonly on the right side; the other is herniation through a patent foramen of Bochdalek[67] which represents the embryonic pleuro-peritoneal canals; it is usually left-sided and is frequently filled with loops of small intestine or colon. Also sometimes to be seen in the chest film are enlargement of liver or spleen, free gas under the diaphragm or absent or distorted gastric gas shadow due to hiatus hernia, large spleen or a tumour of the stomach.

Plain X-ray of the Abdomen

Certain structures should be routinely inspected as in the examination of the chest x-ray. The most important are the size of the liver, spleen, kidneys and psoas shadows (which become indistinct if there is fluid in the peritoneum). The plain x-ray allows the lumbar spine, pelvis, sacroiliac joints and sometimes the hip joints to be assessed. The presence of calcification should be noted particularly in relation to gall bladder, kidneys, pancreas, aorta and arteries: phleboliths and calcified lymph glands may be present. Care should be taken not to confuse swallowed radio-opaque pills, particularly those which contain iron or calcium, with pathological calcification. In the pelvis calcification may be seen in large uterine fibroids, ovarian dermoid cysts, vesical calculi, prostate and bladder wall in schistosomiasis.

The plain abdominal x-ray is most frequently required to assist in the diagnosis of an acute abdomen. Apart from the routine inspection of any x-ray the following should be borne in mind with regard to the presence and diagnosis of an acute abdomen:

1. **Fluid in the peritoneal cavity** (ascites or peritonitis).—Fluid in the peritoneal cavity results in a general loss of definition of the shadows seen in the x-ray particularly of gas-filled bowel and psoas shadows. In the erect film the gas-filled bowel floats upwards and occupies a position under the diaphragm and in the supine film the gas shadows usually appear more in the centre of the abdomen. Gas-filled loops of the bowel may be separated by a greater distance than normal.

2. **Gas in the peritoneal cavity.** — This is usually seen as a radiotranslucent crescent under the diaphragms. As well as perforation, gas will be found in the peritoneal cavity following laparotomy, pneumoperitoneum and paracentesis abdominis.

3. **Distension of part of the gut with or without fluid levels.**—The radiological signs of obstruction are excessive dilatation with accumula-

66. Giovanni Battista Morgagni (1682–1771). Padua anatomist and pathologist.
67. Vincenz Alexander Bochdalek (1801–1883). Prague anatomist.

tion of fluids in the dilated loops of bowel. Fluid levels will be seen in x-rays taken in erect or lateral positions but not in the supine position. The gas that accumulates in obstructed bowel is probably due to swallowed air. In general, paralytic ileus involves much of the alimentary tract and fluid levels are numerous.

4. **Abnormal calcification.**—This may be helpful in the case of cholecystitis, impacted gall-stone causing intestinal obstruction or ureteric calculus as the cause of the abdominal pain.

5. **Enlarged viscus or intra-abdominal mass.**—If seen on the plain film an intra-abdominal mass may be the clue to the diagnosis.

Two conditions give rise to localised paralytic ileus which is manifested by local dilatation of loops of bowel, these are arterial occlusion to part of the gut and localised peritonitis, e.g. following acute appendicitis, cholecystitis, pancreatitis, salpingitis or ruptured ectopic pregnancy.

The approximate site of intestinal obstruction can sometimes be determined from the plain film. Large-bowel obstruction produces gas-filled loops of bowel around the edge of the x-ray although, of course, later the changes of small intestinal obstruction will become superimposed as the effects of the obstruction alter function higher in the intestines. The ileum generally occupies the central portion of the abdomen and the jejunum the upper left quadrant. In ileal obstruction there are likely to be more dilated loops than in jejunal obstruction. The appearances of the gas-filled bowel may give an indication of the site of the obstruction. The jejunal mucosal folds lie very close together at right-angles to the long axis and are easily seen when the jejunum is filled with gas. In the ileum the mucosal folds are sparse and flat and may not be seen.

Fibreoptic Endoscopy

The rapid improvement and increasing robustness of fibreoptic endoscopes in the last 10 years has led to their rapid introduction into routine gastro-enterological practice. There can be little doubt that their use is now mandatory for the correct management of many gastro-intestinal conditions. Their very usefulness and the relative ease and comfort with which they can be passed poses logistic problems. The orthodox routine indications for endoscopy are still controversial but it is generally accepted that about 30 per cent of patients with negative barium meals may have a significant lesion discovered by endoscopy. The available evidence suggests that endoscopy is generally unnecessary in patients who have a radiologically confirmed duodenal ulcer, but all patients with a gastric ulcer should have an endoscopic biopsy for fear that the ulcer is malignant.

Endoscopy should now be considered with radiology as an essential investigation in patients with acute gastro-intestinal bleeding and anastomotic ulcer symptoms. Radiology is unable to detect acute gastric erosions and about half of all anastomotic ulcers escape detection.

Gallium Scanning

There is now evidence that malignant tumours of the colon and rectum take up labelled gallium much more than normal tissue and Gallium[67] scans may be of value in identifying malignant large-bowel tumours.

PEPTIC ULCER

Incidence

In this country the incidence of duodenal ulcer is increasing; duodenal ulcers are at least three times as common in men as in women, and are much commoner in the higher social classes. The increase in duodenal ulcer is mainly between 45 and 65 years of age. Duodenal ulcers are uncommon in women before the menopause.

The incidence of gastric ulcer has declined over the last 50 years, the sex incidence is approximately equal, they are commoner in the lower social classes and the incidence increases steadily with increasing age.

Pathogenesis

1. Race: in every country where studies have been made the incidence of duodenal ulcer is always higher than gastric ulcer. However, in some countries the incidence of gastric ulcer is higher than in this country, e.g. Japan, parts of India and Finland. Chronic peptic ulcers are almost unknown in the South African Bantus.

2. Known aetiological factors:

    (i) Zollinger-Ellison syndrome.
   (ii) Cushing's syndrome.
  (iii) Hyperparathyroidism.
   (iv) Cirrhosis—portal and biliary.
    (v) Drugs: salicylates, steroids in
            high doses, phenylbutazone,
            colchicine and tolbutamide.
   (vi) Severe burns.
  (vii) Septicaemia.
 (viii) Coma.

3. Increased incidence in other diseases, e.g. emphysema, chronic bronchitis, pulmonary tuberculosis, rheumatoid arthritis and atherosclerosis.

4. Heredity: there is often a strong family history in cases of peptic ulceration. Ulceration in the same site is common in the same and succeeding generations. Blood group O plus non-secretion of blood group substances in the exocrine secretions is associated with a higher incidence of duodenal ulceration; this applies particularly to anastomotic ulcers following partial gastrectomy or vagotomy plus drainage. Carcinoma of the stomach is associated with non-secretion in blood group A people.

5. Smoking: the incidence of peptic ulcers is lower in non-smokers.

6. Personality: the incidence of duodenal ulcers is higher in anxiety-prone personalities and in people with responsible jobs.

7. Gastric acidity and mucosal resistance: it is believed that the stomach and the duodenum are protected from autodigestion by mucus, a rapid turnover of epithelial cells and a limited acid production. Breakdown of one of these protective mechanisms will result in too rapid a destruction of mucous membrane and ulceration.

Gastric ulcers are associated with a lower than normal acid secretion and they are more common if there is chronic gastritis and are *much* commoner if there is a coexisting duodenal ulcer. This may be because the duodenal ulcer delays gastric emptying, promoting stasis and damage to the gastric epithelium resulting in gastric atrophy and loss of mucosal resistance. Distortion of the pylorus by the duodenal ulcer may also lead to reflux of bile into the stomach which can also damage the gastric mucosa. Because duodenal ulcers promote gastric stasis which may lead to reflux oesophagitis, symptoms of reflux oesophagitis are common with a chronic duodenal ulcer.

Duodenal ulcers are usually associated with a higher than normal gastric acid output which may be due to an increased number of acid-producing parietal cells or an increased drive (e.g. by gastrin) in a normal number of parietal cells. Those cases of duodenal ulcer where gastric acid output is in the normal range presumably have a deficiency in mucosal protection.

Treatment of Peptic Ulceration

Medical treatment of peptic ulceration is mainly symptomatic and largely empirical since the primary cause is usually not known. Duodenal ulceration is usually associated with hyperchlorhydria and an increased parietal cell mass; this is not so in the case of gastric ulcer. Gastric ulcers are commoner in the older age groups and are occasionally complicated or caused by carcinoma of the stomach. Any ulcer in the stomach which is not situated on the lesser curve should be assumed to be malignant until proved otherwise (by negative occult bloods, gastric cytology, gastroscopy or gastric photography or evidence of complete healing on barium meal). Gastric ulcers due to drugs (aspirin and phenylbutazone) usually occur on the greater curve. All gastric ulcers should be checked by repeat barium meal for complete healing; this does not apply to duodenal ulcers: chronic scarring of the duodenal cap means that no ulcer crater, oedema or fresh scarring can usually be demonstrated on a barium meal in an acute exacerbation of duodenal ulcer symptoms.

No medical measures have been shown to prevent relapse of peptic ulceration; medical treatment is directed towards symptomatic relief and promotion of healing. The main forms of medical treatment are:

1. **Bed rest.**—Symptoms of both gastric and duodenal origin disappear more rapidly with bed rest; however, only gastric ulcers have been shown to heal more rapidly with bed rest, there is no evidence that duodenal ulcers are affected (Doll and Pygott, 1952).

2. **Smoking.**—There is some evidence that stopping smoking promotes the healing of gastric ulcers. There is no evidence with regard to duodenal ulcer or whether stopping smoking prevents relapse of ulcers.

3. **Diet.**—Milk undoubtedly gives symptomatic relief in peptic ulceration. For this reason milk diets have long been given in treatment, combined with diets low in "roughage" and protein to prevent excessive stimulation of gastric acid. Such diets were given at frequent intervals in an attempt to keep the acidity of the stomach down. However, the evidence is that milk and milk products are no more beneficial than a diet of the patient's own choosing (Lennard-Jones and Babouris, 1965). Maximum acidity occurs when meals are taken at hourly or four-hourly intervals; the optimum interval between meals is about two hours. These findings have been confirmed by others (Lawrence, 1952; Truelove 1960).

4. **Antacids.**—Most of the effective antacids only reduce the acidity of the stomach for about twenty minutes, although they usually relieve the pain of peptic ulceration for much longer. Sodium bicarbonate is the most effective alkali—its main disadvantage is that it is absorbed from the stomach and may give rise to alkalosis. Calcium carbonate does not cause systemic alkalosis but may cause hypercalcaemia and the "milk-alkali" syndrome. Magnesium oxide is the third most effective antacid but magnesium salts produce diarrhoea; this can be counteracted by giving calcium salts at the same time which tend to constipate. Other antacids are much less effective; magnesium trisilicate is about one-tenth as effective as sodium bicarbonate and 300 ml of aluminium hydroxide gel is equivalent to about 5 g of sodium bicarbonate.

Traditionally a "milk drip" is used for recalcitrant non-healing ulcers. The available evidence is that it does not affect the rate of healing of gastric ulcers (Doll et al., 1956). There is no evidence as to its effect on the rate of healing of duodenal ulcers.

Prolonged medical treatment of peptic ulcers with high doses of alkalis and milk (which contains large amounts of calcium) may lead to renal damage with retention of calcium, albuminuria and a raised blood urea which are the hallmarks of the milk-alkali syndrome. There is usually nephrocalcinosis and sometimes nephrolithiasis; polyuria may occur due to the raised calcium and blood urea. Associated nausea and vomiting with ulcer pain may suggest an exacerbation of the peptic ulcer.

5. **Anticholinergic drugs.**—These drugs are atropine-like in their activity and act on the stomach by reducing its motility and preventing vagal induced acid secretion. They often effectively relieve ulcer symptoms but do not accelerate the healing of ulcers (Lennard-Jones, 1961). There are three absolute contra-indications to the use of anticholinergic drugs namely, a history of acute glaucoma, prostatism and pyloric stenosis. Side-effects are those of atropine, i.e. blurred vision, dry mouth, tachycardia and paralytic ileus.

6. **Carbenoxolone (Biogastrone).**—This has been shown to be effective in the healing of gastric ulcers (Doll *et al.*, 1962). It usually causes fluid retention and potassium depletion which should be treated with a thiazide diuretic and liberal potassium supplements. It is generally agreed that a gain in weight of over 4 lb in six weeks is an indication for diuretic treatment. The drug should not be used in the presence of renal disease, hypertension or cardiac failure. A specially coated form of carbenoxolone is available for the treatment of duodenal ulcers.

The surgical treatment of peptic ulcer is the emergency treatment of the complications or an elective operation for chronic ulceration. Complications of peptic ulcers include:

Haematemesis and melaena.
Perforation.
Pyloric stenosis.
Penetration and fistulae.
Malignant change.
Milk alkali syndrome.

Management of Haematemesis and Melaena

About a quarter of peptic uclers are complicated by haemorrhage. The tendency to bleed is greatest in the first year after an ulcer develops; thereafter, the likelihood of haemorrhage is the same throughout the disease. The mortality from haemorrhage is higher in chronic than acute ulcers and is much higher over the age of 50. Over 95 per cent of bleeding from the upper gastro-intestinal tract is due to peptic ulceration; however, most of the problems of management involve the exclusion of causes other than chronic ulceration.

The bleeding which follows salicylate ingestion is due to acute gastric erosion. The chance of bleeding with salicylates is no greater in patients with a peptic ulcer or a previous history of dyspepsia. Some haemorrhage is said to occur in 50–70 per cent of patients taking aspirin. Bleeding is much less with enteric-coated tablets but absorption is delayed so that they are only useful for long-term treatment—they will not relieve pain quickly which is the commonest reason for taking aspirin. The treatment of haemorrhage due to salicylates includes the administration of vitamin K, because salicylates lower the blood level of prothrombin as well as reducing the platelets.

The main diagnostic difficulty in the management of haematemesis is the exclusion of oesophageal varices. The history is sometimes helpful, apart from a history of alcoholism or recurrent liver failure, exposure to many industrial chemicals results in liver damage and portal hypertension. A previous history of chronic dyspepsia is important in helping to decide the site of bleeding; however the incidence of peptic ulcers in cirrhotics is higher than in the general population. The finding of splenomegaly or other signs of portal hypertension is the most useful pointer to bleeding varices; associated signs of hepatocellular failure should always be looked for. A barium meal should be performed as early as practicable following an upper gastro-intestinal haemorrhage. The ease with which this can be done varies from hospital to hospital but it should be considered essential in the event of a large bleed over the age of 50 and always in the event of a second haemorrhage. If necessary it can be done using a portable x-ray. There is no evidence that an emergency barium meal predisposes to further haemorrhage. Oesophageal varices are demonstrated in about 70 per cent of cases in which they are present. In doubtful cases a BSP excretion test may be helpful; if it shows normal excretion bleeding is most unlikely to be due to varices. If BSP excretion is impaired it is of little diagnostic value since anaemia and recent haemorrhage as well as hepatocellular damage also delay BSP excretion. In about a quarter of cases in which bleeding is due to a peptic ulcer a barium meal does not reveal an ulcer crater. If this negative barium meal is accompanied by a short or absent history of previous dyspepsia in a patient under the age of 50 then it is very likely that the bleeding is due to acute ulceration, which is accompanied by a low mortality when treated conservatively. Long-standing peptic ulcers (particularly chronic gastric ulcers) are associated with a higher mortality when treated conservatively. The treatment of severe haemorrhage whatever the cause is immediate blood transfusion, sedation, bed rest and feeding small frequent meals after a period of 24 hours after bleeding has stopped. If haemorrhage from the stomach is continuous or repeated it may be helpful to pass a Ryle's tube; occasionally bleeding continues because the stomach is distended with clot. This should be evacuated with ice-cold water. Rarely in a desperate situation adrenaline and thrombin in methyl cellulose instilled into the stomach may stop bleeding.

If bleeding has been severe it is wise to set up a central venous pressure line; a fall in CVP may be the first sign that a second bleed has occurred.

The problems of transfusions of large amounts of blood should be borne in mind namely:

1. Circulatory overload.
2. Potassium intoxication.
3. Hypocalcaemia (due to citrate anticoagulant in the blood chelating the calcium in the body).
4. Hypocoagulable states.
5. Serum hepatitis and other infections.
6. Air embolism.
7. Allergic and febrile reactions.
8. Mismatched blood.

Acute bleeding ulcers in patients under the age of 50 are usually treated conservatively. In patients over the age of 50 who have chronic ulcers and recurrent or sustained bleeding emergency laparotomy is performed. The procedure carried out at laparotomy varies; all the procedures involve over-sewing a small ulcer or removing or over-sewing a large ulcer. The three forms of treatment currently in vogue for both bleeding duodenal and gastric ulcers are (Duthie, 1967):

1. Partial gastrectomy.
2. Vagotomy and antrectomy (to remove the gastrin-secreting portion of the stomach and pylorus).
3. Vagotomy and pyloroplasty,

If at operation no ulcer or single bleeding point is seen or palpated, the stomach and duodenum are inspected internally either by performing a gastrostomy or by inserting a sigmoidoscope and inflating the stomach. If the bleeding is due to acute erosions and is not life-threatening no further operation is performed; if no bleeding points are seen partial gastrectomy is usually carried out.

Perforation.—There are three phases of the clinical picture following perforation. The first is the dramatically sudden onset of intense abdominal pain accompanied by rigidity and guarding; the pulse rate and blood pressure are normal and bowel sounds are absent. The second stage of "stage of delusion" develops when abdominal pain subsides and the patient seems to be improving—the abdomen remains rigid. The third stage is that of generalised peritonitis. Two factors modify the clinical picture, the first is a small perforation which becomes localised by omentum or adhesions; the second is perforation in the elderly in whom the clinical picture may be less severe in the early stages. Once the diagnosis has been made laparotomy should be performed without delay. If the perforation is small it can be sutured; if large, a partial gastrectomy is usually performed. Careful conservative treatment of acute perforation in highly selected cases is occasionally used; with correct selection of patients the mortality is much the same as for emergency laparotomy (Herman Taylor, 1957).

Pyloric stenosis.—Pyloric stenosis is almost invariably due to scarring secondary to a duodenal ulcer or to a carcinoma of the stomach, only rarely does a gastric prepyloric ulcer lead to pyloric stenosis. Benign gastric ulcers usually occur on the lesser curve of the stomach hence an ulcer in the prepyloric region should be presumed to be malignant until proved to be benign (by gastroscopy, repeat negative barium meal, or intragastric photography).

With the development of pyloric stenosis the symptoms of duodenal ulcer usually change. The delay in gastric emptying leads to secondary ulceration of the stomach and the increased intragastric pressure may lead to reflux oesophagitis. The symptoms of gastric ulcer and peptic oesophagitis often become superimposed on those of the duodenal ulcer. Repeated vomiting leads to gastric distension and electrolyte changes. The narrowing of the pylorus is due to fibrosis or oedema in relation to the nearby ulcer, in addition, spasm of the muscle of the pyloric canal probably occurs as well. The diagnosis is suggested by the history of changed symptoms, vomiting, recent weight loss and constipation. Physical signs include visible gastric peristalsis and distension, succussion splash, dehydration and alkalosis. The alkalosis may be aggravated by the administration of antacids and may cause a lowering of the ionised calcium in the serum and cause either latent or overt tetany which may be accompanied by a positive Chvostek[69] sign. Tetany may also be caused by potassium loss due to the repeated vomiting. The alkalosis which occurs is due to loss of hydrogen ion in the vomit; secondary uraemia may occur due to dehydration or potassium or sodium depletion damaging the kidneys. Despite the alkalosis the urine may be acid if hydrogen ion is excreted in order to conserve potassium. Anticholinergic drugs are definitely contra-indicated as they reduce gastric motility and hence further impair gastric emptying.

In the management of pyloric stenosis gastric aspiration is performed intermittently or continuously—this reduces the friability of the stomach should operation be necessary. If the volume of juice aspirated after an overnight fast exceeds 500 ml. the diagnosis is confirmed.

If most of the pyloric obstruction is due to inflammatory oedema the symptoms should subside in 2–3 days. Operation is indicated if: (i) the

69. FRANTISEK CHVOSTEK (1835–1884). Vienna surgeon.

vomiting persists more than three days, (ii) more than 500 ml is repeatedly aspirated from the stomach after overnight fasting, (iii) the barium meal reveals a distended stomach with narrowing of the pyloric canal so that the lumen is less than 3 mm (Kirsner, 1967).

Occasionally long-standing pyloric stenosis presents in unusual ways:

1. Diarrhoea—probably due to multiplication of organisms in the poorly emptying stomach.

2. Nephrocalcinosis and tubular damage—due to prolonged alkalosis, hypokalaemia and hyponatraemia.

3. Mental changes due to hyponatraemia.

Penetration.—Chronic peptic ulcers may penetrate any adjacent organ; however, the commonest is the pancreas and the ulcer is usually situated on the posterior wall of the stomach or duodenum. Perforation should be suspected if the ulcer symptoms become severe and continuous. There is usually evidence of pancreatic inflammation (continuous back pain and raised serum amylase). Barium meal may show barium in the penetrating ulcer or fistula.

Malignant change.—This does not occur with duodenal ulcers but occurs occasionally in long-standing gastric ulcers. It is important to note that carcinoma undergoes peptic ulceration and it is frequently impossible to say which came first. Giant gastric ulcers (more than 3 cm in diameter) are seldom malignant (Strange, 1959).

Elective Operation for Peptic Ulceration

The main factors influencing a decision for elective operation for peptic ulcer are:

1. The presence of complications of peptic ulceration weighs heavily in favour of surgery. Following haemorrhage operation is advisable over the age of 50; below this age it is acceptable to wait to see if bleeding recurs. Perforated ulcers which have been sutured require elective surgery if there is recurrence of ulcer symptoms. Organic pyloric stenosis and a long ulcer history are strong indications for surgery.

2. "Failed medical treatment."—Recurrence of symptoms after a prolonged course of medical treatment, no further relief of pain with alkalis, interruption of sleep, frequent time off work, or a long history of frequent relapse favour surgery. Medical treatment should have included sedation, bed rest, milk drip, and abstinence from tobacco.

3. Chronic gastric ulcers particularly if there is doubt as to whether they are benign or malignant.

There is considerable variation as to what operation should be performed to promote healing and prevent recurrence of ulcers. Duodenal ulcers are associated with a high output of hydrochloric acid which is controlled by gastrin secretion from the antrum of the stomach and by the vagi. If the acid output by the stomach is very high both section of the vagi (vagotomy) and removal of the gastrin-producing part of the stomach (antrectomy) are necessary. Lesser degrees of hyperchlorhydria can be treated by vagotomy alone; however, section of the vagi reduces the motility of the stomach and the operation must be accompanied by some form of "drainage procedure". The drainage may be by enlarging the pyloric canal (pyloroplasty) or a side-to-side anastomosis between the stomach and the jejunum (gastro-jejunostomy). The advantage of pyloroplasty or antrectomy over gastro-jejunostomy is that there is no "blind loop", although it is not always possible to perform a pyloroplasty or antrectomy if there is severe scarring; they are less suitable procedures than gastro-jejunostomy for very sick patients. The recurrence rate of duodenal ulcer following any vagotomy and drainage procedure is higher than with partial gastrectomy; in addition there are ill effects from sectioning the vagi, viz., diarrhoea which is usually but not always temporary and disturbances of the motility of stomach and oesophagus which leads to a feeling of fullness, belching and dysphagia in some patients.

Which Vagotomy?

There are three types of vagotomy:

(a) Truncal

(b) Selective (i.e. branches supplying the stomach are cut)

(c) Proximal gastric (i.e. only fibres supplying the acid-secreting mucosa are cut).

The proximal gastric vagotomy is more difficult and time-consuming to perform but because innervation of the remainder of the stomach is kept intact the operation need not be accompanied by a drainage procedure. Recurrent ulceration may be more frequent with this type of operation but post-operative diarrhoea and metabolic disturbances appear to be less frequent.

Many surgeons still prefer to perform a Pólya[70] partial gastrectomy for duodenal ulcer in which the gastric stump is sutured to a jejunostomy and there is a "blind loop" through which bile can drain. The difference between a Pólya partial gastrectomy and a gastro-jejunostomy is that in the gastro-jejunostomy a side-to-side anastomosis is performed but the pylorus and duodenum are left intact, so that stomach contents can either pass through the duodenum or straight from the stomach to jejunum. In the Pólya gastrectomy the first part of the duodenum together with the distal stomach is removed and the remainder of the stomach is anastomosed to jejunum and the duodenum closed proximal to the ampulla of Vater[71] so that bile can still reach the intestines. Re-

70. Eugene Jenö Alexander Pólya (1876–1944). Budapest surgeon.
71. Abraham Vater (1684–1751). Wittenberg anatomist and botanist.

section of part of the stomach and the "blind loop" have their own problems but the rate of recurrence of duodenal ulceration is much less; the duodenal ulcer itself is resected and vagotomy can always be performed later if necessary.

For gastric ulcers a Billroth[72] I partial gastrectomy is favoured by most surgeons. The first part of the duodenum, pylorus and antrum are removed and a gastro-duodenal anastomosis performed. Anastomotic or recurrent ulcers do not usually occur after partial gastrectomy for gastric ulcer but are more likely after partial gastrectomy for duodenal ulcer—the incidence is 1–2 per cent.

Complications of Partial Gastrectomy

The immediate complications are those of any abdominal operation. Within a few weeks of the operation other complications may occur.

1. **Early dumping syndrome.**—After a meal there is a sensation of epigastric fullness and nausea accompanied by faintness, sweating and palpitations. Many mechanisms have been held to be responsible for these symptoms. The main ones are:

(i) Rapid distension of the jejunum.

(ii) Hypovolaemia caused by rapid flow of water from the extra-cellular fluid as a result of rapid transit of gastric contents with a high osmotic pressure into the jejunum. Attempts have been made to infuse fluid intravenously at the time fluid is being lost into the jejunum in order to maintain the blood volume. Also insulin (or tolbutamide) has been given before the meal to lower the blood sugar and encourage more rapid absorption of carbohydrate from the jejunum, thus preventing the outpouring of fluid into the jejunum (Le Quesne *et al.*, 1960).

(iii) Failure of peripheral arterioles to constrict in response to rapid diversion of blood flow to splanchnic areas (Cox and Allen, 1961).

2. **Late dumping syndrome.**—This is due to hypoglycaemia. Soon after food reaches the jejunum there is rapid absorption of carbohydrates leading to an increase in blood sugar which stimulates insulin secretion. If too much insulin is secreted there will be an overswing and hypo-glycaemia will occur. The attacks usually occur 2–4 hours after a meal but may appear much earlier. They generally diminish in severity in the course of time.

3. **Afferent or blind loop syndrome.**—This consists of a feeling of full-ness and nausea relieved by vomiting almost pure bile. It is suggested that there is transient obstruction of the blind loop into which the bile and pancreatic ducts open. The obstruction is due to mechanical distortion and is relieved when vomiting of the contents of the blind loop occurs. Sometimes the dumping syndrome is superimposed on the blind loop

72. CHRISTIAN ALBERT THEODOR BILLROTH (1829–1894). Vienna surgeon.

syndrome. The treatment is surgical and usually consists in converting the operation to a Billroth I type gastrectomy and adding a vagotomy.

4. **Stomal (anastomotic) ulceration.**—The incidence varies from 1–15 per cent in different series and depends on the type of partial gastrectomy. It is much less with a Pólya than with a Billroth I partial gastrectomy. The presenting features are pain induced by food, haematemesis and melaena or iron deficiency anaemia, with persistently positive occult bloods in the stools. Sometimes pain is entirely absent. It is usually difficult to demonstrate an ulcer crater on the barium meal although gastroscopy occasionally helps. The stoma may be more rigid than normal due to local scarring; diagnosis is often very difficult if pain is absent or slight and the barium meal reveals no abnormality. The finding of persistent occult blood is highly suggestive. Anastomotic ulcers do not usually heal by medical means; operation is technically much more difficult than the original partial gastrectomy. The operation usually consists of vagotomy with or without attention to the stoma. When anastomotic ulceration recurs following vagotomy the completeness of the vagotomy can be tested by the insulin test. Measurement of the gastric acid also helps—if the acid output is high anastomotic ulceration is more likely.

5. **Weight loss.**—Most patients lose weight following a partial gastrectomy. It is more marked following a Pólya partial gastrectomy and vagotomy with drainage than following a Billroth I partial gastrectomy (Neale and Hoffbrand, 1967). The most important cause is probably a diminished intake of food. Because of the reduced size of the stomach the patient feels full after only a small meal; the dumping syndrome may make the patient afraid to eat. Chronic iron deficiency anaema and superficial gastritis following partial gastrectomy both reduce the appetite (Cox *et al.*, 1963; Palmer, 1954). Occasionally malnutrition of protein leading to a kwashiorkor-like state may dominate the clinical picture (Neale *et al.*, 1967).

6. **Malabsorption and steatorrhoea.**—The main causes for malabsorption of fat following partial gastrectomy are:

(i) Imperfect mixing of pancreatic juice with contents of jejunum.

(ii) Too rapid a delivery of food to the small intestine with too rapid transit.

(iii) Reduced pancreatic and biliary flow (Butler, 1961).

(iv) By-passing of upper duodenum (in the case of a Pólya partial gastrectomy).

(v) Stagnant loop syndrome. Several strains of bacteroides group of bacteria which may colonise a stagnant loop can deconjugate bile salts. Deconjugated bile salts are less efficient at emulsifying fats (Hoffman, 1965) and they are also toxic to the mucosa of the small bowel (Tabaqchali and Booth, 1966).

7. **Iron deficiency.**—Over 50 per cent of patients develop iron deficiency anaemia following partial gastrectomy; this is usually preceded by a low serum iron and a raised iron-binding capacity. There are several reasons why iron deficiency occurs: pre-operative haemorrhages deplete the iron stores, intermittent blood loss may continue after operation, the upper duodenum is the main site of iron absorption and this may be by-passed. Achlorhydria is associated with diminished absorption of iron, but this may be reversed by ascorbic acid and other reducing substances (Williams, 1959).

8. **Vitamin B_{12} deficiency.**—The incidence of megaloblastic anaemia following partial gastrectomy is about 7 per cent and incidence of a low serum B_{12} about 15 per cent (Deller and Witts, 1962). Occasionally, subacute combined degeneration occurs in the absence of anaemia or megaloblastic changes in the bone marrow. The usual cause of B_{12} deficiency is failure of absorption of B_{12} due to lack of intrinsic factor because of atrophy of the remaining part of the stomach; occasionally it is due to a stagnant loop. Very rarely the diet is deficient of vitamin B_{12}. Patients who have a low serum B_{12} or megaloblastic bone marrow without anaemia should be given regular B_{12} because there may be an improved sense of well-being and a gain in weight as well as a reversal of the megaloblastic marrow.

9. **Folic acid deficiency.**—This is much rarer than iron deficiency and B_{12} deficiency following partial gastrectomy; it is probably due to inadequate intake of folate. This may improve if the appetite is increased with iron and B_{12}.

10. **Bone disease.**—Osteomalacia is commoner than osteoporosis and occurs in 1–3 per cent of patients following a partial gastrectomy. The distinction between osteoporosis and osteomalacia is difficult, particularly as the two frequently coexist. Pseudo-fractures only occur in osteomalacia as do biochemical disturbances; so that diminished calcium and phosphorus levels in the serum (with a raised urinary excretion of phosphorus if there is secondary hyperparathyroidism) and an elevated serum alkaline phosphatase indicate osteomalacia; however, osteomalacia can be present even if the blood biochemistry is normal. In addition bone biopsy may show widening of the osteoid seams.

Osteoporosis should only be diagnosed on x-ray—a lateral x-ray of the lumbar spine is by far the most useful. Osteoporosis may follow a long-continued negative calcium balance (Nordin, 1961). The main causes of post-gastrectomy bone disease are:

(i) Decreased intake of calcium, vitamin D and protein.
(ii) Steatorrhoea.
(iii) Altered pH of duodenum—calcium absorption is favoured by an acid pH.

Treatment consists of prophylaxis with calcium and vitamin D and yearly check-ups at a post-gastrectomy clinic. Treatment of the established condition is with calcium, vitamin D and anabolic steroids. A satisfactory way of dealing with post-gastrectomy problems is for all patients to be seen yearly at a post-gastrectomy clinic and to be given courses of iron, vitamin D, folic acid and vitamin B_{12} for one month every year (the most suitable month is the one in which the patient's birthday falls).

GASTRITIS

The two most important forms of gastritis clinically are acute gastritis due to ingested irritants and atrophic or chronic gastritis. Two rare forms of gastritis are "acute infective" due to invasion of the stomach walls by organisms and "giant rugal hypertrophy" (Menetrier's disease). One condition which frequently gives rise to confusion is "hypertrophic gastritis"; this term is usually given to a radiological appearance in which the mucosal folds of the stomach appear prominent and it is usually associated with the presence of a duodenal ulcer. Histologically the abnormally large mucosal folds are normal, although occasionally such coarse folds are seen in patients suffering from dyspepsia in whom no ulcer is found.

Acute Gastritis

This consists of rapid exfoliation of surface epithelial cells accompanied by infiltration with inflammatory cells. It is not usually accompanied by bleeding in the case of alcoholic gastritis. Similar changes occur in the gastric mucosa in some febrile illness and in staphylococcal gastro-enteritis. Acute gastritis may be accompanied by haemorrhage when it is due to aspirin ingestion.

Atrophic (Chronic) Gastritis

In its most severe form this is seen in pernicious anaemia. It is also common in people over 40 particularly in cigarette smokers, in people who drink hot fluids, in association with heavy alcohol consumption and in gastric carcinoma. The incidence of gastric ulcer is higher in patients with atrophic gastritis than in the normal population. The exact relationship between atrophic gastritis and iron deficiency anaemia is not settled. The incidence of iron deficiency in patients with atrophic gastritis is higher than normal but patients with atrophic gastritis are more liable to bleed. In a few patients with atrophic gastritis, achlorhydria and iron deficiency anaemia, correction of the anaemia results in return of the gastric mucosa to normal and normal secretion of acid. It is now generally accepted that atrophic gastritis probably predisposes to iron deficiency anaemia.

The radiological appearances of atrophic gastritis are (Laws *et al.*, 1966):

1. Tubular stomach with the greater and lesser curves roughly parallel.
2. "Bald" fundus—with absent mucosal folds.
3. Thin mucosal folds on the greater curvature.
4. Active peristalsis.
5. Normal duodenal cap.

Hiatus Hernia

These are of three types:

1. Sliding: the whole oesophago-gastric junction moves up into the chest. The symptoms are those of reflex oesophagitis—the size of the hernia is no guide to the severity of the symptoms.
2. Para-oesophageal: the fundus of the stomach herniates into the chest alongside the gastro-oesophageal junction which remains in the normal position. The main symptom is dysphagia.
3. Mixed sliding and para-oesophageal: this is commoner than the pure para-oesophageal. The symptoms are those of reflux oesophagitis and dysphagia.

The pain of hiatus hernia usually comes on when the patient is lying flat or bending forwards. It is almost invariably made worse by drinking hot fluids and this has been used as the basis of a clinical test for the presence of a hiatus hernia—"the hot tea test". Relief of the pain with liquid alkalis is an important diagnostic feature. Like cardiac pain there may be relief with trinitrin. A large para-oesophageal hernia may displace the heart and give rise to ECG changes.

Complications include stricture formation, aspiration pneumonia, gastric ulceration within the hernia, and oesophageal ulceration. Bleeding from the hiatus hernia may be chronic and insidious or profuse. The indications for surgical treatment of hiatus hernia are (Atkinson, 1967):

1. No systematic relief of the symptoms of oesophagitis after six months conservative treatment. The size of the hernia is of no importtance.
2. Development of a gastric ulcer in a hernia after six months treatment.
3. Development of a stricture.
4. Recurrent bleeding in a young person. In an old person conservative management of recurrent bleeding is usually satisfactory.
5. Occurrence of aspiration pneumonia.
6. Incarceration or strangulation of the hernia.

Dyspeptic Symptoms

As with pain arising from any other site certain specific questions should be answered with abdominal pain or discomfort:

1. Site
2. Intensity
3. Duration
4. Character
5. Constancy (whether continuous or colicky)
6. Radiation
7. Relieving factors
8. Precipitating factors
9. Periodicity (exacerbation and remissions)
10. Associated features.

Oesophageal reflux is suggested by "heartburn", burning pain on drinking hot fluids or dysphagia. A variety of symptoms has been described in duodenal ulcers, gastric ulcers and "non-ulcer dyspepsia". The majority of patients with "non-ulcer dyspepsia" have either atrophic gastritis or a normal mucosa. Attempts to assess the objective diagnostic value of various symptoms have been made.

The most useful distinguishing symptoms are (Edwards and Coghill, 1968):

Peptic Ulcer

Gnawing or *aching* pain
Pain could be severe
Pain occurring at least 2 hours after food
Pain frequently severe at night
Attacks lasting at least 2 weeks
Relief of pain with food.

Non-Ulcer Dyspepsia

Hot or *burning* pain
Bloated feeling; discomfort only
Pain appearing within 1 hour of food
Attacks last less than 1 week
Food causes or aggravates pain
Remissions less than 1 month
Decrease in symptoms since onset.

Gastric Ulcer

Remissions variable in length
Attacks last at least 4 weeks
Food aggravates symptoms
Pain occurs within ½ hour of meal
Waterbrash
Anorexia.

Duodenal Ulcer

Remissions more constant in length
Attacks last less than 4 weeks
Pain lasts until next meal
Food eases symptoms
Pain occurs at least an hour after a meal.

Salicylates

Several series show that 60–70 per cent of normal people have gastro-intestinal bleeding when they take salicylates. The available evidence suggests that this blood loss is much the same for all types of salicylate preparation except that it may be less with enteric-coated aspirin. There is, of course, considerable delay between taking enteric-coated aspirin and absorption, hence they are not suitable for rapid relief of pain (which is the purpose for which most people take an aspirin). Further-more absorption is variable; enteric-coated salicylates are usually suitable for patients on long-term salicylates provided that the degree of absorption is checked by a blood salicylate level at an appropriate time. There is no doubt that acute erosions can occur where particles of salicylate come into contact with the gastric mucosa, that the incidence of gastric ulcers is higher in women who habitually take salicylates and that the incidence of perforation of ulcers is higher in patients who habitually take salicylates (Salter, 1968). It is also likely that patients who have a severe gastric haemorrhage after taking a small dose of salicylates have a hypersensitivity to them. Bleeding may occur from a large area of the gastric mucosa and is probably not always caused by simple erosions due to direct contact of particles of salicylate.

One series has shown that the amount and frequency of bleeding following ingestion of salicylates is no greater in patients who have an established peptic ulcer (Parry and Wood, 1967). Salicylates can produce gastro-intestinal bleeding when given parenterally. They can also cause thrombocytopenia and hypoprothrombinaemia. Vitamin K should always be given to patients whose gastric haemorrhage is assumed to be due to salicylates.

Corticosteroids

There is a widespread clinical belief that patients on long-term corticosteroids have a higher-than-usual incidence of gastro-intestinal haemorrhage and gastric perforation. However, many careful clinical surveys have failed to confirm these views, although it is agreed that patients with rheumatoid arthritis on steroids (and other ulcerogenic drugs) have a higher incidence of gastro-intestinal haemorrhage. The surveys also agree that although gastric perforation is no commoner than in normal people, the symptoms and signs of perforation are masked by steroids and this may lead to dangerous delay in making the diagnosis.

GASTRO-ENTERITIS AND INFECTIVE DIARRHOEA IN
ADULTS IN THE U.K.

The most important infective causes of diarrhoea in adults are:

1. Salmonella.
2. *Shigella* (bacillary dysentery).
3. Virus infections—probably the commonest cause of outbreaks of infective diarrhoea from which bacteria are not isolated.
4. Amoebic dysentery.
5. Pathogenic strains of *E. coli*—these are virtually confined to children under the age of 1 year.
6. Rarities such as cholera.
7. Bacterial contamination of food, e.g. staphylococcal and *Cl. botulinus* toxins. One common trap is to assume that a sudden onset of diarrhoea is infective in origin—remember diarrhoea may be "spurious" —small amounts of liquid stool may be passed in a patient (not necessarily elderly) suffering from chronic constipation. Other important causes of diarrhoea are:

1. Purgative abuse.
2. Ulcerative colitis (or proctocolitis).
3. Crohn's disease.
4. Diverticulitis.
5. Spastic colon.
6. Carcinoma.

Management of Diarrhoea

Before starting symptomatic or specific treatment it is essential to try to establish the definitive cause or to try and exclude certain possible causes if the precise cause cannot be found. This means that every case of sporadic diarrhoea of sudden onset for which no cause is known should have stools examined for ova, cysts and amoebae, and the stools cultured. In the majority of cases sigmoidoscopy should be performed particularly if the patient has lived abroad—amoebic dysentery is notorious as a cause of episodic attacks of diarrhoea. The amoebae may be excreted in the stool when the patient has no diarrhoea or the amoebae may not be seen although diarrhoea is severe. Sigmoidoscopy will often show the characteristic shallow ulcers in the colon.

Symptomatic Treatment of Diarrhoea

1. Absorbents—claimed to absorb the "toxins" in the bowel lumen, examples kaolin or pectin.
2. Opiates—reduce peristalsis in the colon, examples codeine phosphate, morphia.
3. Anticholinergic drugs—also reduce peristalsis in the colon.

The most suitable drugs for symptomatic treatment of diarrhoea are:

1. Mist. kaolin et morph. BPC 15–30 ml 6-hourly.
2. Codeine phosphate 15–16 mg 6-hourly.

There is no convincing evidence that proprietary drugs such as Lomotil have any advantage over the older and simpler remedies.

Specific Treatment

The most frequent clinical problems are patients with diarrhoea who have:

1. A stool culture which grows a *Salmonella* ("enteric fever") or a *Shigella* (bacillary dysentery) without evidence of systemic spread (fever, malaise, leucocytosis, elevated ESR) or complications such as severe dehydration.

2. Negative stool culture.

There is now general agreement, that, except for *Salmonella typhi*, *Shigella shigae* and *Sh. flexneri*, whatever organism is grown from the stool the patient should not receive antibiotics *unless there is evidence of systemic spread*. Antibiotics are potentially dangerous—they do not usually control the infection, they prolong the carrier state and they increase the chance of a subsequent relapse (Aserkoff and Bennet, 1969). The use of proprietary antibiotic-containing remedies such as Ivax, Neovax, Neo Sulfazon and Entero-vioform is usually no more effective than symptomatic treatment and these preparations may be potentially dangerous (Christie, 1969).

Systemic infection with *any* of the Salmonella organisms including *S. typhi*, *S. paratyphi*, *S. typhimurium*, etc. should be treated with chloramphenicol or ampicillin.

Systemic infection with any of the Shigella organisms should be treated with sulphonamides (sulphadimidine 2 g followed by 1 g 6-hourly) if the organism is sensitive (in the U.K. most strains of Shigella are now resistant to the sulphonamides). Other useful drugs are streptomycin, neomycin, nalidixic acid and the tetracyclines.

Diarrhoea may be severe enough to produce dehydration and electrolyte deficiencies; these should be treated with adequate replacement therapy.

The decision not to treat Shigella or Salmonella enteritis with antibiotics may be modified in the case of severely debilitated and old patients or in infection with rare virulent forms of Salmonella or Shigella.

In the event of an outbreak of infective diarrhoea (usually due to Shigella) scrupulous cleanliness is the most effective prophylactic treatment. There is nothing to be gained by giving prophylactic antibiotics to uninfected neighbouring patients.

Conclusion.—When diarrhoea persists or recurs following an acute attack of gastro-enteritis consider the possibility of persisting infection or acquired disaccharide intolerance. Post-dysenteric diarrhoea is very common. Patients who have had proven amoebic dysentery in the past or who have lived in endemic areas and who develop diarrhoea which is persistent and for which no other cause can be found can justifiably be given a therapeutic trial of emetine if symptomatic treatment is not working. Infective diarrhoea should be treated symptomatically. Antibiotics should not be given, if infection is localised to the gastro-intestinal tract, for the majority of infections with Salmonella or Shigella organisms.

INTESTINAL MALABSORPTION

This is one of the conditions where a "high index of suspicion" is essential. Steatorrhoea is not a *sine qua non* of malabsorption—only the more severe cases have any alteration in frequency or consistency of their stools or an increased excretion of faecal fat. Deficient absorption of single substances may lead to isolated symptoms, and for this reason intestinal malabsorption should be suspected in any of the following:

1. Iron deficiency anaemia particularly if it is unresponsive to iron therapy.
2. Loss of weight.
3. Hypoproteinaemia.
4. Raised alkaline phosphatase.
5. Recurrent aphthous ulceration or soreness of the tongue.
6. Osteoporosis, osteomalacia or tetany.
7. Macrocytic anaemia.
8. Diarrhoea and abdominal discomfort.
9. Hypokalaemia.
10. Following partial gastrectomy.

Two screening tests which are used most frequently to exclude malabsorption are the xylose excretion test and the estimation of faecal fat excretion. Following a 25 g oral dose of d-xylose at least 5 g should be excreted in the urine in the next five hours. In malabsorption usually less than 2 g is excreted; the test is of less value if there is delay in gastric emptying, renal impairment or if there is severe diarrhoea and a very rapid transit time through the small intestine. It is not valid in people over the age of 65. In a few patients the 25 g dose gives rise to diarrhoea so that a 5 g dose is sometimes advocated. Xylose is not digested in the gut and is absorbed by passive diffusion, there is no active phosphorylation and it is not absorbed across a concentration gradient.

A normal person on a normal diet rarely excretes more than 6 g of fat per day in the stools (Cooke, 1958). For this reason the daily faecal fat excretion in the stools collected for a 3-day period on a ward diet is a reasonably reliable indication as to the presence of steatorrhoea. These are the most acceptable screening tests although other investigations may be necessary to confirm the diagnosis:

1. **Barium meal follow-through.**—A non-flocculating form of barium is best. The main features in steatorrhoea are a delayed transit time, dilatation of loops in the small bowel (calibre of jejunum more than 3·0 cm is abnormal); in later films the barium does flocculate despite its "non-flocculating" character or it may appear:

(i) *"Scattered"* in which small amounts of barium are seen dispersed throughout most of the small intestine.

(ii) *"Clumped"* in which larger amounts of barium coalesce and remain in the small intestine for longer than normal.

(iii) *"Moulage sign"* in which the barium remains in the small intestine and has the appearance of solid casts of the loops of the ileum (Lumsden and Truelove, 1965).

Flocculation, clumping and scattering are due to excessive amounts of mucus in the small intestine. The purpose of using non-flocculating barium is because similar appearances may be seen in normal people if ordinary barium is used.

2. **Peroral jejunal biopsy.**—Abnormal appearances are:

(i) *Subtotal villous atrophy* in which there is almost total loss of villi and all that remains is the crypts between the villi.

(ii) *Partial villous atrophy* is intermediate between subtotal villous atrophy and normals.

There is often *no* correlation between the severity of the mucosal lesion as judged histologically and the degree of malabsorption. It is important that other histological features suggesting malabsorption should be present before implicating reduced villous height as evidence of malabsorption. These are:

1. Increased mucosal thickness.
2. Decreased epithelial surface cell height.
3. Inflammatory cell infiltration of mucosa and submucosa.

Other investigations are necessary to establish the extent to which different substances are not being absorbed and the general nutritional status of the patient. The most important ones are:

(i) Serum levels of iron, vitamin B_{12} and folic acid.

(ii) Tests of ability to absorb vitamin B_{12} (Schilling test), and folic acid (FIGLU test).

(iii) Serum level of bone alkaline phosphatase, calcium and phosphate. X-ray of bones to find evidence of osteoporosis or osteomalacia. Tetany may occur if the level of ionised calcium falls critically.

(iv) Serum proteins.

(v) Faecal nitrogen content (normally less than 2 g per day).

(vi) Serum electrolytes of which potassium is the most important. Rarely hypokalaemia may lead to secondary paralytic ileus.

(vii) Glucose tolerance test. The curve is flat in intestinal malabsorption, it is very occasionally of diabetic type if malabsorption is due to pancreatic failure and loss of islet cells.

(viii) Prothrombin time to detect malabsorption of vitamin K.

CAUSES OF MALABSORPTION

Loss of Functional Epithelium (Villous Atrophy)

1. Gluten sensitive enteropathy.
2. Idiopathic steatorrhoea.
3. Disaccharide intolerance.
4. Stagnant loop syndrome.
5. Coeliac syndrome.
6. Infestations which destroy the mucosa, e.g. *Giardia lamblia* and *ankylostoma duodenale*.
7. Drug damage: phenindione, neomycin and other antibiotics, phenolthalein, colchicine, PAS, folic acid antagonists and irradiation.

Infiltration of the Wall of the Small Intestine

1. Crohn's disease.
2. Scleroderma.
3. Amyloid disease.
4. Whipple's[73] disease.
5. Reticulosis.

Damage to Vascular Supply or Disturbance of Motility

1. Superior mesenteric artery occlusion.
2. Polyarteritis nodosa.
3. SLE.
4. Diabetes.
5. Congestive heart failure.
6. Constrictive pericarditis.

Short circuiting of Small Intestine

Gastrocolic fistula.

Resection of Small Intestine

Diminished Splitting of Food due to Lack of Digestive Juice

1. Pancreatic insufficiency.

73. GEORGE HOYT WHIPPLE (b. 1878). Baltimore pathologist.

2. Obstructive jaundice or liver failure.

Diminished Splitting of Food due to Inadequate Mixing with Digestive Juices

Partial gastrectomy.

Diminished Splitting of Food due to Inactivation of Digestive Juice

Zollinger-Ellison syndrome.

Disaccharide Intolerance

Deficiency of enzymes which split disaccharides into their constituent monosaccharides may occur as an inborn error of metabolism. The disaccharide most frequently involved is lactose, whose constituent monosaccharides are glucose and galactose. Disaccharides cannot be absorbed unless they are split into monosaccharides. The undigested disaccharides are fermented by intestinal bacteria producing irritant organic acids; these, together with the osmotic effect of the sugar leads to diarrhoea which is very acidic. The symptoms are diarrhoea with a high content of lactic acid, abdominal distension and colic. Disaccharide intolerance in children does not usually heal spontaneously.

The diagnosis is made by a lactose tolerance test in which the rise in blood sugar (glucose) is compared after an oral dose of 100 g of lactose and 50 g glucose, the rise in blood sugar should be the same following both. The pH of the stools is tested. The amount of disaccharidase in the jejunal mucosa can be measured in specimens obtained at peroral biopsy. It is essential to know the site of the biopsy if the mucosal cell content of disaccharidase is used to confirm the diagnosis because the disaccharidase content of cells varies according to their position. It is lower in surface cells of the jejunum than of the ileum. Flocculation and clumping may be seen in the barium meal follow-through if lactose is mixed with the barium. This may be compared with the normal appearance of the follow-through when the barium is given without lactose in a lactose-deficient patient.

Lactase deficiency may be a common cause of "functional" diarrhoea (McMichael et al., 1965). Lactase deficiency may also be acquired as a result of other gastro-intestinal conditions, e.g. partial gastrectomy, gastro-enteritis, coeliac disease, malnutrition and ulcerative colitis. The lactase deficiency may improve as the associated condition improves; furthermore some of the symptoms of the primary condition may be alleviated if lactose is excluded from the diet. Lactose is the main sugar in milk so that exclusion of milk from the diet may be beneficial. In ulcerative colitis the situation is even more complex as there is evidence that the proteins in milk may also aggravate the condition. About one in four patients with ulcerative colitis may be helped by a milk-free diet

(Wright and Truelove, 1965). Other disaccharidase deficiencies occur but are very rare.

Acquired lactose intolerance is a possible explanation for the chronic diarrhoea which may follow treated bacterial or viral gastro-enteritis.

The Coeliac Syndrome

This term is used to describe patients whose intestinal mucosa is abnormal and who have malabsorption. Hindle and Creamer (1965) distinguish three groups.

Group I   Patients with coeliac disease which developed in infancy.

Group II   Patients with a flat intestinal mucosa without other associated disease.

Group III   Patients with a flat intestinal mucosa and an associated disease. This group is further subdivided into (a) those in whom the associated disease preceded the onset of malabsorption and (b) those in whom malabsorption appeared first.

These authors believe that in general the associated conditions may cause the mucosal abnormality, although the number of people in the well population who also have a flat mucosa is not known; for this reason the significance of a flat mucosa in the presence of other diseases is doubtful. Other workers do not accept that a large number of diseases can cause a flat mucosa. They emphasise that a similar proportion of patients in the three groups respond to a gluten-free diet. Pancreatic insufficiency should always be considered in patients who respond poorly to a gluten-free diet. Corticosteroids may be of value in patients with the coeliac syndrome not due to pancreatic insufficiency which fails to respond to gluten withdrawal.

It is now widely accepted that the coeliac syndrome can be pre-malignant. The commonest malignancy is a lymphoma of the small intestine or draining mesenteric glands, the next commonest carcinoma of the oesophagus, and thirdly carcinoma or lymphoma elsewhere. Nearly all patients who develop a malignancy after the coeliac syndrome have had malabsorption for more than 10 years (Harris et al., 1966). Features which should alert one to the possibility that the coeliac syndrome is complicated by a malignancy are a long history, profound sudden weight loss, abdominal pain and anorexia. The coeliac syndrome may occur with skin disorders, particular psoriasis, rosacea and dermatitis herpetiformis. The skin condition as well as the malabsorption may respond to a gluten-free diet. Before deciding that a patient is not responding to gluten withdrawal it is essential to wait at least 6 months and to ensure that the patient is not occasionally taking gluten-containing foods.

Stagnant Loop Syndrome

The upper small intestine is normally sterile; the presence of large numbers of coliform and bacteriodes organisms may lead to malabsorption. Excessive numbers of bacteria may be present if there is any slowing of transit through the small intestines, e.g. in the presence of a stricture or Crohn's disease; excess bacteria may be present if they are allowed to multiply excessively, e.g. in a diverticulum or blind loop following a partial gastrectomy. Excessive numbers of coliform organisms cause malabsorption by splitting bile salts into substances which are ineffective in the splitting of fat and which are toxic to the mucosa of the small intestine (Tabaqchali and Booth, 1966). The organisms also utilise vitamin B_{12} in competition with the host.

The diagnosis can be made by performing bacterial counts on the contents of the jejunum; this is obtained by a special capsule which avoids contamination with any other part of the gut. The coliform organisms break down tryptophane to indole and then indican, this is absorbed and excreted in the urine. The urinary indican level is high if there are excessive numbers of coliform and bacteroides organisms in the jejunum. The absorption of vitamin B_{12} will also be abnormal in the stagnant loop syndrome. The diagnosis can be clinched by demonstrating a reduction in jejunal organisms, a decrease in urinary indican, and diminished faecal fats and an improvement in vitamin B_{12} absorption following treatment with broad-spectrum oral antibiotics. The serum folate is often abnormally high in the stagnant loop syndrome because the organisms are able to manufacture folate which is then absorbed.

A recent biochemically elegant confirmatory test for excessive overgrowth of intestinal bacteria is the labelled carbon-glycocholic acid breath test. The bile acids, cholic and chenodeoxycholic acids, are linked by an amide bond to their glycine or taurine conjugates and this bond may be broken down only by the action of bacterial enzymes. In the test C^{14}-labelled glycocholic acid is given by mouth. Bacterial deconjugation of the C^{14} glycine from the cholic acid caused by excessive bacteria (or by the normal colonic bacteria should the enterohepatic circulation of conjugated bile salts be interrupted by ileal resection) causes release of C^{14}-labelled glycine which is converted into C^{14}-labelled CO_2 which is exhaled. The amount of C^{14} labelled CO_2 in the breath is a direct reflection of the amount of bacterial deconjugation of bile salts which has occurred (James et al., 1973).

Chronic Intestinal Ischaemia

Chronic incomplete narrowing of the superior mesenteric artery may result in intestinal ischaemia, and this may also occur with chronic venous congestions as in congestive heart failure or constrictive pericarditis. The main symptoms are "abdominal angina"—abdominal pain developing soon after a meal and relieved before the next meal, weight loss and sometimes malabsorption (Heard et al., 1963).

Narrowing of the mesenteric vessels may result in ischaemia of the colon. The important clinical features are sudden abdominal pain, rectal bleeding and signs of left-sided peritonitis. The attacks may be transient, or may lead to gangrene; in a third group the ischaemia results in stricture formation, which are most frequent in the region of the splenic flexure and are often surprisingly extensive. The main distinction is from Crohn's disease, in which other lesions are usually present, and carcinoma, which usually causes a shorter structure. The characteristic feature of intestinal ischaemia on the barium enema is "thumb printing" of the outline. This is due to local oedema in folds of mucosa. It can occasionally be seen at sigmoidoscopy and usually disappears when collateral circulation is established in 4–6 weeks.

The disease may occur in early adult life when it usually presents as haemorrhagic colitis and is frequently right-sided. Stricture formation is unusual when the disease occurs in this age group.

Protein-losing Gastro-enteropathy

Low serum albumin may result from diminished synthesis as in cirrhosis, excessive breakdown as in post-operative states, Cushing's syndrome or excessive loss from the body as in the nephrotic syndrome, severe burns and exfoliative dermatitis. Decreased intake of protein may also be responsible; however, occasionally hypoalbuminaemia occurs in the presence of normal absorption and *increased* synthesis. Some conditions are associated with exudation of protein into the gut— this has been demonstrated by recovering plasma protein from the intestinal contents by direct intubation (Holman et al., 1959).

From a practical clinical point of view in order to detect the presence of excessive protein loss into the gut albumin is labelled with [131]I. Following an injection of radio-active labelled albumin the level in the serum declines rapidly as albumin is distributed to the total protein pool—this takes 5 days; after this the serum level falls slowly as the radio-active labelled albumin is metabolised and is replaced by recently synthesised albumin. This later rate of decline is a measure of the rate of albumin synthesis and albumin loss. The serum level falls rapidly if there is excessive loss into the gut. Fortunately for clinical purposes this test is sufficiently accurate. However, for research purposes attempts have been made to assess the exact amount of protein lost. One of the problems is that when radio-active labelled albumin is lost into the gut the albumin is digested and the radio-active iodine is reabsorbed. In an attempt to circumvent this problem a technique using a resin which would bind radio-active iodine was introduced. The resin was fed by mouth at the same time as an intravenous dose of ^{131}I-labelled albumin was given.

A further improvement was suggested using a synthetic substance which is metabolised in much the same way as albumin except that once in the gut the radio-active iodine is not split from it, this substance is ^{131}I labelled polyvinyl pyrrolidone (PVP). The main conditions causing protein exudation into the gut are (Dawson, 1965):

1. Giant rugal hypertrophy of the stomach (Menetrier's disease).
2. Ulcerative lesions of the gut.
3. Neoplasms of the gut.
4. Idiopathic steatorrhoea.
5. Crohn's disease.
6. Stagnant loop syndrome.
7. Radiation.
8. Intestinal lymphangiectasia.
9. Cardiac failure or constrictive pericarditis.
10. Idiopathic hypoproteinaemia.

CROHN'S DISEASE (REGIONAL ILEITIS)

The disease usually begins in early adult life and in the majority, onset is gradual—symptoms have often been present for several years before the patient attends his doctor. Diarrhoea is the commonest early symptom, pain comes later and is often worse before defaecation. The pain is usually colicky and is often localised to the right lilac fossa. Other features which may be present are fever, anaemia, weight loss, iritis, erythema nodosum, clubbing and arthritis. Complications include fistulae, obstruction, malabsorption and ischiorectal abscess. The presence of a chronic anal fissure with fever or abdominal pain should suggest the probability of Crohn's disease. The perianal skin is often a bluish-red colour and swollen and sometimes ulcerated skin tags are present.

Widespread involvement of the terminal ileum will result in a megaloblastic anaemia as this is the part of the ileum from which vitamin B_{12} is absorbed. It should be noted that diarrhoea does not invariably occur but sometimes diarrhoea is profuse and is accompanied by blood and mucus; under these circumstances the colon is usually but not invariably involved.

Crohn's disease most commonly affects the ileocaecal region or terminal ileum, however, any part of the gut from the duodenum to the anus may be affected. About 10 per cent of cases of Crohn's disease affect the large bowel alone while in 20 per cent of the remainder the large bowel is involved to a variable extent. The incidence of pathological anal skin tags is much higher when the colon is involved.

The x-ray appearances consist of narrowing of the lumen—"the string sign"; the lesions are usually separated by normal bowel—"skip lesions". If the mucous membrane is swollen and oedematous there may be a "cobble-stone" appearance. Small fissures may be seen as spikes of barium projecting at right angles from the lumen, sometimes a fistula may fill with barium. In the colon the x-ray appearances may resemble those of ulcerative colitis except that there is often a segment of normal bowel between two affected areas, strictures are very uncommon in ulcerative colitis; the ascending colon is more frequently involved in Crohn's disease. Narrowing of the terminal ileum with changes in the colon is highly suggestive of Crohn's disease rather than ulcerative colitis.

Comparisons between Crohn's disease and ulcerative colitis.—Both conditions tend to run in families, some members suffering from one and some from the other. Occasional patients have typical Crohn's disease of the terminal ileum with typical changes of ulcerative colitis in the colon. There are documented instances of the same patient developing both diseases.

In their classical form there are distinctive pathological differences. Crohn's disease consists of non-caseating granulomata with giant cells, involving the submucosa of the terminal ileum. There is oedema and fibrosis involving the whole of the bowel wall with enlargement of the regional lymph glands. The fibrosis predisposes to stricture formation; the swollen oedematous loops of bowel adhere to each other and predispose to fistula formation.

In ulcerative colitis the mucosa is primarily affected, firstly in the sigmoid colon or upper rectum. The mucsosa becomes hyperaemic and infiltrated with inflammatory cells, ulceration of the mucosa occurs which later spreads into the submucosa; the ulcers often heal by granulation tissue which becomes epithelialised forming pseudopolyps.

Treatment of Crohn's Disease

Certain aspects of treatment are uncontroversial, viz:

1. Affected patients who are symptom-free need no treatment.
2. Steroids are indicated for severe systemic manifestations (fever, eye, skin or joint involvement).
3. Steroids are indicated when small bowel involvement is extensive.
4. Steroids are indicated in patients who have a recurrence of the disease after having more than one small bowel resection.
5. Surgery is indicated for surgical complications, such as fistulae, perforation, ischiorectal abscess or bowel stenosis.
6. Laparotomy may be indicated in rare instances of doubt about the diagnosis. Ileocaecal tuberculosis still occurs although the Mantoux

test will then be positive. The Mantoux test is frequently negative in Crohn's disease.

Treatment of the Acute Attack

1. Bed rest.
2. Sulphonamides (phthalylsulphathiazole) followed by sulphasalazine and possibly broad-spectrum antibiotics.

Corticosteroids by mouth usually result in symptomatic and objective improvement. Steroids never cure the ileal lesion and they may need to be given continuously to suppress the disease. If the disease is apparently limited to a small length of the ileum, surgical resection should be considered in the hope that steroids can be withdrawn. However, following resection there is a high recurrence rate. It has been estimated that symptomatic relapse at five years occurs in about one-third and at ten years in about half the patients. The proportion requiring further resection is about one-sixth at five years and a quarter at ten years. The probability of recurrence following a second recurrence is probably twice as high (Lennard-Jones and Stalder, 1967).

For Crohn's disease of the colon resection is usually performed; ileo-rectal anastomosis is possible in a much higher percentage of patients with Crohn's disease of the colon than with ulcerative colitis. Recurrence of the disease in the terminal ileum following colectomy for colonic involvement is probably less common than recurrence when a localised segment of Crohn's disease has been removed from the ileum. Crohn's disease of the colon may heal when a temporary bypass ileostomy is performed (Kivel *et al.*, 1967).

Immunosuppressives.—Several small series have shown that immunosuppressive drugs may induce a remission (Bean, 1966; Bowen *et al.*, 1966). Azathioprine (Imuran) has been the most used immunosuppressive and may induce a remission when steroids have failed (Jones, 1969).

ULCERATIVE COLITIS

The disease usually starts in the upper rectum and sigmoid colon and then spreads proximally. The rectum is usually, but not invariably, involved. It is uncommon for the appearances at sigmoidoscopy to be normal provided a good view is obtained.

The first symptom is usually bright red blood passed per rectum following defaecation, later the stools become more liquid and more frequent and are accompanied by blood and mucus. Abdominal pain is also a common early symptom as in Crohn's disease. When the disease is limited to the rectum (granular or distal proctitis) constipation is usual. Occasionally the disease presents in an acute fulminating form or rarely with one of its complications. In a patient who has evidence of ulceration and bright red blood passed per rectum for the first time it is essential to exclude other causes of rectal bleeding. The main alternative conditions which should be considered are:

1. Infections, particularly due to:
   Entamoeba histolytica
   Dysentery (*Shigella*)
   Staphylococci
   Viruses
   Salmonella
   Pathogenic *E. coli*
   Tuberculosis.
2. Crohn's disease.
3. Granular proctitis (which is a form of ulcerative colitis).
4. Carcinoma.
5. Haemorrhoids.
6. Ischaemic colitis.
7. Spastic colon.
8. Purgative abuse.
9. Post-dysenteric diarrhoea.

Sigmoidoscopy

Sigmoidoscopy should *always* be performed on patients admitted with diarrhoea or with loss of bright red blood per rectum. In an interesting survey Watts and his colleagues (1966*b*) found that there are only four characteristics of the rectal mucosa which are recognised consistently by different skilled observers:

1. The overall impression of normality or abnormality.
2. The presence or absence of a vascular pattern.
3. The presence or absence of contact bleeding.
4. The presence or absence of oedema.

Important appearances in the rectum which may suggest ulcerative colitis are:

1. Abnormally red or abnormally pale mucosa.
2. Absent vessel pattern.
3. Contact bleeding.
4. Granularity.
5. Oedema.
6. Ulceration.
7. Rigidity.
8. Free blood, liquid faeces.

Local Complications
1. Haemorrhage.

2. Perforation.
3. Acute dilatation of the colon.
4. Paracolic abscess.
5. Ischiorectal abscess.
6. Fistula.
7. Stricture.
8. Pseudopolyposis.
9. Carcinoma.

Radiological Signs

The reliable radiological signs of ulcerative colitis seen on the barium enema are (Geffen *et al.*, 1968):

1. Narrowing of the bowel.
2. Shortening of the bowel.
3. Decreased distensibility.
4. Decreased tone.
5. Ulceration.
6. Loss of haustrations.
7. Fine serration.
8. Polyps.
9. Longitudinal folds after evacuation.
10. Double outline.

Remote Complications

1. *Skin disorders.*—Erythema nodosum, erythema multiforme and purpura are the commonest. Pyodermia gangrenosum is a skin lesion only seen in ulcerative colitis, and despite its name it is not due to pyogenic organisms. The lesion consists of bulla formation which usually involves the legs and results in ulceration and necrosis of the skin. The lesions are usually sterile and closely resemble pressure sores except that they often occur in areas other than pressure areas. Many of the drugs used in treatment of ulcerative colitis may result in skin rashes. Aphthous ulcers in the mouth are also common.

2. *Liver damage* (Mistilis and Goulston, 1965).—The liver is frequently involved in severe ulcerative colitis. The types of liver disease are:

(i) Fatty infiltration.
(ii) Pericholangitis with the inflammation around the bile canaliculi within the liver. This is probably due to portal pyaemia which is a frequent finding in ulcerative colitis. Portal hypertension may ensue.
(iii) Chronic active hepatitis.
(iv) Cirrhosis.
(v) Sclerosing cholangitis.

The liver damage does not depend on the severity of the colitis and may progress even though the colitis is in remission or has been cured by a colectomy.

3. *Eye complications.*—Conjunctivitis, iritis and episcleritis occur. When eye complications are present there are usually other systemic manifestations of the disease. The eye complications usually improve when the condition is treated surgically but not so frequently with conservative treatment.

4. *Arthritis.*—A rheumatoid type of arthritis may develop; however, there are several differences from classical rheumatoid arthritis, it is usually a recurrent monoarticular arthritis affecting a large joint of the lower limbs, the rheumatoid factor is absent, nodules do not occur and the arthritis is cured when the colon is cured. Ankylosing spondylitis and sacro-iliitis also occur more commonly than in the general population. The spondylitis may precede the colitic symptoms and may continue to progress when the colon is cured. Unlike classical ankylosing spondylitis the spondylitis of ulcerative colitis is equally common in both sexes.

5. *Nutritional deficiencies and anaemia.*

6. *Renal calculi.*—Several series have shown an increased incidence of renal calculi in patients with ulcerative colitis. The incidence probably increases if the patient has an ileostomy. The postulated causes are many, viz. dehydration, low urinary sodium and increased oxalate excretion.

Course of Ulcerative Colitis

The natural history of ulcerative colitis follows two distinct pathways. Some patients are free of symptoms between the acute attacks—chronic intermittent type; while others are never free of symptoms once the disease has presented—chronic continuous type (Truelove, 1967). The mortality of ulcerative colitis is greatest in patients under the age of 20 or over 60, and it increases with the number of attacks. The mortality is much higher if the whole of the colon is involved (Watts *et al.*, 1966*a*).

It has been suggested that the long-term prognosis of ulcerative colitis depends on the severity of the first attack (Edwards and Truelove, 1963). However, more recent work suggests that the long-term prognosis is not related to the severity of the first attack, although the outcome of the first attack alone is related to its severity. The outcome of the first and all other attacks is related to the age of the patient, severity of the attack and extent of the colon involved. Patients over the age of 60 have a poorer prognosis than younger patients (Watts *et al.*, 1966*a*).

Management of the Acute Attack

1. Bed rest.
2. Correction of dehydration and electrolyte depletion.
3. Correction of anaemia.
4. High calorie and protein intake. If there is vomiting parenteral feeding with aminosol, alcohol and fructose can be used to supply enough calories and proteins. The colon should be "rested" by reducing the volume of indigestible roughage. If necessary methyl cellulose can be given two or three times a day.
5. Corticosteroids. Prednisone 40–60 mg daily with local application to the colon through a rectal drip or by retention enemata. Some series have shown that ACTH drip is more effective than parenteral steroids alone. There is no evidence that steroids increase the incidence of perforation or affect subsequent surgical mortality, although they undoubtedly mask the signs of perforation.
6. Sulphasalazine (Salazopyrin). 0·5 g tablets in a dose of 1–3 g 3–6 times a day. This drug is chemically allied to the salicylates and sulphonamides and has been shown to be beneficial in shortening an acute attack of colitis.
7. Antibiotics are usually given—they should be administered *parenterally* so as not to sterilise the colon which predisposes to superinfection with staphylococci.
8. Daily abdominal x-rays to detect acute dilatation of the colon. This can be suspected clinically if there is a sudden decrease in the number of stools, loss of gut sounds with a markedly distended and tympanitic abdomen and abdominal pain.

Features Suggesting an Acute Exacerbation

1. More than six bowel actions per day.
2. Macroscopic blood in the stool.
3. Fever and tachycardia.
4. Anaemia.
5. Raised sedimentation rate.
6. Lowered serum albumin.
7. Colon greater than 6 cm in diameter on plain x-ray of the abdomen.

Surgical Treatment of the Acute Attack

The mortality of an emergency colectomy is much higher than that of an elective one; however, the mortality in an acute attack of colitis treated medically is closely related to its severity and duration. Some argue that it is better to persist with medical treatment in the hope that the patient will improve enough for "elective" operation; others argue that it may be better to operate early in an acute attack after a short period of intensive medical treatment. The mortality of severe attacks treated medically is over 10 per cent; when severe cases are treated with early colectomy, the mortality is just over 1 per cent. Early operation means within 2–3 days in the elderly and within 4–5 days in younger patients (Goligher *et al.*, 1967). Despite differences with regard to its timing most would agree that the indications for surgery in the acute attack are:

1. Involvement of the whole colon.
2. Severe haemorrhage.
3. Perforation.
4. Acute dilatation of the colon.
5. Sudden deterioration under medical treatment.
6. Failure to improve after *three* days in patients over 60 years of age.
7. Failure to improve after *six* days in young patients.

Long-term Management

Not all acute attacks of ulcerative colitis are severe enough to present the dilemma of surgical or medical treatment; many are of moderate severity and can nearly always be controlled by the medical regime.

Recurrence of acute attacks can seldom be prevented by therapeutic doses of corticosteroids; the risks of steroids in therapeutic doses usually outweigh the possible advantages. Small doses of steroids are totally ineffective in preventing recurrences. It is *not* now recommended that steroids be used when the patient is in remission (Lennard-Jones *et al.*, 1965), although the occasional patient is seen who appears to relapse when steroids are withdrawn. It is reasonable to make a general working rule to withdraw steroids when a patient goes into remission but to bear in mind that there are occasional exceptions to the working rule. Sulphasalazine is much more effective than steroids in preventing relapses.

Diet.—There is some evidence that a proportion of patients with ulcerative colitis are sensitive to the proteins of cows' milk. In these patients the colitis improves when milk is withheld but relapse occurs if the milk is reintroduced (Truelove, 1961).

Patients with attacks of ulcerative colitis may have a deficiency of lactase in the affected colon so that they suffer from intolerance to the disaccharide lactose which is present in milk. There is evidence that withdrawal of lactose from the diet of some patients with ulcerative colitis leads to an improvement (Frazer *et al.*, 1966). The deficiency of lactase becomes less marked when the disease goes into remission.

Factors Favouring Surgery

1. Increasing frequency of acute attacks (whether severe or moderate).

2. Chronic continuous type of ulcerative colitis with continuing symptoms.

3. Involvement of the whole colon.

4. Severe remote complications particularly iritis and liver damage.

5. Prevention of carcinoma. The main factors associated with the development of carcinoma are a history of over 10 years involvement of the whole of the colon and an onset in childhood. The appearance of a stricture on the x-ray should be assumed to be carcinomatous until proved otherwise. Pseudopolyps indicate severe disease but are not pre-malignant.

The operation performed is a colectomy with either an ileostomy or an ileorectal anastomosis if the rectum is not involved. Some surgeons recommend an ileorectal anastomosis even if the rectum is mildly involved (Aylett, 1966). Ileorectal anastomosis is not widely used and is criticised on the grounds that patients may continue to have severe diarrhoea, that they are still exposed to the risk of developing carcinoma of the rectal stump and that if a subsequent ileostomy is necessary the operation is much more difficult.

Spastic Colon

This term is used to signify abnormal colonic function as a result of emotion, anxiety or mental stress. The symptoms are abdominal pain with constipation which may alternate with diarrhoea. There are a large number of synonyms for the condition many of which are misnomers; these include irritable colon, nervous diarrhoea and colonic spasm. The term mucous colitis is also a synonym and refers to the large amounts of mucus which very occasionally accompany the stools.

Pressure recordings from different positions in the lumen of the colon show that there may be localised increased intraluminal pressure during emotional stress—the hyperactivity can be reduced by anticholinergic drugs. The barium enema appearances reflect the hyperactivity of the colon—the lumen is diminished, haustral markings are prominent and numerous; these changes can usually be reversed with anticholinergics (Truelove and Reynell, 1963).

The pain is usually worse before defaecation after which it generally disappears. The pain may be felt anywhere over the course of the colon; when it occurs in relation to the splenic flexure it is sometimes known as the "splenic flexure syndrome". Sometimes palpation of the caecum produces pain in the transverse and descending colon. Patients with this condition often complain of excessive abdominal gurgling—in some patients the small bowel is also hypermotile. Constipation is commoner than diarrhoea although often the two alternate; the stools are usually small no matter what their consistency. Clinical features identical to those of spastic colon occur after attacks of dysentery, after vagotomy and in ulcerative colitis. The mandatory sigmoidoscopy also frequently reproduces the patient's symptoms.

Treatment is with anticholinergic drugs and psychotherapy if the symptoms are severe and protracted.

ENDOCRINE CAUSES OF DIARRHOEA

Diarrhoea may be caused by disorders of the major endocrine glands:

1. Addison's disease.
2. Thyrotoxicosis.
3. Hypoparathyroidism (and hypocalcaemia).
4. Diabetes.
5. Phaeochromocytoma.

Diarrhoea may also be produced by other humoral agents:

1. Non-beta-cell tumours of the pancreatic islets (Zollinger-Ellison syndrome).
2. Carcinoid tumours.
3. Ganglioneuromas in children.
4. Medullary carcinoma of the thyroid.
5. Bronchial carcinoma.

Zollinger[74]-Ellison[75] Syndrome

In 1955 Zollinger and Ellison described a syndrome consisting of a triad of peptic ulceration at an unusual site or recurrent anastomotic ulcers, gastric hypersecretion and a non-insulin-secreting islet cell tumour of the pancreas. In about half the cases there is a profuse watery diarrhoea and sometimes steatorrhoea, which is probably due to intestinal hurry as a result of inability of the pancreas to neutralise the excessive quantities of acid gastric juice. The diarrhoea may be present for several years before other manifestations of the syndrome are apparent. A substance has been isolated from the tumours which resembles gastrin (the acid-stimulating hormone normally produced by the antrum of the stomach).

About 10 per cent of patients with the syndrome have adenomata in other endocrine glands, the commonest being the parathyroids and

74. ROBERT M. ZOLLINGER. Contemporary Professor of Surgery, Columbus, Ohio.
75. EDWARD HOMER ELLISON. Contemporary surgeon, Columbus, Ohio.

adrenals—the "pluriglandular" syndrome. There is a high familial incidence of the "pluriglandular" syndrome and the Zollinger-Ellison syndrome.

The diagnosis is suggested by the presence of multiple peptic ulcers particularly if they are in unusual sites such as the postbulbar region of the duodenum or in the jejunum. In the stomach there is usually giant hypertrophy of the mucous membrane. Excessive gastric acidity should be demonstrated in a 12-hour nocturnal collection of the gastric juice— more than 100 mEq per 12 hours is highly suggestive. The pentagastrin test is of less value. The most important diagnostic finding is a high level of serum gastrin. With regard to treatment there are several important factors to be considered: two-thirds of the tumours are in the body or tail of the pancreas; 10 per cent are in aberrant pancreatic tissue; about 30 per cent are multiple; approximately half the tumours are malignant and of these about a third have metastasised by the time diagnosis is made. However, the metastases are always very slow growing so that it is usually worthwhile to remove the primary tumour if this can be found. Total gastrectomy carries a better prognosis than operations on the pancreas. There is evidence that some pancreatic tumours regress and serum gastrin levels return to normal after operations on the stomach.

Carcinoid Syndrome

The carcinoid syndrome consists of a variable combination of flushing, diarrhoea, asthma and valvular heart lesions. The syndrome is usually caused by humoral substances produced by the metastases of tumours arising from the ileum. The cells of the tumours stain with silver salts hence the alternative name—argentaffinomas. The primary tumour and its metastases contain large quantities of 5-hydroxytryptamine (5HT) and this is excreted in the urine as 5-hydroxyindole acetic acid (5HIAA). 5HT is synthesised from tryptophan which is an essential amino acid and is a precursor of nicotinamide (vitamin B_6). There may be a deficiency of the vitamin leading to pellagra if excessive 5HT is produced. Many but not all the clinical features of the carcinoid syndrome are produced by release of the 5HT into the circulation. Other substances are produced by carcinoid tumours (Grahame-Smith, 1968):

1. *5-hydroxytryptophan*—this is a precursor of 5HT and is produced by carcinoids arising from the embryological foregut.

2. *Histamine*—this is occasionally produced by carcinoids arising from the stomach.

3. *Bradykinin*—some carcinoid tumours produce a proteolytic enzyme, kallikrein, which splits a circulating α_2-globulin (kininogen) to produce bradykinin.

The type of flush varies from patient to patient depending on which humoral substance predominates. 5HT alone rarely produces a flush—when it does the flush is cyanotic; bradykinin tends to produce an erythematous flush. The flushes may be provoked by cheese, alcohol or emotion.

The diarrhoea is almost certainly due to 5HT and can usually be controlled with a 5HT antagonist such as methysergide. The cardiac effects of the carcinoid syndrome are an increase in cardiac output due to vasodilatation and endocardial fibrosis which leads to tricuspid and pulmonary stenosis in many instances of liver metastases. In the rare instance of a pulmonary carcinoid the valve lesions may be in the left side of the heart. Asthma may occur during attacks of flushing.

The clinical diagnosis of the carcinoid syndrome is confirmed by demonstrating the primary tumour and metastases by radiology and by demonstrating a high urinary excretion of 5HIAA. Flushing may be provoked by small intravenous injections of noradrenaline.

Treatment (Grahame-Smith, 1968).—The carcinoid syndrome usually only develops after metastases have occurred; however, these are usually very slow growing. Methysergide is a 5HT antagonist and may control the asthma and diarrhoea (side-effects include vascular spasm and retroperitoneal fibrosis).

The stimulating effects on the tumours of catecholamines may be prevented with α-methyldopa (Aldomet) and the peripheral effects of the humoral substances produced by the tumour may sometimes be inhibited by an α adrenergic blocking drug such as phenoxybenzamine.

REFERENCES

ASERKOFF, B., and BENNETT, J. V. (1969). *New. Engl. J. Med.*, **281**, 636.

ATKINSON, M. (1957). *Brit. med. J.*, **3**, 218.

AYLETT, S. O. (1966). *Brit. med. J.*, **1**, 1001.

BEAN, R. H. (1966). *Brit. med. J.*, **1**, 1081.

BOWEN, G. E., IRONS, G. V., RHODES, J., and KIRSNER, J. B. (1966). *J. Amer. med. Ass.*, **195**, 460.

BUTLER, T. J. (1961). *Ann. roy. Coll. Surg. Engl.*, **29**, 300.

CHRISTIE, A. B. (1969). *Infectious Diseases*. Edinburgh: E. & S. Livingstone.

COOKE, W. T. (1958). *Brit. med. J.*, **2**, 261.

COX, E. V., WILLIAMS, J. A., and JONES, C. T. (1963). In *Partial Gastrectomy. Complications and Metabolic Consequences*. Eds. Stammers, F. A., and Williams, J. A. London: Butterworth & Co.

COX, H. T., and ALLAN, W. R. (1961). *Lancet*, **2**, 672.

DAWSON, A. M. (1965). In *Recent Advances in Gastroenterology*. Eds. Badenoch. J., and Brooke, B. N. London: J. & A. Churchill.

DELLER, D. J., and WITTS, L. J. (1962). *Quart. J. Med.*, **31**, 89.

DOLL, R., HILL, I. D., HUTTON, C. F., and UNDERWOOD, D. J. (1962). *Lancet*, **2**, 793.

DOLL, R., PRICE, A. V., PYGOTT, F., and SANDERSON, P. H. (1956). *Lancet*, **1**, 70.

DOLL, R., and PYGOTT, F. (1952). *Lancet*, 1, 171.

DUTHIE, H. L. (1967). *Brit. med. J.*, 2, 790.

EDWARDS, F. C., and COGHILL, N. F. (1968). *Quart. J. Med.*, 37, 337.

EDWARDS, F. C., and TRUELOVE, S. C. (1963). *Gut*, 4, 299.

FRAZER, A. C., HOOD, C., MONTGOMERY, R. D., DAVIES, A. G., SCHNEIDER, R., CARTER, P. A., and GOODHART, J. (1966). *Lancet*, 1, 503.

GEFFEN, N., DARNBOROUGH, A., de DOMBAL, F. T., WATKINSON, G., and GOLIGHER, J. C. (1968). *Gut*, 9, 150.

GOLIGHER, J. C., de DOMBAL, F. T., GRAHAM, N. G., and WATKINSON, G. (1967). *Brit. med. J.*, 3, 193.

GRAHAME-SMITH, D. G. (1968). *Hosp. Med.*, 2, 558.

HARRIS, O. D., COOK, W. T., THOMPSON, H., and WATERHOUSE, J. A. (1966). *Gut*, 7, 710.

HEARD, G., JEFFRIES, J. D., and PETERS, D. K. (1963). *Lancet*, 2, 975.

HINDLE, W., and CREAMER, B. (1965). *Brit. med. J.*, 2, 455.

HOFFMAN, A. F. (1965). *Gastroenterology*, 48, 484.

HOLMAN, H., NICKEL, W. F., and SLEISENGER, M. H. (1959). *Amer. J. Med.*, 27, 963.

JAMES, O. F., AGNEW, J. E., and BOUCHIER, I. A. (1973). *Brit. med. J.*, 3, 191.

JONES, F. A. (1969). *Proc. roy. Soc. Med.*, 62, 499.

KIRSNER, J. B. (1967). In *Textbook of Medicine*. Eds. Beeson, P. B., and McDermott, W. Philadelphia: W. B. Saunders.

KIVEL, R. M., TAYLOR, K. B., and OBERHELMAN, H. (1967). *Lancet*, 2, 632.

LAWRENCE, J. S. (1952). *Lancet*, 1, 482.

LAWS, J. W., MOLLIN, D. L., and COGHILL, N. F. (1966). *Lancet*, 1, 510.

LENNARD-JONES, J. E. (1961). *Brit. med. J.*, 1, 1071.

LENNARD-JONES, J. E., and BABOURIS, N. (1965). *Gut*, 6, 113.

LENNARD-JONES, J. E., MISIEWICZ, J. J., CONNELL, A. M., BARON, J. H., and JONES, F. A. (1965). *Lancet*, 1, 188.

LENNARD-JONES, J. E., and STALDER, G. (1967). *Gut*, 8, 332.

LE QUESNE, L. P., HOBSLEY, M., and HAND, B. H. (1960). *Brit. med. J.*, 1, 141.

LUMSDEN, K., and TRUELOVE, S. C. (1965). *Radiology of the Digestive System*. Oxford: Blackwell Scientific.

MCMICHAEL, H. B., WEBB, J., and DAWSON, A. M. (1965). *Lancet*, 1, 717.

MISTILIS, S., and GOULSTON, S. (1965). In *Recent Advances in Gastroenterology*. Eds. Badenoch, J., and Brooke, B. N. London: J & A. Churchill.

NEALE, G., ANTCLIFF, A. C., WELBOURN, R. B., MOLLIN, D. L., and BOOTH, C. C. (1967). *Quart. J. Med.*, 36, 469.

NEALE, G., and HOFFBRAND, A. V. (1967). *Hosp. Med.*, 1, 402.

NORDIN, B. E. (1961). *Lancet*, 1, 1011.

PALMER, E. D. (1954). *Medicine (Baltimore)*, 33, 199.

PARRY, D. J., and WOOD, P. H (1967). *Gut*, 8, 301.

SALTER, R. H. (1968). *Amer. J. dig. Dis.*, 13, 38.

STRANGE, S. L. (1959). *Brit. med. J.*, 1, 476.

TABAQCHALI, S., and BOOTH, C. C. (1966). *Lancet*, 2, 12.

TAYLOR, H. (1957). *Gastroenterology*, 33, 353.

TRUELOVE, S. C. (1960). *Brit. med. J.*, 2, 559.

TRUELOVE, S. C. (1961). *Brit. med. J.*, 1, 154.

TRUELOVE, S. C. (1967). *Hosp. Med.*, **2**, 128.

TRUELOVE, S. C., and REYNELL, P. C. (1963). *Diseases of the Digestive System.*
Oxford: Blackwell Scientific.

WATTS, F. M., de DOMBAL, F. T., WATKINSON, G., and GOLIGHER, J. C.
(1966*a*). *Gut*, **7**, 16.

WATTS, J. McK., THOMPSON, H., and GOLIGHER, J. C. (1966*b*). *Gut*, **7**, 288.

WILLIAMS, J. (1959). *Clin. Sci.*, **18**, 521.

WRIGHT, R., and TRUELOVE, S. C. (1965). *Brit. med. J.*, **2**, 138.

4

LIVER AND PANCREAS

FUNCTIONS OF THE LIVER

1. Excretion of bilirubin.
2. Excretion of bile salts and cholesterol.
3. Synthesis of glycogen.
4. Synthesis of albumin and urea.
5. Storage of vitamins A, D and B_{12}.
6. Detoxication of hormones such as aldosterone, oestrogens and antidiuretic hormone.
7. Detoxication of drugs such as opiates, barbiturates, salicylates, quinine and heavy metals.

Excretion of bilirubin.—Bilirubin is a waste product resulting from destruction of worn out red cells or their precursors. The iron and protein (globin) of the haemoglobin are metabolised and re-used, the remainder of the haemoglobin is a waste product and becomes bilirubin. The destruction of red cells takes place throughout the reticulo-endothelial system, including the bone marrow. Bilirubin is carried to the liver attached to serum albumin—in this form it is insoluble in water. In the liver bilirubin is removed from the albumin and conjugated with glucuronic acid. Once it is removed from the albumin and conjugated it becomes soluble in water. This difference in solubility before and after passage through the liver is the basis of the van den Bergh[76] reaction. Water-soluble conjugated bilirubin changes the colour of the diazotised sulphanilic acid; water-insoluble bilirubin (unconjugated) will not change the colour until it has been removed from the serum albumin by the addition of alcohol—unconjugated bilirubin is, therefore, referred to as indirect-acting bilirubin. Conjugated bilirubin is referred to as direct-acting.

In the gall bladder the bile is concentrated by the removal of water, thence conjugated bilirubin passes down the small intestine unchanged. In the colon it is reduced by coliform and other organisms to stercobilinogen which when oxidised gives the brown colour to the faeces. Some stercobilinogen is absorbed, some of it is excreted in the urine as urobilinogen and some is re-excreted by the liver (enterohepatic circulation).

In obstructive jaundice, direct-acting (conjugated) bilirubin is forced

76. ALBERT ABRAHAM HUJMANS VAN DEN BERGH (1869–1943). Utrecht physician.

back through the liver cells into the blood as a result of increased pressure in the biliary system. In haemolytic jaundice indirect-acting (unconjugated) bilirubin accumulates in the blood because red cells are being broken down faster than the liver can excrete the bilirubin. In addition, increased amounts of stercobilinogen are present, more is absorbed from the colon but the ability to re-excrete urobilinogen is limited, therefore, more has to be excreted in the urine accounting for the increased urinary urobilinogen which appears in haemolytic anaemias.

In hepatocellular jaundice two things are happening; one is that damaged liver cells cannot conjugate bilirubin in the normal amounts so that there is a rise in indirect (unconjugated) bilirubin in the blood and the other is that the damaged liver cells swell and block the bile canaliculi causing intrahepatic biliary obstruction which will cause a rise in direct-acting (conjugated) bilirubin, provided the liver cells are still capable of conjugating some bilirubin. In hepatocellular damage due to infective hepatitis the obstructive element generally comes first and is followed by failure of the liver cells to conjugate bilirubin.

Excretion of bile salts and cholesterol.—Bile salts are the end-product of cholesterol metabolism; however, they are essential for the emulsification and hence absorption of fats (and the fat-soluble vitamins A, D and K), and they also activate pancreatic and intestinal lipase. In obstructive jaundice the excretion of bile salts is prevented, they accumulate in the serum and are responsible for the skin irritation of obstructive jaundice. Cholesterol exists in the serum as free cholesterol or as cholesterol esters—this esterification takes place in the liver. In hepatocellular damage the liver loses its ability to esterify cholesterol; hence the proportion of esterified to free cholesterol in the serum falls. In chronic biliary obstruction there is usually a marked rise in serum cholesterol.

Bile salts are almost completely reabsorbed in the distal ileum and take part in an enterophepatic circulation. Diseases which affect the distal ileum will prevent reabsorption of bile salts which are, therefore, not re-excreted—this may cause failure of emulsification of fats and exaggerate the effects of malabsorption.

Synthesis of glycogen and carbohydrate.—Glycogen is stored in the liver cells and can be synthesised from and metabolised to glucose. In hepatocellular damage this ability is impaired and may result in hyperglycaemia if glycogen is not formed quickly enough, or hypoglycaemia if glycogen is not broken down to glucose quickly enough.

Synthesis of albumin and urea.—Urea is the waste product of amino acid metabolism within the liver. Severe liver damage is associated with impaired production of urea, a low blood urea and increased amino acids in the blood leading to aminoaciduria.

Albumin is manufactured by the liver, whereas most of the globulins are produced by the reticulo-endothelial system. Other proteins are manufactured in the liver; the most important of these are prothrombin and other protein factors concerned with blood coagulation. In obstructive jaundice the serum lipids are raised, many of them are attached to β globulins so that in obstructive jaundice there may appear to be an increase in β globulins.

Bilirubin is transported attached to the plasma albumin; many drugs are also transported in the same way. Substances which are bound to the plasma proteins are not pharmacologically active, and it is the concentration of the free drug in the plasma which determines its activity. Some substances are more readily displaced from protein-binding sites than others. In newborn babies there are relatively small amounts of plasma albumin and all the binding sites are occupied by bilirubin. If sulphonamides are given to premature babies, bilirubin is displaced from the albumin and is then free in the serum to enter the brain and cause kernicterus. For this reason neonates should never be given sulphonamides or salicylates.

There are many examples of one drug displacing another from the albumin-binding sites giving rise to toxic concentration of the displaced drug in the serum.

The following list (Brodie, 1965) shows drugs which are attached to plasma albumin; phenylbutazone will displace most of the others. The most important examples clinically are potentiation of anticoagulants in patients given phenylbutazone and potentiation of tolbutamide causing hypoglycaemia by most of the others in this list:

1. Phenylbutazone.
2. Warfarin.
3. Salicylates.
4. Sulphonamides.
5. Penicillin.
6. Tolbutamide.

Several hormones are transported attached to plasma proteins, e.g. thyroxin, corticosteroids and insulin. Many of the antirheumatic drugs may cause their effect by displacing corticosteroids from their binding plasma protein. Tolbutamide may act in a similar way with regard to insulin. It has been noted that patients with rheumatoid arthritis may improve if they develop obstructive jaundice, probably as a result of displacement of corticosteroids from their binding sites by bilirubin (Hench, 1952).

Storage of vitamins.—Patients with cirrhosis sometimes develop night blindness due to deficiency of vitamin A. A macrocytic anaemia occurs in cirrhosis but is probably not related to inability to store vitamin B_{12}—by far the commonest causes of anaemia in cirrhosis are iron deficiency or haemolysis.

Detoxication of hormones.—Failure to detoxicate hormones results in features of hormone excess—the most important of which are oestrogens, ADH and aldosterone.

Detoxication of drugs.—Liver damage results in a reduced ability to excrete those drugs normally handled by the liver. This results in serious overdosage if these drugs are inadvertently used.

Liver Function Tests

The patient's description of alteration of colour of his urine and stools is still one of the most useful pointers in the diagnosis of liver disorders. The urine should always be examined for bilirubin before embarking on formal biochemical tests of liver function. The main tests are:

1. Serum bilirubin.
2. Urinary urobilinogen.
3. Excretion tests.
4. Serum proteins.
5. Serum enzymes.
6. Plasma prothrombin and fibrinogen.
7. Amino acids in blood and urine.
8. Blood ammonium.
9. Serum lipids.
10. Galactose tolerance.

Serum bilirubin.—Indirect-acting (unconjugated) bilirubin increases in haemolytic jaundice. Direct-acting (conjugated) bilirubin accumulates in obstructive jaundice.

Urinary urobilinogen.—This will be increased in haemolytic jaundice and absent in complete obstruction of the bile ducts. The reappearance of urobilinogen in the urine in infectious hepatitis is a good prognostic sign, because it means that the swelling of the liver cells is subsiding allowing some bile through the bile canaliculi. Urobilinogen is found in the urine mainly in the afternoon or evening, hence early morning specimens of urine are not so suitable for estimation of urinary urobilinogen.

Excretion tests.—Bromsulphthalein (BSP) is a dye which is more or less completely excreted by the liver in 45 minutes. Retention of more than 5 per cent of the original dose at this time indicates some impairment of liver function. The test will always be abnormal in the presence of obstructive jaundice. A number of other conditions may give false high readings at the end of 45 minutes, e.g. congestive heart failure, anaemia (by causing hepatic anoxia), fever, recent meal, shock and chronic debilitating diseases.

Serum proteins.—The serum albumin is usually reduced in liver damage. The γ globulin is sometimes raised in cirrhosis. The flocculation tests of liver functions depend on alterations in the proportions of the various plasma proteins.

Serum enzymes.—Hepatocellular damage causes leakage of intracellular substances into the blood, and these include iron and various enzymes. The main enzymes are the transaminases and the dehydrogenases (glutamic oxaloacetic, glutamic pyruvic transaminases, SGOT and SGPT and lactic and iso-citrate dehyrdogenases, LDH and ICD). SGPT and ICD are the most sensitive as indicators of liver impairment.

Alkaline phosphatase is excreted by the liver cells and by the mucosal cells of the biliary tree. The serum level is generally higher in biliary obstruction than in hepatocellular damage. Levels above 150 iu/l indicate biliary obstruction.

Carcinoma of the biliary epithelium results in extremely high levels of alkaline phosphatase in the serum. Alkaline phosphatase is also found in bone and in the gastro-intestinal tract. It is possible to differentiate the different alkaline phosphatases biochemically. An enzyme similar to alkaline phosphatase, 5-nucleotidase, is specific for liver disease.

Plasma prothrombin and fibrinogen.—Plasma prothrombin may be reduced because the hepatocellular damage is so severe that it cannot be synthesised, or because vitamin K from which it is formed is not absorbed because of lack of bile salts. Lack of fibrinogen may also be responsible for excessive bleeding.

Amino acids in blood and urine.—There is increased aminoaciduria in severe cirrhosis, particularly of cystine. The raised level of amino acids in the blood may be partly responsible for hepatic coma.

Blood ammonium.—There is some correlation between the blood ammonium level and hepatic coma; however, the exact cause of hepatic coma remains obscure.

Serum lipids.—The serum cholesterol is increased in obstructive jaundice. The proportion of esterified cholesterol may fall in liver impairment.

Galactose tolerance.—The rate at which galactose is metabolised to glycogen is measured by the rate of decrease in serum levels of galactose following a loading dose.

JAUNDICE

Increase in Unconjugated Bilirubin.

1. Increased production as in haemolytic anaemias.
2. Impaired handling of bilirubin by the liver.
(*a*) Impairment of entry of bilirubin into hepatic cells (Gilbert's[77]

---

77. NICHOLAS AUGUSTIN GILBERT (1858–1927). Paris physician.

disease). This is characterised by mild fluctuating jaundice which is present from childhood. The condition may be exacerbated by acute infections, the increased bilirubin is always the unconjugated type; it is the commonest of the congenital hyperbilirubinaemias. Nevertheless, it should only be diagnosed by exclusion of all other causes of a raised bilirubin, particularly haemolysis. Liver biopsy is always normal.

(*b*) Failure of conjugation of bilirubin inside the hepatic cell (Crigler-Najjar syndrome). This condition is always fatal in infancy.

(*c*) Impairment of excretion of conjugated bilirubin by the hepatic cells (Dubin Johnson and Rotor syndrome). These are benign, rare conditions associated with an increase of conjugated bilirubin in the serum. Liver biopsy shows brown pigmentation of the liver cells.

Gilbert's disease can be positively confirmed by the rise in unconjugated bilirubin which occurs with reduced calorie intake (Owens and Sherlock, 1973).

Jaundice due to Increased Conjugated Bilirubin

This is always due to obstruction of the biliary tree which may be intrahepatic in the case of "drug cholestasis" or extrahepatic in the case of obstruction to the bile duct.

Jaundice due to Increased Conjugated and Unconjugated Bilirubin

This means liver cell damage as well as biliary tree obstruction and is exemplified by virus hepatitis.

Jaundice Caused by Drugs

Drugs may produce jaundice in the following ways:

1. Liver cell necrosis which is usually fatal.

Examples are chloroform, carbon tetrachloride, heavy metals, hypothermia and hyperthermia.

2. Hepatitis-like syndrome. This usually improves if the drugs are withdrawn. There may be evidence of generalised hypersensitivity (urticaria, asthma and eosinophilia).

Examples are iproniazid, phenindione (Dindevan), PAS, sulphonamides, phenylbutazone and barbiturates.

3. Hypersensitivity cholestasis, i.e. intrahepatic biliary obstruction occurs in hypersensitive patients only and is not dose dependent.

Examples are phenothiazines, chlorpropamide, tolbutamide and erythromycin.

4. Non-hypersensitivity cholestasis, i.e. biliary obstruction will occur in anyone who takes drugs for long enough.

Examples are methyltestosterone and norethandrolone.

5. Haemolytic jaundice. In glucose 6-phosphate-dehydrogenase deficient subjects haemolytic crises develop with some drugs.

Examples are primaquine, aspirin, sulphonamides, methyldopa, Furadantin and phenacetin.

6. Hepatitis transmitted by blood transfusion or unsterile syringes.

VIRUS HEPATITIS

The virus causing infective hepatitis has not yet been isolated although there have been reports of transmission of hepatitis by cell-free filtrates. The practical implication of failure to culture the virus is that it is impossible to isolate an antigen against which to test circulating antibody in cases of naturally acquired hepatitis. This would be useful from the point of view of diagnosis and epidemiological studies. The disease has a world-wide distribution and is spread by contamination of food, by infected blood, stools or urine; faecal contamination is probably the commonest.

The incubation period is two to six weeks and the illness starts with four to five days malaise, anorexia and aversion to cigarettes. There is generally a fever and sometimes a slight skin rash. With the onset of jaundice the stools become pale and the urine dark, indicating that there is intrahepatic biliary obstruction. Before the onset of jaundice, bile may be found in the urine. Urinary urobilinogen is also increased early in the illness, the damaged liver cells are unable to excrete the stercobilin which has been absorbed from the gut, and this appears in the urine as an excess of urobilinogen. The intrahepatic bile ducts become obstructed, no bile reaches the intestine, no stercobilin is absorbed and urobilinogen, therefore, disappears from the urine. During recovery the obstruction of the bile ducts is reduced, bile once more enters the intestines and urobilinogen once again appears in the urine. Similarly, when the pale stools again become brown, the obstructive element of the disease is subsiding. Occasionally cholestasis is prolonged giving rise to great diagnostic difficulty particularly in the middle-aged and elderly. The liver is usually enlarged and tender and the spleen frequently enlarged but not usually tender, in contradistinction to glandular fever in which the spleen is usually enlarged and tender and the liver enlarged but not tender. The disease is not always accompanied by overt jaundice if the liver is only mildly affected—nonicteric hepatitis. The transaminases may remain elevated for several months after clinical recovery without adversely affecting the ultimate prognosis. It is generally assumed that the stools may remain infective 7–10 days after jaundice has developed. Infected patients should be given their own cutlery and their excreta disinfected.

The incidence of Australia (hepatitis) antigen varies according to different series. It is certainly present much more frequently in serum hepatitis and may persist for years, hence can be a useful screening test to detect unsuitable blood donors. Australia antigen is detectable in the blood late in the incubation period and in the acute stage of serum hepatitis. The antigen occurs in about 0·1 per cent of normal healthy people in this country, but in about 5 per cent of normals in the tropics. Antigen-positive hepatitis can be transmitted by insects, during dental treatment and possibly by inhalation.

There are occasionally relapses and occasionally vague malaise and ill-health after an attack has completely subsided. Rarely, infective hepatitis is fulminating and fatal; a small proportion develop post-hepatic cirrhosis.

Protection by Gamma Globulin

Immunoglobulin has been shown to be effective in preventing infectious hepatitis in contacts provided it is given early in the incubation period (Public Health Laboratory Services, 1968). The dose is 500 mg; the half-life of the immunoglobulin is approximately 20 days, hence the larger the dose the longer a protective amount of immunoglobulin will be present. With this dose immunity lasts for about 6 months. There is evidence that although immunoglobulin prevents the overt manifestations of infectious hepatitis the liver is frequently infected even after immunoglobulin has been given. As judged by liver function tests subclinical hepatitis may be equally common in contacts who receive immunoglobulin as in those who do not (Krugman, 1963).

Immunoglobulin should be given to close contacts of cases of infectious hepatitis and to travellers abroad who are likely to come into contact with the disease. Normal immunoglobulin is not effective in protecting against Australia antigen-positive hepatitis; however immunoglobulin from antigen-positive donors is effective.

ACTIVE CHRONIC HEPATITIS

Hepatitis in Haemodialysis Units

Numerous outbreaks of hepatitis have occurred in patients and staff in haemodialysis units. All the serious outbreaks have been of Australia antigen-positive hepatitis and it is now universal practice to exclude from dialysis units patients who are Australia antigen-positive.

The diagnostic features are (Mackay *et al.*, 1965):

1. Persistent elevation of SGOT above 100 units/100 ml.
2. IgG in excess of 2·0 g per cent.
3. Lymphocyte or plasma cell infiltration of the liver as seen in the biopsy.

Clinically there is often splenomegaly, recurrent fevers, polyarthralgia and pleural effusions. The disease is commoner than cryptogenic (idiopathic) cirrhosis in younger patients and the incidence in women is higher. Other conditions are associated more often than would be expected by chance, e.g. ulcerative colitis, thrombocytopenia, haemolysis, glomerulonephritis, Hashimoto's disease and thyrotoxicosis.

A feature of active chronic hepatitis is the number of circulating antibodies which include antinuclear, smooth muscle, antimitochondrial antibodies and rheumatoid factor; in addition the autoimmune complement fixation test and Coombs' tests are frequently positive. It is most important to note that these same antibodies may be present in primary biliary cirrhosis and to a lesser extent in cryptogenic cirrhosis. Some series have demonstrated the Australia antigen in cases of active chronic hepatitis.

Treatment

Both corticosteroids and immunosuppressives have been shown to induce remissions (Mackay and Wood, 1963; Mackay et al., 1965). However a recent controlled trial (Murray-Lyon et al., 1973) has shown that prednisone is more effective than azathioprine; nevertheless if there is no improvement in three months with prednisone it is worth adding azathioprine. It is not usually worth giving azathioprine alone. If azathioprine is used it may need to be given in higher doses than normal because it is converted in the liver to its active metabolite 6-mercaptopurine and if there is liver damage this conversion is impaired. If improvement does occur the drug producing it should be continued in the lowest dose which maintains the improvement (Mackay, 1968).

The indices of improvement are:

1. Well-being of the patient.
2. Improvement in biopsy appearances.
3. Reduction in transaminases.
4. Reduction in IgG.
5. Increase in serum albumin.
6. Improvement in BSP excretion.

The value of steroids is not universally agreed; Read and his colleagues (Read et al., 1963) consider that steroids should only be used in active chronic hepatitis if the patient feels ill.

In cryptogenic cirrhosis steroids do not improve survival except possibly in females without ascites (Lancet, 1969a). They are sometimes indicated for their transient diuretic effect.

THE HALOTHANE PROBLEM

Hepatic necrosis occurs occasionally in the post-operative period. Chloroform was known to do this particularly after repeated administration. Halothane was suspected of doing the same but less frequently —nevertheless its continued use was more than justified by the fact that it is in other ways a safe anaesthetic agent. Once the drug was suspected the question arose whether the drug was causally related to the hepatic necrosis or only an associated factor. In order to try and resolve the problem the National Halothane Study was established in the U.S.; in a retrospective survey it could not be established that halothane is causally related to post-operative hepatitis (*Lancet*, 1966*b*). However, the case against halothane as a very rare cause of hepatitis still remains —particularly after repeated administration. There are proven instances of halothane (and other anaesthetic agents) producing acute hepato-cellular damage (*Lancet*, 1969*b*). Despite analysis of nearly a million cases the National Halothane Study still stress the need for collecting more information on the subject. However, the fact that the case against halothane is so difficult to bring to court implies that the dangers of its use are remote and its safety in other respects justify its continued use. There is no evidence to suggest that the dangers of post-operative hepatic necrosis are greater when operations are performed on the biliary system.

OTHER INFECTIONS

The liver may be involved in septicaemia and almost all viraemias; the most important are yellow fever, glandular fever, Q fever, influenza and Coxsackie infections. The liver is usually involved in Weil's disease, which is due to *Leptospira icterohaemorrhagiae* acquired from contact with infected rat's urine. A similar illness may be caused by *Lept. canicola* acquired from dogs. The important clinical features of lepto-spirosis are abdominal pain, muscle pains, meningitis, conjunctivitis, haemorrhagic tendency, nephritis and carditis. The clinical diagnosis can be confirmed by demonstrating and culturing the spirochaetes from the blood, a rising antibody titre and intraperitoneal guinea-pig inoculation. The leptospiroses are treated with penicillin or tetracycline.

The two commonest infective diseases affecting the liver are malaria and schistosomiasis. Schistosomiasis gives rise to "pipe stem" cirrhosis in which the lesions are predominantly in the portal tracts. It is the commonest cause of presinusoidal portal hypertension.

The liver is the site of election for many parasitic infections; particu-larly amoebiasis (*Entamoeba histolytica*) and hydatid disease (*Echino-coccus granulosus*) acquired from the excreta of dogs who have eaten infected sheep. Amoebiasis is said never to result in cirrhosis although there may be impairment of liver function tests. Liver function tests are often abnormal in infections remote from the liver. Liver histology in these cases shows "non-specific reactive hepatitis". Where liver function tests are abnormal due to infection within the liver the serum B_{12} is often raised (Neale *et al.*, 1966).

CIRRHOSIS

The liver in common with many other organs can only react in a limited number of ways to disease processes. Liver cells may become damaged and necrotic and replaced by fat and fibrous tissue; the portal tracts and central zones may become infiltrated with fibrous tissue and inflammatory cells. The architecture of the liver is dislocated by fibrous tissue and the hepatic cells cease to function because they are directly damaged by the disease, compressed by fibrous tissue and deprived of their blood supply. The liver cells are capable of considerable regeneration, but unfortunately this tends to occur in localised areas and although liver cells may regenerate, the architecture of the liver is not restored. These regeneration nodules may in turn become necrotic if their blood supply is not adequate. The fibrosis and distorted architecture constricts the portal venules, causing a rise in pressure in the portal veins. In the absence of normal liver cells blood is able to flow direct from the portal vein through the sinusoids into the central veins, without coming into contact with viable liver cells causing a shunt between the portal and systemic veins. These changes explain the main manifestations of liver disease:

1. *Portal hypertension* due to obstruction of portal venules within the liver.

2. *Hepatocellular failure*—due to loss of functioning liver cells.

3. *Porta-systemic encephalopathy* due to shunting of blood from the portal vein into the hepatic vein and thus the systemic circulation.

4. *Ascites* due to a combination of portal hypertension and hepatocellular failure.

PORTAL HYPERTENSION

The portal vein is formed by union of the splenic and superior mesenteric veins. The inferior mesenteric vein drains into the splenic vein. There are several situations where there is a capillary connection between the portal and systemic venous systems. At these sites capillaries and venules become dilated if the pressure in the portal system rises. The most important sites are the lower end of the oesophagus and the anus. The superficial veins on the anterior abdominal wall also dilate; in the normal person the direction of flow in these veins is always away from the umbilicus. The direction of flow is *not* altered in portal hypertension but the veins are dilated and easy to see. If there is obstruction of the inferior vena cava the direction of flow in the veins below the umbilicus is towards the umbilicus and in the veins above the umbilicus the direction of flow remains normal, i.e. upwards. In the rare instances of thrombosis of the portal vein blood reaches the liver through remnants of the umbilical vein (the falciform ligament) and the direction of flow in all the dilated veins is towards the umbilicus. Increased flow of blood in these veins may result in a venous hum.

The spleen enlarges as a result of increased portal vein pressure and congestion. An enlarged spleen from any cause may result in hypersplenism which is characterised by a pancytopenia in the peripheral blood with a normoblastic bone marrow; occasionally only one of the cellular elements of the blood is reduced.

Portal hypertension should rarely be diagnosed unless the spleen is palpable or seen to be enlarged on x-ray. In the extremely rare instance of thrombosis of the splenic vein the spleen may not enlarge. It may also be small and fibrotic as a result of repeated splenic infarcts.

The intrasplenic pressure accurately reflects portal vein pressure; percutaneous splenic puncture is a convenient way of measuring the portal venous pressure, which should not normally exceed 10 mm Hg. It is also a convenient way of performing portal venography to demonstrate the anatomy of the portal venous system or the site of a blockage.

Obstruction of the hepatic vein is known as Chiari's[78] syndrome, the appearances of the liver are those of severe congestion. The same appearance occurs in "veno-occlusive disease", a condition caused by ingesting brews containing Senecio (ragwort) or bush teas commonly drunk in Jamaica. Occlusion of the hepatic veins may be caused by invasion by tumour, thrombophlebitis migrans and thrombosis secondary to polycythaemia or inferior vena cava thrombosis. Two clinical features are important: one is the presence of gross ascites and the other is the absence of hepatojugular reflux due to obstruction of the hepatic vein.

Portal hypertension results from obstruction of the portal venous system inside or outside the liver; extrahepatic portal obstruction is rare in this country. Within the liver the block may be before the portal blood reaches the sinusoids or after the sinusoids (pre- or post-sinusoidal portal hypertension). Portal cirrhosis results when obstruction is post-sinusoidal. The commonest example of pre-sinusoidal portal hypertension is the fibrosis which results from schistosomiasis. It is possible to distinguish between pre- and post-sinusoidal block by measuring the hepatic vein wedge pressure. A catheter wedged tightly in the hepatic vein will measure the pressure in the sinusoids, hence in post-sinusoidal block the wedge pressure will be high and in pre-sinusoidal block the wedge pressure will be low.

78. HANS CHIARI (1851–1916). Prague and Strasbourg pathologist.

Management of Bleeding Oesophageal Varices

Although bleeding from oesophageal varices is usually severe, death is often due to hepatocellular failure and electrolyte disturbances which the loss of blood will almost inevitably produce in a patient with portal hypertension and barely adequate liver function. In this country extra-hepatic portal hypertension is a rare cause of oesophageal varices. Patients with cirrhosis causing portal hypertension and oesophageal varices may bleed from a chronic peptic ulcer to which they are more prone than normal people or occasionally they may bleed from alcoholic gastritis.

The first essential is to restore blood volume and to institute treatment of hepatocellular failure at the same time. Vitamin K should be given in case there is prothrombin deficiency. The patient may need sedation; the most suitable drugs are chloral, phenobarbitone or chlorpromazine. Paraldehyde, opiates and short-acting barbiturates should not be used.

Control of Haemorrhage

1. *Vasopressin* (*Pitressin*).—Posterior pituitary extract lowers portal venous pressure by constricting splanchnic arterioles, it is useful in reducing portal blood flow and promoting haemostasis. Pitressin is given intravenously, 20 units in 5 per cent dextrose are given over 20 minutes, and it is effective for about an hour. Widespread arteriolar constriction occurs resulting in pallor, a rise in blood pressure and narrowing of the coronary arteries; it should, therefore, be used with caution in patients with coronary artery disease. Another effect is to cause colic and stimulation of the colon which results in diarrhoea. As well as reducing blood flow in the portal vein it also reduces hepatic artery flow which may lead to further anoxia of the liver and hepatocellular damage. Prolonged use of Pitressin results in tachyphylaxis—repeated doses have to be increased in order to have the same effect. The therapeutic dose is the same as the dose which produces side-effects, hence the drug is probably not fully effective until pallor of the skin and colic have been produced.

2. *Sengstaken oesophageal tube* (oesophageal tamponade).—The bleeding veins are compressed by an oesophageal balloon kept in place by a balloon in the stomach. Asphyxia and aspiration pneumonias as well as ulceration of the stomach and oesophageal mucosa are common complications.

3. *Gastric hyphothermia.*—This is available in some centres and may control bleeding.

4. *Emergency surgery.*—The main operations used are:

   (i) Ligations of varices.

   (ii) Emergency portacaval shunt.

   (iii) Oesophageal and gastric transections.

In transection operations oesophagus or stomach are cut across and resutured. The dilated veins are thereby divided, reducing the pressure at the site at which they are bleeding. Unfortunately new varices develop very quickly.

   (iv) Injection of varices with sclerosing substances. This procedure is particularly useful for bleeding varices due to extrahepatic portal hypertension (Johnson, 1963).

   5. *Elective portacaval shunt.*—Anastomosis of the portal vein to the inferior vena cava will reduce the pressure in the portal veins and oesophageal varices may disappear. The most favoured operation is anastomosing the end of the portal vein to the side of the inferior vena cava. Before the operation a splenoportagram is performed to demonstrate the presence of a patent portal vein. Careful selection of patients for this elective operation is essential. Important features to be considered with regard to operation are:

   (i) Serum albumin over 30 g/l.

   (ii) Serum bilirubin below 17 μmol/l.

   (iii) Age under 50.

   (iv) Absent neurological signs during haemorrhage.

Portacaval anastomosis undoubtedly reduces the incidence of further bleeding from varices. However, there is a high incidence of porta-systemic encephalopathy—probably about 20 per cent (Grace *et al.*, 1966) even with rigid selection for operation; the 5-year survival is about 50 per cent. Nevertheless, there is still some doubt whether a portacaval shunt materially improves the mortality rate as compared with conservative management of well-compensated cirrhosis with portal hypertension. The mortality following the first haemorrhage from oesophageal varices is much higher than following subsequent bleeds—in other words a patient who survives his first bleed has already had his most dangerous haemorrhage (Hislop *et al.*, 1966). Prophylactic shunt operations do not influence survival and they carry the risk of porta-systemic encephalopathy although they do reduce the frequency of bleeding (Grace *et al.*, 1966).

HEPATOCELLULAR FAILURE

The main features of hepatocellular failure relate to the main functions of the liver:

   1. **Jaundice** due to failure to conjugate and excrete bilirubin. Severe

jaundice is unusual in chronic liver failure except as a terminal event. Many causes of cirrhosis are complicated by a haemolytic anaemia which will exaggerate the retention of bilirubin.

2. **Impaired synthesis of proteins, glycogen and glucose** leading to weight loss, loss of muscle bulk, hypoglycaemia and a low plasma albumin. Other plasma proteins such as prothrombin and other coagulation factors are also affected, leading to a haemorrhagic tendency. This may be exaggerated if associated portal hypertension causes splenomegaly and hypersplenism with a reduction in platelets.

3. **Endocrine changes** due to inability to detoxicate hormones. The principal hormones detoxicated by the liver are oestrogens, aldosterone and ADH. The effects of excess oestrogens are gynaecomastia, testicular atrophy, spider naevi and palmar erythema. Failure to detoxicate aldosterone and ADH results in retention of salt and water.

4. **Hyperkinetic circulation** due to:

(i) Increased blood volume.

(ii) Associated anaemia which may be caused by haemorrhages, impaired conversion of folic acid into effective folinic acid and impaired metabolism of vitamin B_{12}. The serum levels of folic acid and B_{12} may be normal. Haemolysis may also contribute to the anaemia.

(iii) Arteriovenous shunting within the lungs.

(iv) Excessive vasodilator material (VDM) causing peripheral vasodilatation—possibly due to failure of detoxication by the damaged liver (Shorr et al., 1951).

(v) Associated alcoholism may cause beri beri with peripheral vasodilatation and high cardiac output. The hyperkinetic circulation may result in tachycardia, warm peripheries and an ejection-type systolic murmur at the aortic area.

5. **Fever.**—A low grade fever is very common in chronic liver damage, but the exact cause is not known; it has been postulated that the liver fails to detoxicate a pyrogenic steroid or that damaged liver cells release a pyrogen (Tisdale and Klatskin, 1960). Gram-negative septicaemias are more common in severe liver disease due to shunting of blood direct from the portal system to the systemic circulation.

6. **Ascites** is due to a combination of hepatocellular failure and portal hypertension. The principal mechanism of formation of ascites is:

(i) Increase in portal vein pressure.

(ii) Decrease in osmotic potential of plasma, due to decreased serum albumin.

(iii) Increased production of lymph by the liver.

(iv) Sodium retention due to hyperaldosteronism from failure of the liver to detoxicate aldosterone.

(v) Increased water retention due to failure to detoxicate antidiuretic hormone.

(vi) Reduced renal blood flow.

(vii) Intrarenal shunting.

Ascites is often accompanied by a pleural effusion. Ascitic fluid contains 1–2 g/100 ml protein, in contrast to ascites due to malignant
disease and tuberculosis which usually contains at least 3 g per cent of
protein. In a patient with cirrhosis, the presence of a raised protein
content and blood staining of the ascitic fluid may be due to a hepatoma.
There is a rapid interchange between ascitic fluid and the extracellular
fluid. Ascites should not be tapped unless the patient is distressed;
removal of large amounts of ascitic fluid will deplete the patient's
already reduced protein pool, it will also remove a large amount of
sodium. Albumin infusions and steroids may be necessary to induce a
diuresis and tide the patient over a temporary episode of liver impairment. They are of little value for long-term use.

7. **Porta-systemic encephalopathy.**—Severe liver cell damage enables
portal blood arriving at the liver to pass through the liver sinusoids
directly into the hepatic vein. With the development of portal hypertension there are additional communications between the portal and
systemic venous systems. Portal blood contains toxic substances which
are normally metabolised in the liver; with extensive porta-systemic
shunting these substances pass direct into the systemic circulation.

The clinical features range from minimal mental deterioration to deep
coma. The picture is often a mixture of neuropsychiatric manifestations; however, in the early stages the mental changes may predominate, they include personality change, disturbance of sleep rhythm,
intellectual deterioration and slurred speech.

The most common neurological abnormality is the "hepatic flap"
which is a coarse tremor of the outstretched arms—it is not specific for
liver disease. Other neurological abnormalities seen in porta-systemic
encephalopathy are:

(i) Cerebellar and basal ganglia disturbances.

(ii) Paraplegia.

(iii) Motor neuropathy.

(iv) Epilepsy.

(v) Cortical degeneration.

(vi) Muscle spasms.

Some of these improve with treatment of the primary condition, but
others are due to permanent damage and will not improve. The two
which usually do not improve are the paraplegia and the focal cortical
degeneration.

The CSF may show an increase in protein and the EEG may show
slowing of the normal waves. In the normal the dominant wave in the
EEG is the α wave with a frequency of 8–13 per second. In porta-

systemic encephalopathy the speed is about 3–5 per second (delta waves). These changes are also seen in other conditions causing coma but their appearances in a conscious patient is virtually diagnostic. The EEG is useful in assessing the influence of treatment (Sherlock, 1968*a*). One of the best ways of recording progression of cerebral changes is to record the patient's ability to make certain shapes out of match sticks or to draw symmetrical objects, e.g. making a star out of match sticks or drawing a clock face in the notes. Encephalopathy generally leads to constructional apraxia.

The toxic substance producing encephalopathy is not known but there is some correlation with increased blood ammonium levels, although occasionally both blood and CSF ammonium levels are normal in the presence of deep coma.

Peripheral neuropathy occurs in primary liver disease with surprising frequency if carefully looked for. In some instances it is impossible to be certain that the neuropathy is not caused by the frequently associated alcoholism, uraemia or diabetes.

Hepatocellular failure may be precipitated by:

   (i) Gastro-intestinal haemorrhage.
  (ii) High-protein diet.
 (iii) Infections.
 (iv) Anaesthesia and operations.
  (v) Hypnotic drugs.
 (vi) Diuretic therapy and hypokalaemia.
(vii) Paracentesis abdominis.

Treatment of Hepatocellular Failure and Porta-systemic Encephalopathy

1. *Bed rest.*
2. *High-calorie and low-protein diet with vitamin supplements.*
3. *Correction of electrolyte disturbances.*—Hypokalaemia may occur as a result of reduced dietary intake, diuretics and purgation; hypokalaemia may precipitate liver failure by causing an increase in blood ammonium (Baertl *et al.*, 1963).

Patients with ascites and oedema may have a low serum sodium due to excessive retention of water. Despite the low serum sodium they should not be given sodium, but should be treated with sodium and water restriction and an osmotic diuretic. This is followed by oral diuretics; in general it is better to combine a diuretic which acts on the proximal renal tubule, such as the thiazides or frusemide, with one which acts on the distal tubule and conserves potassium such as spironolactone. However, patients with hyponatraemia *without* ascites and oedema may be sodium-depleted and require hypertonic saline. Paracentesis abdominis may precipitate hyponatraemia. A rise in blood urea may occur and is often associated with hypotension or gastro-intestinal haemorrhage. However, the pressure of ascites on renal veins may be responsible for the rise in blood urea in which case some improvement may be obtained by removing some of the ascitic fluid (Bradley and Bradley, 1947).

Following prolonged use the effectiveness of the standard diuretics may decline; in some cases it is possible to obtain a diuresis with prednisone or salt-free albumin infusion (Dykes, 1961), although prolonged albumin injections are of no value (Wilkinson and Sherlock, 1962).

4. *Avoidance of precipitating factor.*—Drugs which are excreted by the liver such as morphia and the short-acting barbiturates are never used.

5. *Purgation* to remove nitrogen-containing products from the colon.

6. *Antibiotics* to sterilise the colon and destroy ammonia-producing organisms. The antibiotic most commonly used is neomycin in a dose of 4 g daily. It should be noted that enough neomycin may be absorbed to cause damage to the eighth nerve.

Colonisation of the colon with non-ammonia-producing organisms which are resistant to neomycin.—Enpac consists of a dried preparation of *Lactobacillus acidophilus* and has been used for this purpose (Read *et al.*, 1966).

7. *Milk and cheese diet.*—The proteins in milk and cheese do not cause as much elevation of blood ammonia as other proteins because they undergo less degradation by ammonia-producing colonic organisms. Milk and cheese are also rich in non-ammonia-producing organisms which tend to displace the ammonia-producing organisms from the colon (Fenton *et al.*, 1966).

8. *Lactulose.*—This is a synthetic disaccharide which is split into lactose and lactic acid. The lactose acts as an osmotic purgative and induces diarrhoea and the lactic acid decreases the pH, inhibiting ammonia-producing organisms (Bircher *et al.*, 1966).

9. *Surgical colectomy.*—This has been advocated but the operative mortality is prohibitive.

10. *Liver transplantation and exchange transfusion.*—Liver transplantation has been performed in animals and humans (Sicular and Kark, 1965). Exchange transfusions and crossed circulation techniques have been used in human patients with encouraging results (*Lancet*, 1966a).

CLASSIFICATION OF CIRRHOSIS

Cirrhosis is best classified as follows:
1. Portal.
2. Biliary.
3. Cardiac.

Portal Cirrhosis

Portal cirrhosis is so called because the pathological changes are mainly in the portal tracts. In the majority of cases no antecedent cause for the cirrhosis can be found; however, known causes of portal cirrhosis include:

1. Alcohol.
2. Virus hepatitis (post-necrotic cirrhosis).
3. Malnutrition.
4. Haemochromatosis.
5. Wilson's disease.

The liver has a limited number of ways in which it can react to injury. There are no specific histological features which distinguish alcoholic from post-necrotic portal cirrhosis. Both types have a diffuse disorganising fibrosis, liver cell necrosis and regeneration nodules. There are minor pathological differences between some cases of portal cirrhosis which are suggestive but not diagnostic of alcoholic cirrhosis:

1. The liver is more uniformly affected.
2. Nodules are finer.
3. Fatty change is more pronounced.
4. Cytoplasmic eosinophilic inclusion bodies are commoner (Mallory[79] bodies). There is a tendency for alcoholic and post-necrotic cirrhosis to present initially in different ways. Alcoholic cirrhosis tends to present with features of hepatocellular failure and hepatomegaly, whereas post-necrotic cirrhosis tends to present with portal hypertension with splenomegaly and oesophageal varices.

The incidence of alcoholism among cirrhotics is about 50 per cent (Ratnoff and Patek, 1942), and the incidence of cirrhosis among alcoholics is about 10 per cent (Jolliffe and Jellinek, 1941). No particular liquor is more hepatotoxic than any other.

Nutritional liver disease such as occurs in kwashiorkor has many similarities with the liver disease which occurs in alcoholics. Both are characterised by fatty infiltration and portal cirrhosis although fatty infiltration is much commoner than cirrhosis in malnutrition. Many alcoholics exist on a diet which is vitamin deficient and low in proteins; this is probably the cause of the fatty liver in most alcoholics. However, the fatty change in the livers of alcoholics has never been shown to proceed to cirrhosis and furthermore cirrhosis can develop in an alcoholic who has never had a fatty liver (Sherlock, 1968a).

Alcoholic cirrhosis is reputed to be more commonly associated with a number of extrahepatic manifestations than other forms of cirrhosis.

79. FRANK BURR MALLORY (1862–1941). Boston pathologist.

These are: parotid gland enlargement, gynaecomastia, Dupuytren's[80] contracture and leuconychia. Other manifestations of alcoholism are likely to be present in alcoholic cirrhosis—these include peripheral neuropathy with tender calves, gastritis, pancreatitis, myopathy and cardiomyopathy.

In the case of a fatty liver or very mild cirrhosis the liver may revert to normal if the patient totally abstains from alcohol. Abstention from alcohol should be supplemented with B vitamins and a high-protein diet, provided there is no evidence of hepatocellular failure.

Acute alcoholic hepatitis.—The liver may be affected acutely by a high intake of alcohol. There is a sudden onset of hepatocellular failure accompanied by a tender enlarged liver, fever, leucocytosis and cholestasis. Pre-existing cirrhosis need not be present, the condition may occur in a previously normal liver.

Zieve's[81] syndrome.—In 1958 Zieve defined a syndrome which consists of jaundice, haemolytic anaemia and hyperlipaemia or hypercholesterolaemia. The syndrome develops following a bout of alcoholic drinking and is commoner in males; it always recedes with abstinence from alcohol; the histology of the liver may be normal or may show fatty infiltration or mild portal cirrhosis. There may be a pyrexia but the transaminases are usually normal. From a practical point of view the syndrome is important because the presence of jaundice with hypercholesterolaemia is highly suggestive of biliary obstruction and secondly because the haemolytic anaemia may not be recognised and an unrewarding search be made for bleeding from the gut.

Post-necrotic (Post-hepatitic) Cirrhosis

The incidence of post-necrotic cirrhosis following virus hepatitis varies from series to series. Most reports agree that it is probably not more than 1 per cent although there is some variation in different epidemics. Several large series have failed to demonstrate any cases of cirrhosis following hepatitis. The usual course is for portal hypertension to occur about five years after the initial attack and for hepatocellular failure to occur after a further five years. The incidence is higher in women (Sherlock, 1968a).

Other complications of portal cirrhosis include:

1. Peptic ulcer.
2. Intercurrent infections.
3. Thrombosis of the portal vein.
4. Primary hepatoma.
5. Gram-negative septicaemias.
6. Haemochromatosis.

80. BARON GUILLAUME DUPUYTREN (1777–1835). Paris surgeon.
81. LESLIE ZIEVE. Contemporary Minneapolis physician.

Haemochromatosis

Iron is carried in the blood bound to a beta 1 globulin (transferrin). Transferrin can transport about 350 µg/dl of iron. Normally the serum iron is about 125 µg/dl. The transferrin is only transporting one-third of the amount of iron that it is potentially capable of carrying, i.e. it is normally 33 per cent saturated. In iron deficiency anaemia the serum iron is low, the percentage saturation of transferrin is low, but the iron-binding capacity (amount of transferrin) is normal. In haemochromatosis there is increased iron absorption and the serum iron is high, the percentage saturation is increased but the iron-binding capacity is normal.

Some conditions are associated with an iron deficiency anaemia even though enough iron is being ingested—the main ones are uraemia, carcinomatosis and rheumatoid arthritis. The reason for this is that there is in these conditions either a reduction in the iron-binding capacity or there is a reduced ability to remove iron from the transferrin.

In haemochromatosis, excessive iron is absorbed from the gastro-intestinal tract and is deposited intracellularly as ferritin in certain sites, particularly liver, pancreas and heart and skin. Its deposition is accompanied by fibrosis and an increase in lipofuscin which is partly responsible for the "bronzed" appearance of the skin which gave this condition its original name of "bronzed diabetes". The incidence of mild iron and lipofuscin deposition in the siblings of patients with haemochromatosis is high. Patients with alcoholic cirrhosis also absorb more iron and have a higher serum iron than normal. Excessive iron storage is, therefore, associated with both an inherited defect in the intestinal mucosa and an acquired disease. The controversy about the relative importance of genetic or environmental causes in the development of haemochromatosis has not yet been resolved.

Haemosiderosis is the condition which results from excessive iron ingestion in the presence of a normal small bowel mucosa, such as occurs in Bantus who cook in iron vessels, or chronic haemolytic anaemias and multiple blood transfusions (usually more than 100). The distribution of ferritin is usually similar to that of haemochromatosis; it may, however, be confined to the reticulo-endothelial system which in the liver is represented by the Kupffer[82] cells.

Clinical features.—The disease is rare but not unknown in women; it does not occur before the menopause unless menstruation has stopped for some other reason. There is a higher incidence of the disease among siblings of affected patients. Occasionally the serum iron is normal and liver biopsy is often necessary to confirm the diagnosis and to check progress. Haemosiderin is frequently found in the liver in cirrhosis and

82. KARL WILHELM VON KUPFFER (1829–1902). Munich anatomist.

is increased following portacaval shunt operations. The sites most frequently affected are the liver, pancreas, skin and endocrine glands, particularly pituitary, adrenals and testes. Abdominal pain occurs and may be due to stretching of the capsule of the liver. Patients frequently die in shock due to widespread arteriolar dilatation caused by release from the liver of ferritin which has strong vasodilator properties. Haemochromatosis is one cause of cardiomyopathy, the myocardium becomes fibrotic; involvement of the conducting tissue leads to conduction defects and arrhythmias.

Diagnosis.—Important diagnostic tests are:

1. Serum iron.
2. Saturation of transferrin.
3. Biopsy appearances of liver, skin and bone marrow.
4. Demonstration of increased iron absorption.
5. Increased urinary excretion of iron with iron-chelating agents.
6. Screening of relatives.

Treatment.—Still the most effective method of removing iron is by repeated phlebotomy. On average the body contains about 50 g of iron in haemochromatosis. One pint of blood contains 250 mg iron. For severe cases, a pint of blood is removed at weekly intervals, until the haemoglobin and serum iron begin to fall. Treatment may have to continue for two years.

Iron-chelating agents (*Gk.* chele—a claw) such as desferrioxamine can only remove about 15 mg of iron per day. Nevertheless, desferrioxamine is a useful adjunct to phlebotomy; its main use, however, is in the treatment of iron overdosage in children who accidentally swallow iron tablets.

Wilson's[83] Disease

Hepatolenticular degeneration is characterised by deposition of copper in liver, basal ganglia and cornea, increased copper secretion in the urine, aminoaciduria, glycosuria and phosphaturia. In the plasma there is a deficiency of the copper-carrying protein caeruloplasmin, an alpha globulin; in its absence copper is loosely bound to albumin and easily deposited in the tissues. Deposition of copper in the cornea is in the form of copper containing pigment in Descemet's[84] membrane in the posterior surface of the cornea. The deposition is in the form of a ring, separated from the limbus (the corneoscleral junction) by a small zone of clear iris. This clear zone distinguishes Kayser[85]-Fleischer[86] rings

83. SAMUEL ALEXANDER KINNIER WILSON (1877–1937). London neurologist.
84. JEAN DESCEMET (1732–1810). Paris surgeon.
85. BERNHARD KAYSER (b. 1869). Stuttgart ophthalmologist.
86. BRUNO FLEISCHER (b. 1874). Erlangen ophthalmologist.

from arcus senilis. Portal hypertension is commoner than in haemo-chromatosis.

Diagnosis.—Important diagnostic tests are:

1. Low serum copper.
2. Low caeruloplasmin.
3. High urinary copper after penicillamine.
4. Copper content of liver or muscle biopsy.
5. Aminoaciduria.
6. Screening of relatives.

Treatment is with penicillamine (dimethyl cysteine) and must continue for at least two years. Toxic effects are similar to those of penicillin. Wilson's disease should be considered as a cause in any patient who develops cirrhosis under the age of 30.

<h3 style="text-align:center">CHRONIC INTRAHEPATIC CHOLESTASIS (CHRONIC CHOLANGITIDES)
(SHERLOCK, 1968b)</h3>

Sclerosis of the intrahepatic cholangioles may be due to ascending infection from the extrahepatic bile ducts. The ducts begin by being dilated due to the biliary obstruction; infection may persist despite complete and successful removal of the obstructing gall-stone; some years later the persisting infection results in widespread stricture formation in the intrahepatic cholangioles. Other causes of intrahepatic cholestasis are:

Ulcerative colitis.
Primary biliary cirrhosis.
Chlorpromazine (and all its analogues).
Carcinoma of intrahepatic ducts.

It is usually possible to distinguish intra- and extrahepatic biliary obstruction on the liver biopsy specimen; the jaundice of extrahepatic obstruction does not usually fluctuate in the way that the obstructive jaundice of intrahepatic biliary obstruction may.

Another rare cause of cirrhosis particularly (but not exclusively) in children is α_1, antitrypsin deficiency. This is a glycoprotein synthesised in the liver which normally inhibits trypsin and other proteases. There are a number of phenotypes for α_1, antitrypsin deficiency; the homozygotes have almost complete absence of α_1 globulins and usually associated cirrhosis and pulmonary emphysema. The heterozygotes may have a slight deficiency in the amount of serum α_1 antitrypsin and may have no pulmonary or hepatic abnormality. However some of the heterozygotes develop either a milder form of emphysema or develop emphysema later in life. It behoves these people rigorously to avoid smoking—if they do, disabling lung damage may be further delayed.

Management of Chronic Biliary Obstruction

Bile salts are necessary for the emulsification of dietary fat. Chronic biliary obstruction leads to steatorrhoea and consequent malabsorption of fat-soluble vitamins. The steatorrhoea can be prevented by a low-fat diet; the fat-soluble vitamins (in particular D and K) may need to be given parenterally. Medium (length) chain triglycerides can be absorbed when given by mouth without bile acids or pancreatic lipase.

Pruritis can be alleviated in partial biliary obstruction by giving an ion exchange resin, cholestyramine, by mouth. Cholestyramine binds acid substances including the bile salts. It will also bind acid drugs such as chlorothiazide, phenobarbitone, phenylbutazone, or tetracycline which should be given an hour before the resin. In the case of complete biliary obstruction pruritus can usually be relieved by methyltesterone 25 mg daily in men or norethandrolone 30 mg daily in women. A trial of ampicillin which is excreted in the bile should be given in cases of chronic biliary obstruction in which it is thought that ascending infection may be playing a part.

Primary Biliary Cirrhosis

Biliary cirrhosis is always due to some form of obstruction of the biliary system. Primary biliary cirrhosis refers to cirrhosis due to obstruction of the intrahepatic cholangioles and secondary biliary cirrhosis to cirrhosis due to obstruction of the larger extrahepatic bile ducts, such as bile-duct atresia, impaction of a gall-stone, or stricture formation.

In most cases the aetiology of primary biliary cirrhosis is unknown; however, three factors are occasionally known to cause proliferation of the epithelium of the bile canaliculi, namely infective hepatitis, arsenic ingestion and haemochromatosis.

Some drugs such as methyltesterone constantly cause cholestatic jaundice if used for long enough. Primary biliary cirrhosis occurs almost exclusively in women and is characterised by obstructive jaundice, xanthomata, gross hepatomegaly and later portal hypertension. There may be steatorrhoea and malabsorption as a result of bile failing to reach the intestines. The serum bilirubin and alkaline phosphatase are invariably raised, there is often evidence of hepatocellular damage. Electrophoresis of the plasma proteins shows a marked rise in the β globulins due to an increase in β lipoproteins which transport the increased cholesterol and other lipids which accumulate in the blood.

There are certain serological tests which have been used to help distinguish primary from secondary biliary cirrhosis. The distinction is important as there may be a surgically remediable cause in secondary biliary cirrhosis, whereas any sort of operation is hazardous in primary biliary cirrhosis. Antibodies against bile ductules and non-organ specific antimitochondrial antibodies are present in primary but not secondary biliary cirrhosis (Walker *et al.*, 1965).

Corticosteroids are definitely contra-indicated as they have not been shown to affect the primary condition and they aggravate the osteoporosis resulting from malabsorption.

ACUTE PANCREATITIS

In most cases the aetiology of an attack of acute pancreatitis is not known, but there is an association between attacks of acute pancreatitis and a number of known factors. These are:

1. Cholelithiasis.
2. Alcoholism.
3. Pancreatic duct obstruction.
4. Trauma.
5. Vascular insufficiency.
6. Hyperparathyroidism.
7. Steroid therapy.
8. Hypothermia.
9. Septicaemia.
10. Virus infections, such as mumps.

Clinical Features

In the classical case there is a sudden onset of severe epigastric pain which is constant in intensity but may be relieved by the patient leaning forward or by kneeling forward on the bed. The pain does not always radiate to the back, it is not usually relieved by opiates and is accompanied by vomiting. The physical signs depend on the stage of the disease. In the early stages there may be a resemblance to acute cholecystitis with upper abdominal pain and guarding; at this stage there is no ileus and bowel sounds may be normal. Some hours later the patient becomes shocked, there is peritonitis with widespread rigidity and absent bowel sounds. In the early stages the diagnostic clue may be mild tenderness in the flanks, which usually becomes obvious in the later stages.

The level of serum amylase is helpful but it is essential to realise that raised serum amylase is not diagnostic. Levels over 1000 Somogyi[87] units are highly suggestive but do occur in other causes of peritonitis possibly as a result of associated pancreatic damage. Conditions in which a raised serum amylase may occur are perforated ulcer, paralytic ileus, acute cholecystitis, cirrhosis, mumps, parotitis and renal failure.

87. MICHAEL SOMOGYI. Contemporary biochemist, St. Louis, U.S.A.

The rise in serum amylase may be transient but the urinary amylase is raised for longer; in addition, the serum lipase shows a more sustained rise than the amylase in acute pancreatitis.

Other clinical features which may be present are hyperglycaemia, tetany—due to a reduction in the serum calcium possibly as a result of combination with liberated fats in the peritoneum—electrocardiographic changes and an x-ray appearance of an isolated distended loop of small intestine. The other condition in which an isolated distended loop may be seen is localised ischaemia due to occlusion of a branch of the mesenteric artery.

Treatment

If possible laparotomy should be avoided if the diagnosis is reasonably certain as the mortality of acute pancreatitis is increased following an operation. Pain is treated with analgesics which will not constrict the sphincter of Oddi[88] or cause contraction of the gall bladder. Vagal stimulation of the pancreas can be prevented by blocking the vagi with atropine or propantheline. Continuous gastric suction will prevent gastric contents causing hormonal stimulation of the pancreas by means of secretin and pancreozymin.

Pain may also be relieved by epidural or paravertebral block. Broad-spectrum antibiotics are usually given; corticosteroids are justified if all else seems to be failing.

Trasylol is a proteolytic enzyme inhibitor and there has been one double blind controlled trial which has confirmed that Trasylol improves mortality and may reduce the severity of the illness (Trapnell et al., 1974). Nevertheless the mortality in the controlled group was 25 per cent which seems unusually high, although the mortality in the treated group was 7·5 per cent which would suggest that when used according to the scheme advocated by these authors Trasylol may be beneficial.

Glucagon

Glucagon produced by the islet α-cells is known to reduce both the volume and enzyme content of exocrine pancreatic secretion. Furthermore glucagon levels are raised in acute pancreatitis. It is suggested that following any acute injury to the pancreas there is a rise in glucagon levels which protects the pancreas against auto-injury—only when endogenous glucagon levels fall does pancreatic damage progress. This would account for the delay frequently noted between pancreatic injury and the onset of pancreatic symptoms and signs. It is suggested that on this basis glucagon infusion is logical and worthwhile in the management of acute pancreatitis (Knight et al., 1972).

88. RUGGERO ODDI. 19th century Bologna surgeon.

CHRONIC PANCREATITIS

The commonest features are constant dull upper abdominal or back pain and weight loss, rarely jaundice, diabetes or pancreatic cysts occur.

Pancreatic exocrine insufficiency can be confirmed by measuring the volume, bicarbonate and enzyme content of pancreatic juice obtained by duodenal intubation. Secretin causes the pancreas to produce an increased volume of juice with a high bicarbonate content; pancreozymin increases the enzyme content. In the presence of diffuse damage to the pancreas as a result of chronic pancreatitis, secretin and pancreozymin produce a juice of normal volume but of reduced bicarbonate and enzyme content, whereas in the presence of duct obstruction the volume falls off but the concentration of bicarbonate and enzymes remains roughly normal (Dreiling and Janowitz, 1962). The serum levels of amylase and lipase are measured before and after injection of secretin and pancreozymin—a rise in serum enzymes indicates obstruction of the pancreatic duct. A further refinement is to give an agent which will cause spasm of the sphincter of Oddi (such as morphia) and demonstrate a further rise in the serum enzymes. If the pancreas is completely replaced by fibrous tissue there will be no response to secretin and pancreozymin either as measured by the serum enzymes or by duodenal intubation.

REFERENCES

BAERTL, J. M., SANCETTA, S. M., and GABUSDA, G. J. (1963). *J. clin. Invest.*, **42**, 696.

BIRCHER, J., NULLER, J., GUGGENHEIM, P., and HAEMERLI, U. P. (1966). *Lancet*, **1**, 890.

BRADLEY, S. E., and BRADLEY, G. P. (1947). *J. clin. Invest.*, **26**, 1010.

BRODIE, B. B. (1965). *Proc. roy. Soc. Med.*, **58**, 946.

DREILING, D. A., and JANOWITZ, H. D. (1962). In *Exocrine Pancreas*, a Ciba Symposium. London: J. & A. Churchill.

DYKES, P. W. (1961). *Quart. J. Med.*, **30**, 297.

FENTON, J. C., KNIGHT, E. J., and HUMPHERSON, P. L. (1966). *Lancet*, **1**, 164.

GRACE, N. D., MUENCH, H., and CHALMERS, T. C. (1966). *Gastroenterology*, **50**, 684.

HENCH, P. S. (1952). *Ann. intern. Med.*, **36**, 1.

HISLOP, I. G., WATERS, T. E., KELLOCK, T. D., and SWYNNERTON, B. (1966). *Lancet*, **1**, 945.

JOHNSTON, G. W. (1963). *Gut*, **4**, 90.

JOLLIFFE, N. J., and JELLINEK, E. M. (1941). *Quart. J. Stud. Alcohol*, **2**, 544.

KNIGHT, M. J., CONDON, J. R., and DAY, J. L. (1972). *Lancet*, **1**, 1097.

KRUGMAN, S. (1963). *New. Engl. J. Med.*, **269**, 195.

Lancet (1966a), **1**, 695.

Lancet (1966b), **2**, 1061.

Lancet (1969a), **1**, 119.

Lancet (1969b), **2**, 364.

MACKAY, J. R., WEIDEN, S., and HASKER, J. (1965). *Ann. N.Y. Acad. Sci.*, **124**, 767.

MACKEY, I. R. and WOOD, I. J. (1963). *Gastroenterology*, **45**, 4.

MURRAY-LYON, I. M., STERN, R. B., and WILLIAMS, R. (1973). *Lancet*, **1**, 735.

NEALE, G., CAUGHEY, D. E., MOLLIN, D. C., and BOOTH, C. C. (1966). *Brit. med. J.*, **1**, 382.

OWENS, D., and SHERLOCK, S. (1973). *Brit. med. J.*, **3**, 559.

Public Health Laboratory Services (1968). *Brit. med. J.*, **3**, 451.

RATNOFF, O. D., and PATEK, A. J. (1942). *Medicine (Baltimore)*, **21**, 207.

READ, A. E., SHERLOCK, S., and HARRISON, C. V. (1963). *Gut*, **4**, 378.

SHERLOCK, S. (1968a). *Diseases of Liver and Biliary System*. Oxford: Blackwell Scientific.

SHERLOCK, S. (1968b), *Brit. med. J.*, **3**, 515.

SHORR, E., ZWEIFACH, B. W., FURCHGOTT, R. F., and BAEZ, S. (1951). *Circulation*, **3**, 42.

SICULAR, A., and KARK, A. E. (1965). In *Progress in Liver Diseases*. Eds. Popper, H., and Schaffner, F. New York: Grune & Stratton.

TISDALE, W. A., and KLATSKIN, G. (1960). *Yale J. Biol. Med.*, **33**, 94.

TRAPNELL, J. E., RIGBY, C. C., TALBOT, C. H., and DUNCAN, E. H. (1974). *Brit. J. Surg.*, **61**, 177.

WALKER, J. G., DONIACH, D., ROITT, I. M., and SHERLOCK, S. (1965). *Lancet*, **1**, 827.

WILKINSON, P., and SHERLOCK, S. (1962). *Lancet*, **2**, 1125.

ZIEVE, L. (1958). *Ann. intern. Med.*, **48**, 471.

5

AUTOIMMUNE AND JOINT DISEASES

AUTOIMMUNITY

Great confusion has arisen over the word immunity because it implies absolute protection; a much more suitable word would be "sensitivity" (Gell and Coombs, 1968). Sensitivity (or immunity) is the mechanism by which the body attempts to protect itself against an antigen which it regards as foreign. The two main sensitivity (immunity) mechanisms are:

1. The production of antibodies circulating in the blood. These are gamma globulins and are produced by the plasma cells; circulating (or humoral) antibodies are responsible for immediate sensitivity reactions such as anaphylaxis and urticaria.

2. The production of antibodies bound to circulating lymphocytes; these antibodies are responsible for delayed sensitivity reactions (such as the tuberculin test).

Hypersensitivity (allergy) applies to an increased sensitivity to antigens to which the body has previously been exposed. There are four main hypersensitivity or allergic reactions.

Type I: Anaphylactic reactions.—Circulating (humoral) antibody (IgE) becomes attached to certain tissue cells. When antigen is presented an antibody-antigen reaction takes place leading to damage to the cells to which the antibody is attached and release of histamine. The sites where circulating antibody may become attached to cells are:

(*a*) Respiratory tract (leading to asthma).

(*b*) Skin (leading to urticaria).

(*c*) Gastro-intestinal tract (leading to food allergies).

Type II: Cytotoxic reactions.—Some circulating cells contain antigens and the serum contains circulating antibody. The two do not react together until a third substance or "hapten" is present. (A hapten is a substance which is not itself an antigen but it may "catalyse" an antibody-antigen reaction.) The reaction is characterised by destruction of the cells to which the antigen is attached. Examples:

(*a*) Purpura and haemolytic anaemia with drugs (the drug acts as hapten, the red cells as antigen).

(*b*) Blackwater fever with quinine (malaria-infected red cells are the antigen, the serum contains antibody and quinine is the hapten).

(*c*) Transfusion reactions.

(*d*) Haemolytic disease of the newborn.

Type III: Toxic combinations of antigen and antibody.—The combination is toxic because it becomes deposited in the walls of the small arteries resulting in an arteritis. Examples: foreign serum (antigen) may react with circulating antibody forming toxic complexes leading to arteritis (serum sickness).

Type IV: Delayed sensitivity reactions.—Antibody is attached to lymphocytes. Antigenic tissues attract these lymphocytes because of their attached antibody and lymphocytic infiltration of the area occurs, e.g. infiltration by lymphocytes of an area recently infected by tubercle bacilli leading to an inflammatory reaction which goes on to caseation and fibrosis (post-primary tuberculosis).

These are the mechanisms by which all antigen-antibody reactions take place. The examples given for these reactions have all been antigens (or haptens) introduced to the body from outside; some of them are protective against foreign antigens. Under certain circumstances the body forms antibodies against its own tissue (autoimmunity or autosensitivity). Normally, any antigen brought into contact with the antibody-producing mechanism (reticulo-endothelial system) very early in its development does not induce antibody formation if it is again presented to the antibody-forming mechanism later in life. This is known as "immunological tolerance". Autoimmune diseases are a result of breakdown of immunological tolerance, i.e. the antibody-forming mechanism fails to recognise "self".

There are five ways in which a breakdown of immunological tolerance can occur—some involve alteration of antigen and some of them abnormal production of antibody (Waksman, 1962):

1. *Release of antigens normally isolated* ("*segregated antigen*" *disease*).—Immunological tolerance has not been acquired because the antibody-producing system has never before (even in the embryo) come into contact with the antigen. Examples are: Hashimoto's disease, pernicious anaemia and Addison's disease.

2. *Alteration of normal tissues by drugs or infection.*—Examples are thrombocytopenic purpura and haemolysis with drugs (Sedormid and methyldopa). Another example is contact dermatitis.

3. *Exposure to foreign antigen which is sufficiently alike to cause a cross-reaction with normal tissues.*—Examples: antibody produced against certain strains of streptococcus also reacts with normal heart muscle and glomeruli causing rheumatic fever and acute nephritis. Antibody against intestinal bacteria is also effective against colonic mucosa leading to ulcerative colitis.

4. *An acquired alteration of the immunity process.*—Mutation within the reticulo-endothelial system results in abnormal antibodies against

antigens which have always been present and which hitherto have not excited antibody formation because of immunological tolerance. Examples: Hodgkin's disease and lymphomas which may result in antibodies against normal red cells and platelets (autoimmune haemolytic anaemia and thrombocytopenia).

5. *Exaggerated sensitivity of the immunity apparatus to weak antigens which have always been present.*—For some reason there is a breakdown in immunological tolerance to weak antigens which are always present but do not normally excite antibody formation. Examples: systemic lupus erythematosus in which antibodies are produced to weak antigens normally present in the serum the whole time, e.g. red cells, platelets, white cells, plasma proteins responsible for coagulation, cell nuclei and thyroid tissue. This type of breakdown of immunological tolerance generally results in the "toxic" type of antibody-antigen reaction which becomes deposited in small arteries causing an arteritis. Another example is rheumatoid arthritis.

Discussion of Diseases produced by Autoimmunisation

Hashimoto's[89] disease.—In Hashimoto's disease there is lymphocytic infiltration into the thyroid followed by fibrosis and myxoedema. The circulating level of antibodies to thyroglobulin is usually high and often the serum gamma globulin is elevated. Anti-thyroglobulin antibodies are sometimes found in primary myxoedema (i.e. myxoedema due to disease of thyroid and not secondary to pituitary failure). Low titres are often present in the serum of patients with non-toxic goitre and in normal middle-aged women, but they are of no significance.

An abnormally "sensitive" immunity apparatus is suggested by the fact that in Hashimoto's disease there is an increased incidence of Addison's disease, SLE, haemolytic and pernicious anaemias.

Pernicious anaemia.—Pernicious anaemia is invariably accompanied by atrophic gastritis and infiltration of the gastric mucosa with lymphocytes. The circulating level of antibody to parietal gastric cells is often high, suggesting that the gastric atrophy is due to destruction of the mucosa as a result of parietal cell antibodies. The atrophic mucosa is deficient in producing intrinsic factor which is necessary for the absorption of vitamin B_{12} from the terminal ileum. There are often circulating antibodies to intrinsic factor as well.

"Idiopathic" Addison's disease.—The association of Addison's disease with myxoedema and pernicious anaemia and the lymphocytic infiltration frequently seen in the adrenal cortex in Addison's disease suggests an immune basis. Circulating antibodies to adrenal cortex are found in a few cases of "idiopathic" Addison's disease.

In the three diseases mentioned so far the antibodies in the serum are

89. HAKARU HASHIMOTO (b. 1881). Japanese surgeon.

only against antigen produced by one organ, they are, therefore, called organ specific antibodies (or the segregated antigen diseases).

Haemolytic anaemia.—Drugs and infections may alter the antigenic nature of red cells. The antigen of red cells is contained in a coating of globulin on the cell surface; in normal cells this surface globulin does not react with anti-human globulin, surface antigen only reacts if it is combined with antibody or has been altered (e.g. by drugs). It is this surface antibody which is demonstrated in the Coombs[90] test. Anti-human globulin is prepared by injecting human globulin into rabbits. Human red cells which are coated with abnormal antibody will be haemolysed by anti-human globulin—this is the direct Coombs test. The haemolysis occurs because of the antibody-antigen reaction occurring on the surface of the red cells. Some infections (such as primary atypical pneumonia) cause the production of antibodies in the serum which are also effective against normal red cells. Similar antibodies against normal red cells are produced in diseases of the immunity system which produce harmful antibodies by mutation (e.g. Hodgkin's disease and lymphomas). When there are these circulating antibodies in the serum against normal red cells they cannot be demonstrated until they are made to coat the red cells and then exposing them to anti-human globulin—this is the indirect Coombs test. The direct Coombs test detects antibody already on the surface of red cells; the indirect Coombs test detects antibody which is circulating in the serum. Many drugs and infections affect the platelets and white cells in a similar way, i.e. causing leucopenia and thrombocytopenia.

Acute nephritis.—The kidney probably contains an antigen which cross-reacts with antibody formed against certain strains of streptococci. Similar mechanisms probably account for rheumatic fever and ulcerative colitis. It is most important to note that the demonstration of circulating antibodies against an organ does not mean that the organ has been damaged by an immune process. Circulating antibodies may arise as a result of damage to an organ, for example, myocardial antibodies are found following myocardial infarction, anti-kidney antibodies are found following pyelonephritis and anti-thyroid antibodies in mild thyrotoxicosis. Usually the antibody titres in these conditions are much lower than in those conditions thought to be due to an immune process, none the less, the significance of circulating antibodies is not always clear.

Rheumatoid arthritis.—Many features of rheumatoid arthritis suggest that it is an immune disease, e.g. haemolytic anaemias, arteritis, multisystem involvement and increased gamma globulin. The rheumatoid factor is a macroglobulin (MW approx. 1,000,000) which is probably

90. ROBIN COOMBS. Contemporary Cambridge pathologist.

an antibody produced against normal gamma globulin. The concentration of rheumatoid factor in rheumatoid joints is very high; the typical histological feature of rheumatoid arthritis is infiltration of the synovial membrane with lymphocytes suggesting that a local antibody-antigen reaction (rheumatoid factor and normal gamma globulin) is responsible for the damage. Infections associated with an increase in gamma globulin occasionally stimulate the formation of rheumatoid factor. Rheumatoid factor was found in 50 per cent of patients with SBE in one series (Williams and Kunkel, 1962).

Systemic lupus erythematosus.—Numerous auto-antibodies are produced in SLE against cell nuclei, cytoplasm, red cells, white cells and platelets. One of the antibodies against white cell nuclei is the LE factor (another antibody against nuclei is the antinuclear factor or ANF). *In vitro* white cells mixed with the LE factor phagocytose the nuclei of other white cells resulting in the "LE cell".

The toxic type of antibody-antigen combination which takes place in SLE causes an arteritis which is responsible for the widespread manifestation of the disease. In some susceptible people an SLE-like illness may be caused by drugs such as procainamide, hydrallazine and PAS. Because the antibodies produced in SLE react with antigen in many tissues they are called "non organ specific".

Other diseases which may have a partial autoimmune basis are: ulcerative colitis, Crohn's disease, coeliac disease, Graves' disease, multiple sclerosis, carcinomatosis neuropathy, peripheral neuropathy, pemphigus and aphthous mouth ulcers.

Gamma Globulins and Their Disorders

The gamma (γ) globulins are a distinct band of proteins which migrate to one electrode when human serum proteins are placed in an electric field (electrophoresis).

Most antibodies are found in the gamma globulin fraction; *antibodies* in their turn can act as *antigens* and provoke antibodies if injected into a different species. Globulins which can induce an antibody (i.e. immunity) response in other species are immunoglobulins. There are three main groups of immunoglobulins designated immunoglobulins G, M and A or IgG, IgM and IgA. The normal amounts of these in the serum are:

IgG: 700–1500 mg per cent.
IgM: 60–170 mg per cent.
IgA: 150–250 mg per cent.

Structure of Immunoglobulins (*Brit. med. J.*, 1968)

The structure of immunoglobulins can be represented diagrammatically as four chains of polypeptides parallel to each other with the shorter "light" chains enclosing a pair of larger "heavy" chains. All four chains are joined at intervals by sulphydryl bonds (Fig. 10). All the immunoglobulins have the same basic structure except that IgM (macroglobulins) consist of aggregates of 5 of the basic units. There are only two types of light (L) chains known as $\varkappa$ (kappa) and λ (lambda); these are never mixed in the same *molecule*. Normally two-thirds of the immunoglobulins contain $\varkappa$ L chains and one-third contains λ L chains. IgG contains 4 different types of H chain which are antigenically distinct (i.e. when isolated and injected into another species each provokes a sepa-

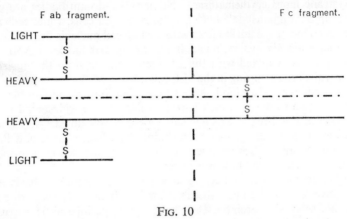

FIG. 10

rate and different antibody response); the 4 antigenically different H chains on IgG are designated a, b, c, and d. IgA contains only one antigenic type of H chain designated an α H chain as does IgM which is designated a μ H chain. It should be noted that there are probably hundreds of different antibodies contained in the few antigenically distinct H chains, thus there are six basic types of H chain containing 300–400 amino acids; the different antibodies are produced by jiggling around with the last, say, dozen amino acids in the chain—the vast bulk of the chain remaining unchanged. It is the vast bulk of the chain which is responsible for producing the recognisable six basic types of H chain.

Individual molecules of immunoglobulins can be split by "papain digestion" as shown in Fig. 10. This produces two fragments which still have antigenic properties and are therefore called the antibody fragment (Fab) and one fragment which crystallizes (Fc).

IgG contains about 80 per cent of the antibodies including antibacterial and antiviral antibodies; IgG alone has other properties which it owes to its Fc component, viz.:

1. Ability to cross the placenta.
2. Ability to initiate complement fixation.

3. Fixation to skin receptor sites for sensitisation in the passive cutaneous anaphylactic reaction.

IgA comprises about 10 per cent of human antibodies which are:

1. Isohaemagglutinins.
2. Anti-brucella.
3. Anti-diphtheria.
4. Anti-insulin.

IgA is found in high concentrations in secretions such as saliva, tears and bronchial mucus. IgA found in secretions contains an additional unit—the T chain which presumably allows it to pass into these secretions. IgA found in secretion is not antigenically identical to serum IgA. Secretion IgA has some antibacterial and antiviral activity.

IgM contains 5–10 per cent of antibody, IgM constitutes about one-third of macroglobulin normally present, the remaining two-thirds are an α_2 and a γ globulin—this α_2 macroglobulin is *not* an immuno-globulin. The antibodies which IgM contain are:

1. Heterophile antibody.
2. Wassermann antibody.
3. Cold agglutinins.
4. Endotoxins of Gram-negative organisms.

It is important to note that there are immunoglobulins other than IgG, IgA and IgM; already IgD and IgE have been discovered.

In normals a small amount of IgG globulin (not IgA or IgM) is found in the urine mainly as Fab fragments.

The immunoglobulins are synthesised in the plasma cells and probably the lymphocytes; each cell can only produce one type of H or L chain.

Disorders of the Immunoglobulins

Increase in the immunoglobulins (plasma cell dyscrasias) may affect all components (i.e. diffuse increase) or it may affect only one component (i.e. local increase). Any local increase in immunoglobulins is known as an M component. This terminology has given rise to confusion; and M component is *not* the same as either macroglobulins or an increase in IgM; an M component merely means a local increase in one of the immunoglobulins whether it be IgA, IgG, IgM, etc. An M component is believed to indicate that only one clone of cells is producing an excess of protein; it is therefore referred to as *mono*clonal "gammopathy". Increase in several proteins (diffuse increase) suggests that several clones are involved, i.e. polyclonal "gammopathy". It should be noted that the protein produced need not be abnormal qualitatively, it may only be increased in quantity.

Diffuse increase in the globulins suggests hyperplasia of the plasma cells and lymphocytes, the ratio of $\varkappa$ to λ light chains remains normal. These can be measured in the serum globulins now that anti-$\varkappa$ and anti-λ antisera are available.

Causes of diffuse increase in globulins:

1. Infection and neoplasia—usually an increase in IgG except in trypanosomiasis in which there is an increase in IgM.

2. Hepatic disease—the increase may be in IgG, IgA or IgM; in cirrhosis there is loss of a clear distinction between the beta and gamma globulins (so-called "beta-gamma bridging").

3. Collagen diseases.

Causes of an M Band (Local Increase in Globulins)

1. *Myeloma* in which approximately 75 per cent of the M components are IgG and 25 per cent IgA although rarely M bands occur in other components. Not all patients with myeloma with an M band have Bence Jones protein in the urine and occasionally in myeloma there may be no M band, the presence of Bence Jones protein in the urine being the only evidence of a protein abnormality. The Bence Jones protein, of course, appears when the urine is warmed and disappears when the urine is brought to boiling point, although this may be difficult to see if there is associated albuminuria. Bence Jones protein consists of light chains, either $\varkappa$ or λ but never both in the same patient; these can be detected by paper electrophoresis and immuno-electrophoresis of the urine. The particular L chain in the urine is the same as those occurring in the protein of the M band. For some entirely unknown reason the conditions causing proliferation of the plasma cells (plasma cell dyscrasias) produce both $\varkappa$ and λ L chain proteins in excess but when there is Bence Jones protein either in the blood or urine excessive amounts of only one type of L chain are produced. This may be important diagnostically: abnormalities of the plasma cells with a good prognosis produce the two types of L chains in the proportion normally found in the body—those plasma cell dyscrasias with a poor prognosis produce only one type of L chain.

2. *Waldenstrom's macroglobulinaemia.*—The plasma cells in this condition more closely resemble large lymphocytes (lymphocytoid cells), the serum contains an M band in the IgM component. Bence Jones protein occurs in 10–15 per cent of patients. Features of the condition are hepatosplenomegaly, lymphadenopathy, anaemia, coagulation disorders, cryoglobulins and increased blood viscosity.

Cryoglobulins are a feature of myeloma and *Waldenstrom's* macroglobulinaemia; they give rise to Raynaud's phenomenon, vascular occlusion and peripheral gangrene. The increased blood viscocity causes heart failure, dyspnoea and localised bulging of the retinal veins which may be associated with retinal haemorrhages and exudates. Transient limb paresis, neuropathies and myelopathies may occur.

Unlike myeloma in Waldenstrom's macroglobulinaemia the following are rare:

1. Renal impairment.
2. Hypercalaemia.
3. Osteolytic bone lesions.
4. Amyloidosis.

The treatment of Waldenstrom's macroglobulinaemia is plasma-phoresis for the viscosity-induced manifestations and corticosteroids for the bleeding disorders, followed by chlorambucil.

Benign M bands (essential paraproteinaemia).—These occur in patients with no evidence of malignant disease; the incidence is 1 per cent over 50 years of age and 3 per cent over 70 (Hällén, 1966). The M band may be permanent or transient (Young, 1969) and associated with a wide variety of diseases other than those causing a diffuse increase in glob-ulins. The main problem of M bands is to decide whether they are truly benign or are a manifestation of myeloma, macroglobulinaemia, plasma cell leukaemia or Hodgkin's disease. Contrary to previous reports there is no evidence that paraproteins are more common in other malignancies than in the general population (Hobbs, 1969).

The factors suggesting that M bands are associated with malignant disease in a particular patient are:

1. Presence of Bence Jones protein in the urine.
2. Diminution in the other immunoglobulins.
3. A high level of paraprotein greater than 1 g/dl for IgA and IgM and greater than 2 g/dl for IgG.
4. A rapid rise in the level of paraprotein.
5. Presence of anaemia; leucopenia or thrombocytopenia.
6. Presence of bone marrow infiltration or osteolytic lesions.

Heavy chain disease (Fc fragment disease).—A few cases have been described of patients with a lymphoma-like illness with an M band and urinary protein consisting of the Fc fragment of IgG.

Immunological Deficiency Syndromes

The main mechanisms protecting against infections are:

1. Antibodies.
2. Cellular mechanisms mediated by lymphocytes.
3. Polymorphs.

There are of course other mechanisms, e.g. interferon and complement. As a very rough working rule antibody deficiency gives rise to infections with the common cocci; impairment of cellular mechanisms gives rise to infections caused by intracellular organisms such as viruses, fungi (e.g. monilia, histoplasma, aspergillus and cryptococcus), and proto-zoa (pneumocystis carinii and toxoplasma); deficiency of polymorphs causes infection with organisms normally of low pathogenicity usually found as commensals in the mouth or large gut. The antibody deficiency diseases are:

Congenital.—1. Agammaglobulinaemia—sex-linked—seen only in male children.

2. Wisckott-Aldrich syndrome: eczema, infections, bleeding.

3. Ataxia telangiectasia.

4. Congenital rubella-induced agammaglobulinaemia.

5. Late onset hypogammaglobulinaemia (higher than normal incidence of hypogammaglobulinaemia in relatives).

Acquired. — Primary hypogammaglobulinaemia — occasionally patients have a thymoma, rarely there may be a high family incidence, usually, IgG, IgA and IgM reduced, occasionally only one immuno-globulin reduced and others increased (a situation known as dysgam-maglobulinaemia).

Secondary immunoglobulin deficiencies (from Hobbs, 1968).—1. Physiological—IgG is low in premature babies; the normal adult levels are usually reached by age 3. Occasionally there is delay in producing IgG (and other immunoglobulins).

2. Excess catabolism—mainly IgG
   Nephrotic syndrome
   Malnutrition
   Protein-losing enteropathy
   Dystrophia myotonica.

3. Marrow disorders—mainly IgG
   Hypoplasia
   Metastases
   Myelosclerosis.

4. Immunoglobulin deficiencies probably due to toxic factors—IgM usually affected first followed by IgA then IgG
   Uraemia
   Corticosteroids
   Cytotoxic drugs
   Gluten-sensitive enteropathy
   Severe infection
   Diabetes
   Thyrotoxicosis.

5. Reticulo-endothelial neoplasia—again IgM first followed by IgA or IgG
   Reticulosarcoma

Mycosis fungoides
Hodgkin's disease
Lymphosarcoma
Giant follicular lymphoma
Lymphatic leukaemia
Myeloma
Macroglobulinaemia.

The lymphoid disorders leading to disturbed cellular immunity are:

1. Acute leukaemia
2. Chronic lymphatic leukaemia
3. Lymphosarcoma
4. Hodgkin's disease
5. Irradiation
6. Antimetabolite and corticosteroid administration
7. Thymoma
8. Thymic aplasia.

The main causes of reduced or abnormal polymorphs are:

1. Myeloid leukaemia
2. Lymphatic leukaemia
3. Hypersplenism
4. Uraemia
5. Toxic drugs
6. Bone marrow depression or replacements.

RADIOLOGY OF BONES AND JOINTS

BONES

Increase in Bone Density (Sclerosis)

Paget's[91] disease.—This may be localised or widespread. The bone involved may become deformed, but the involved area does not project above the surface of the bone—unlike secondary deposits which may grow outside the confines of the bones. The trabecular pattern of the bone is replaced by dense structureless bone. Bone deformity causes bowing of the tibia and a triradiate pelvis. In the skull, Paget's disease may cause an area of rarefaction which is well circumscribed (osteoporosis circumscripta) or platybasia in which the soft skull is indented by the vertebral column. Normally the odontoid process of the axis should not project more than 5 mm above the straight line drawn backwards from the hard palate (Chamberlain's line).

Secondary deposits.—The only common primary carcinoma which produces sclerotic secondaries is prostatic. Rarely sclerotic secondaries

91. SIR JAMES PAGET (1814–1899). London surgeon.

occur from a breast carcinoma or in the reticuloses. Sclerotic second-aries occur mainly in vertebrae, pelvis and ribs, the long bones are rarely involved.

Chronic osteomyelitis.

Myelofibrosis (often but not invariably due to secondary carcinoma).

Avascular area of bone, e.g. infarction, or damage to blood supply (via the periostium) as in a fractured scaphoid.

Marble bone disease (osteopetrosis or Albers-Schönberg[92] disease).

Fluorosis due to ingestion of fluoride usually in drinking water. The vertebrae are usually sclerotic and there is calcification of vertebral ligaments (in contradistinction, the vertebrae in ankylosing spondylitis are rarefied).

In the skull, sclerosis may be due to a meningioma or hyperostosis frontalis (interna or externa) in which the frontal bone is thickened as well as sclerotic.

Skeletal scintiscanning using Strontium[85] may be useful in detecting bone secondaries. There is an increased uptake of the isotope by osteolytic and osteosclerotic secondaries except for multiple myeloma. There is also an increased uptake in osteo-arthritis and Paget's disease.

Osteomalacia and Osteoporosis

In osteomalacia there is loss of mineral from the bone but the protein matrix remains relatively intact. If the mineral loss is sustained the pro-tein matrix may become secondarily diminished and the radiological features of osteoporosis are superimposed. Osteomalacia is exemplified by the bone disorder which occurs due to lack of vitamin D. One of the features of this bone disease is an excess of osteoid tissue. Conditions other than lack of vitamin D can cause an increase in osteoid tissue, e.g. renal failure, renal tubular defects, hyperparathyroidism, hyper-thyroidism and Paget's disease (Morgan and Fourman, 1969). Cases of osteomalacia are nutritional deficiency, partial gastrectomy, mal-absorption and obstructive jaundice.

In osteoporosis there is a decrease in the protein matrix of the bone, but the matrix which remains calcifies normally. Causes of *osteoporosis* are old age, Cushing's syndrome (and corticosteroid treatment), im-mobilisation and thyrotoxicosis. In intestinal malabsorption in which calcium and protein are malabsorbed, osteomalacia and osteoporosis may coexist.

Radiological signs which unequivocally indicate *osteomalacia* are: the Milkman[93] fracture or Looser[94] zone which is a tongue of radio-

92. HEINRICH ERNEST ALBERS-SCHÖNBERG (1865–1921). Hamburg radiologist.
93. LOUIS ARTHUR MILKMAN (1895–1951). Scranton (Pa.) radiologist.
94. EMIL LOOSER (1877–1936). Zürich surgeon.

translucency extending about a centimeter into the bone from the surface; they are most frequently seen in the upper end of the femur and humerus or lower end of the tibia. Bending of the bones usually indicates osteomalacia.

Radiological signs which indicate *hyperparathyroidism* are:

1. *Subperiostial erosions*, usually best seen in the middle phalanges of the fingers and in the femoral necks. The cortex of the phalanges may become fragmented and lace-like.

2. *Multiple bone cysts* which may project from the surface of the bones (von Recklinghausen's[95] disease).

3. *Loss of the lamina dura* round the teeth.

4. *Mottling of the skull*—"pepper-pot skull".

In hyperparathyroidism the radiological appearances of osteomalacia usually appear later.

The changes of *osteoporosis* are most marked in the vertebrae. There is increased translucency of the bones with loss of trabeculae. However, the trabeculae that do remain usually appear sclerotic particularly in lines of stress—thus in the vertebrae the vertical trabeculae appear sclerotic whereas the horizontal trabeculae may be difficult to see. The width of the cortex of the bones is reduced, it is also more irregular than normal, but in contrast with the increased translucency (rarefaction) of the cancellous bone the cortex may appear sclerotic. Osteoporosis usually involves some bones while sparing others, thus wedge-shaped collapse of a few vertebrae is highly suggestive. *Osteomalacia* is a disease which affects the whole skeleton evenly so that any deformity tends to affect all the vertebrae equally. It also tends to cause the "cod fish" spine in which the intervertebral discs indent the surface of the vertebrae more or less equally. Collapse of a single vertebra or localised Schmorl nodes favours *osteoporosis*. As a working rule osteoporosis affects the axial skeleton (spine and limb girdles) more than the long bones, therefore, osteoporosis should only be diagnosed from an x-ray of the lumbar spine (preferably a lateral view).

There are two causes of bone disease secondary to renal disease (renal osteodystrophy). The first is due to renal failure in which the kidneys fail to excrete phosphate. This is accompanied by an acidosis, there is diminished absorption of calcium from the gut and increased resistance to vitamin D. The lowered serum calcium may stimulate the parathyroids causing hyperparathyroidism, thus the bone abnormalities will be those of rickets in children or osteomalacia in adults with the addition of hyperparathyroidism. In addition to the effects of osteomalacia on the spine there are often areas of sclerosis in relation to the intervertebral discs ("rugger-jersey spine").

95. Friedrich Daniel von Recklinghausen (1833–1910). Strasbourg pathologist.

The other type of renal osteodystrophy occurs in tubular defects in which there is a tubular inability to reabsorb phosphate, amino acids and glucose (Fanconi syndrome). The tubular loss of phosphate results in hypophosphataemia and failure to calcify bone resulting in osteomalacia and rickets which is resistant to vitamin D. Both these types of renal osteodystrophy may require large doses of vitamin D.

Causes of Localised Translucency of Bone

1. *In relation to arthritis.*
2. *Simple bone cysts.*—These are usually in the upper end of humerus and are surrounded by a rim of sclerotic bone. The cyst may be divided by bony septa and are usually filled with fluid. If the "cyst" is filled with fibrous tissue it is called fibrous dysplasia. When this condition is seen in many bones it is called polyostotic fibrous dysplasia.
3. *Secondary deposits* particularly from thyroid, bronchus, breast and kidney. They are usually irregular in outline. Myeloma causes widespread areas of translucency which are often well defined.
4. *Reticuloses* usually look like secondaries but leukaemia may cause numerous pin-point translucent areas.
6. *Sarcoidosis* seen particularly in the phalanges.
5. *Histiocytosis X* (lipoidoses).
7. *Tumours of the bone.*

Causes of Periostial Calcification (Periostitis)

1. *Subperiostial haemorrhage* which may be due to trauma or spontaneous bleeding such as in leukaemia or haemophilia.
2. *Following a fracture.*
3. *Bone infections:* pyogenic, tuberculous or syphilitic.
4. *Pulmonary osteo-arthropathy.*
5. *Bone neoplasms and secondary deposits.*

JOINTS

The radiological sign common to all forms of arthritis is narrowing of the joint space. Changes occurring in association with a narrowed joint space are:

Osteophyte formation at the edges of the joint.

Areas of bone resorption which may be erosions of the joint surface or be entirely within the substance of the bones.

Decalcification of bones.

Periostial calcification.

Periarticular thickening of adjacent soft tissues.

Rheumatoid arthritis.—The distribution of joints involved is a valuable pointer. The interphalangeal joints (except the distal I-P joint), second and third metacarpo-phalangeal joints and wrist are involved most frequently. The joint space is narrowed and there are erosions of the joint surfaces and "spindling" of the fingers, due to associated inflammation causing thickening of periarticular structures. A rheumatoid nodule may be seen in the soft tissues. Usually there is decalcification of the bones whose joints are affected. Later in the disease the joint becomes distorted and the joint cavity entirely disappears because of fibrous or bony ankylosis. A very severe form of joint deformity occurs particularly after Still's disease and is known as arthritis mutilans.

Psoriatic arthritis.—This is similar to rheumatoid arthritis except that all the interphalangeal joints (including the distal) are involved, but involvement of metacarpo-phalangeal joints is rare. Rheumatoid nodules, arteritis and neuropathy do not occur. Involvement of the nails with psoriasis is almost always present in psoriatic arthritis.

Arthritis with ulcerative colitis.—The arthritis is similar to rheumatoid except that knees, ankles and sacro-iliac joints are more frequently involved. The rheumatoid factor is absent and the arthritis improves as the primary condition improves.

Reiter's syndrome.—The arthritis is similar to rheumatoid except that periostial calcification is commoner and that calcification of the plantar fascia particularly at its attachment to the os calcis is very common (calcaneal spur).

SLE.—Similar to rheumatoid except that, like psoriatic arthritis, all the interphalangeal joints are often affected.

Ankylosing spondylitis (rheumatoid spondylitis).—Widening of the sacro-iliac joint space occurs because of joint erosion. Later there is narrowing of the joint space and calcification of intervertebral discs and longitudinal ligaments of the spine and kyphosis ("bamboo spine").

Osteo-arthritis.—Narrowing of the joint spaces particularly of hips, knees, and lumbar spine occurs together with osteophytic formation at the joint margins and calcification of synovial membranes and ligaments. Cyst-like areas are often seen near the joint surface but do not become sclerotic in relation to the joint; later bony ankylosis occurs.

Charcot's[96] arthropathy.—This is a severe form of osteo-arthritis with synovial calcification, often calcified intra-articular loose bodies and severe joint deformity. Diminished sensitivity to deep pain is responsible. The condition occurs with tabes dorsalis and peripheral neuropathy in the lower limbs, with syringomyelia and peripheral neuropathy in the upper limbs. An identical x-ray appearance may occur in joints which have been frequently injected with intra-articular steroids.

Gout.—Narrowing of the joint spaces occurs with well-defined "punched-out" circular erosions of the bones in relation to the joint. The

96. JEAN MARTIN CHARCOT (1825–1893). Paris neurologist.

periarticular soft tissues are usually swollen, by inflammation or tophi. Only one joint at a time is affected in acute gout. However, following many attacks of gout, chronic gouty arthritis occurs in which several joints are involved—there are usually tophi in relation to the deformed joints.

Alkaptonuria.—This causes calcification of the intervertebral discs and dark pigmentation of cartilage (seen in the ear) and tendons (seen on the back of the hand).

Infective arthritis.—Early there is slight opacity of the joint space and swelling of soft tissues compared with the opposite side due to intra-articular fluid. The development of an effusion causes widening of the joint space. After about two weeks the surrounding bone becomes de-calcified and periostial calcification begins, bony ankylosis is common. The x-ray appearances are similar in tuberculous arthritis.

RHEUMATOID ARTHRITIS

Predisposing Factors

Age: the mean age of onset is around 40 in men and women (ERC 1950).

Sex: women are three times more commonly affected than men. About 5 per cent of women in this country are affected.

Heredity: the incidence of this disease and the frequency of a positive rheumatoid factor are higher in the relatives of patients than in the general population.

Climate: the disease is very rare in the tropics—probably because of the reduced life-expectancy.

Basic Pathology

The disease begins with hyperaemia, oedema and lymphocyte in-filtration of the synovial membrane followed by an effusion into the joint cavity. Similar changes occur in the joint capsule and surrounding ligaments. The synovial membrane becomes thickened and fibrous but the joint space becomes thinner as a result of damage to cartilage. Later fibrous and body ankylosis occurs.

Rheumatoid Factor

This is a macroglobulin, the Rose-Waaler and Latex fixation tests are two different methods of measuring the rheumatoid factor. One or other test is positive in 85 per cent of cases of definite rheumatoid arthritis. The rheumatoid factor is found less commonly in cases of otherwise typical rheumatoid arthritis occurring in the tropics. A persistently present rheumatoid factor is associated with a poor prognosis, in mild cases the factor is absent from the serum during remissions. LE cells are found in about 15 per cent of patients with pure rheumatoid arthritis.

Diagnosis

The American Rheumatism Association (1959) has devised a useful method of making a "definite" diagnosis. Joint symptoms must be present for at least six weeks and at least five of the following findings must occur:

1. Morning joint stiffness.
2. Pain on movement of a joint.
3. Soft tissue thickening over a joint.
4. Soft tissue thickening over a second joint.
5. Spontaneous symmetrical joint swelling.
6. Subcutaneous nodules.
7. Characteristic x-ray findings.
8. Presence of rheumatoid factor.
9. Characteristic histological changes in the synovial membrane.
10. Characteristic histological changes in the nodule.

The occurrence of so many manifestations outside the joints is responsible for the condition sometimes being called "rheumatoid disease".

Extra-articular Manifestations

1. Anaemia: this may be of three types: hypochromic due to diminished ability to utilise iron, macrocytic or haemolytic.

2. Predisposition to infection particularly leg ulceration in the presence of peripheral neuropathy.

3. Arteritis and Raynaud's phenomenon. The arteritis may be acute and histologically indistinguishable from polyarteritis nodosa; alternatively intimal proliferation of the digital arterioles may occur insidiously.

4. Pericardial and pleural effusions. The effusions may be serous or pseudochylous and are rich in protein and desquamated cells and low in sugar content.

5. Cardiomyopathy with non-specific fibrosis and rheumatoid nodules in the myocardium. Aortic incompetence rarely occurs.

6. Rheumatoid nodules in the lungs. Caplan's syndrome consists of a chest x-ray appearance of discrete nodules in patients with pneumoconiosis which is usually not severe. The nodules may cavitate and disappear, the patient usually has a strongly positive Rose-Waaler test, although joint deformity need not be present. Rheumatoid involvement of crico-arytenoid joints may lead to hoarseness and stridor.

7. Diffuse interstitial pulmonary fibrosis.
8. Proteinuria.
9. Amyloidosis.

10. Peripheral neuropathy and/or entrapment neuropathies. From a clinical point of view it is important *not* to assume that all peripheral nerve lesions in a patient with rheumatoid arthritis are due to a rheumatoid neuropathy—readily remediable compression neuropathies due to deformed and swollen joints and extra-articular soft tissues occur frequently.

11. Carpal tunnel syndrome.

12. Eye complications: kerato-conjunctivitis sicca (Sjögren's[97] disease), corneal ulceration, uveitis, cytoid bodies in the retina and scleromalacia perforans.

13. Lymphadenopathy.

Prognosis

The main factors associated with a good prognosis are asymmetrical joint involvement, short initial attack, rapid response to treatment of the initial attack and a persistently low ESR.

Treatment

In acute attacks rest is still the treatment of choice, specific anti-inflammatory and analgesic drugs are only needed if symptoms fail to subside after a reasonable period of rest. Aspirin is given to relieve the pain, it does not have any specific anti-inflammatory activity but is usually the most effective analgesic. Aspirin may produce gastric bleeding—this is said to occur in about 70 per cent of patients taking the drug. The bleeding does not bear any relation to dyspepsia or previous gastric ulcer. Enteric-coated aspirin causes less bleeding. The main drawbacks to bed rest are hypercalcaemia, weakening of voluntary muscles, loss of proper alignment of joints, loss of cardiac reserve and hypostatic pneumonia.

Splinting of the joints is necessary for the correction and prevention of deformities and at night to relieve pain (by complete immobilisation) of painful joints.

If aspirin in adequate doses fails to relieve the symptoms or if dyspepsia occurs, it is necessary to substitute or add other anti-inflammatory drugs. Indomethacin ("Indocid"), ibuprofen ("Brufen"), naproxen ("Naprosyn"), mefenamic acid ("Ponstan") should be tried roughly in this order. Phenylbutazone is now generally not used until the others have been tried.

Corticosteroids.—The main indications are (ERC, 1962):

1. Patients under 50—with progressive disease of more than two year's duration.

2. Radiological evidence of progressive joint damage.

97. HENRIK SAMUEL CONRAD SJÖGREN (b. 1899). Stockholm ophthalmologist.

3. Patients who are unable to undergo conservative treatment.
4. Severe chronic invalids.

Intra-articular steroids.—These are often beneficial, but should not be repeated too often as the joint may be damaged further. *Gold* is still used. Injections are given at weekly intervals, it is always combined with other forms of treatment. If there is no improvement with one course of gold it is valueless to give further courses. Toxic effects are frequent and include albuminuria, leucopenia, stomatitis and skin reactions.

Felty's[98] **syndrome** is rheumatoid arthritis with splenomegaly and leucopenia.

Sjögren's syndrome is rheumatoid arthritis with kerato-conjunctivitis sicca due to deficient secretion of the lachrymal glands. The salivary glands are also involved.

Still's disease is an acute form of rheumatoid arthritis occurring usually between the ages of 2 and 4. Systemic and constitutional effects are much more in evidence than in rheumatoid arthritis. Lymphadeno-pathy and a leucocytosis are common. Corticosteroids are used much earlier than in adult rheumatoid arthritis.

Palindromic rheumatism.—This term is used to describe recurrent acute attacks of arthritis and inflammation of the periarticular structures. There is no permanent joint deformity even after many attacks. The ESR may be raised but the rheumatoid factor is always absent. A small proportion of patients who have had numerous attacks of palindromic rheumatism will develop true rheumatoid arthritis.

Ankylosing spondylitis (rheumatoid spondylitis).—The sacro-iliac joints are always involved, usually the spine and sometimes the larger peripheral joints of the legs are also affected. The disease is much commoner in men and occurs at an earlier age than rheumatoid arthritis. Presenting symptoms may be low backache, joint pains worse in the morning, and iritis. The main complications are:

Aortitis and myocarditis—leading to aortic incompetence and cardiac failure.

Iritis in 20–40 per cent of patients.

Atlanto-axial subluxation.

Certain accompaniments of rheumatoid arthritis do not occur in ankylosing spondylitis, viz., rheumatoid nodules, rheumatoid factor, arteritis and peripheral neuropathy. In treatment phenylbutazone is the drug of choice as nearly all patients respond to it. Radiotherapy and steroids are only used when a trial of phenylbutazone has failed and the disease is progressing rapidly. There is often a family history of the disease and the incidence of prostatitis is higher than in the general

98. AUGUSTUS ROI FELTY (b. 1895). Hartford, Connecticut, physician.

population. There is also a higher incidence of Reiter's disease and psoriasis in the relatives of affected patients. The sacro-iliac joints are examined by:

1. Pressing the pelvis backwards by pressing on the anterior superior iliac spines.
2. Pressing the pelvis together by pressing on both iliac crests.
3. Pushing the sacrum forwards when the patient is lying face down.

If the sacro-iliac joints are inflamed these manoeuvres will cause pain. In ankylosing spondylitis pain may also be elicited by pressure on the symphysis pubis, ischial tuberosities and greater trochanters.

Reiter's disease.—This consists of urethritis, conjunctivitis and arthritis. It is rare but not unknown in women, usually it follows an attack of non-gonococcal urethritis (which is probably due to a mycoplasma) or an attack of bacillary dysentery or non-specific diarrhoea. The first manifestation is usually urethritis followed by arthritis which is characteristically bilateral and involves knees and ankles. The soft tissues surrounding the joint are often excessively tender. The arthritis may last three months and it relapses in 10 per cent of cases. The arthritis is also associated with plantar fascitis and tendonitis— calcification of the plantar fascia gives rise to the "calcaneal spur" which is virtually diagnostic; iritis and conjunctivitis may not occur in the first attacks. Important diagnostic features are the pain in the feet, low back pain and thickening of the periarticular tissues. The arthritis which is commonest in the knees and ankles may relapse and remit. Rarely, keratoderma blenorrhagica, a skin lesion resembling psoriasis, may appear on the palms and soles and involve the nails, it is commoner in the post-dysenteric variety. The incidence of psoriasis and ankylosing spondylitis is higher in the relatives of patients who have Reiter's disease than in the remainder of the population. A shallow ulcerated lesion on the penis known as circinate balanitis involves the glans and is commoner in the venereal variety. The iritis demands urgent treatment with steroid and atropine drops; the arthritis is treated with rest and analgesics. The cardiac manifestations are similar to those of ankylosing spondylitis namely pericarditis, myocarditis and aortitis.

Unusual Causes of Arthritis include:

Sickle-cell anaemia and haemophilia.
Serum sickness and drug sensitivity.
Brucellosis—generally a monoarticular arthritis involving hip or knee.
Dysentery (amoebic or bacilliary).
Ulcerative colitis and Crohn's disease.
Rubella.
Mumps.

Glandular fever.

Behçet's syndrome (stomatitis, genital ulceration, recurrent iritis, vasculitis and peripheral neuritis).

Intermittent hydrarthrosis.

Meningococcal septicaemia.

Sarcoidosis.

Whipple's disease (lymphadenopathy, skin pigmentation, steatorrhoea and arthritis).

Familial Mediterranean fever (FMF).

Primary hypercholesterolaemia.

Angiokeratoma corporis diffusum.

Alkaptonuria.

Haemochromatosis.

Hyperparathyroidism.

Acromegaly.

Myxoedema.

OTHER COLLAGEN DISORDERS

There is some clinical overlap between the collagen disorders, for example patients with classical rheumatoid arthritis sometimes develop polyarteritis or SLE and those with polyarteritis may develop dermatomyositis or rheumatoid arthritis. None the less the most common course of each of them is along fairly well-defined, distinct pathways. It is worthwhile from diagnostic, prognostic and therapeutic points of view to think of them as distinct clinical entities but to bear in mind that they may have a common pathogenesis.

Polyarteritis Nodosa

The medium and small arteries are mainly involved and the lesions may be seen in any tissue or organ; however, there are certain clinical features which are useful pointers to the diagnosis. Unlike all the other collagen disorders polyarteritis is commoner in men; the characteristic nodes in relation to the arteries occur in only about a third of patients. As a general rule the collagen disorders are multisystem diseases, but there are exceptions to this rule—one system may be involved for years before the disease becomes generalised. This is important in polyarteritis because the lung lesions may present first and prompt diagnosis and treatment with steroids at this stage may prevent the fatal renal lesions developing. The lung lesions consist of transient patchy shadowing in the lung fields which may not be limited by interlobar septa; asthma and a peripheral blood eosinophilia usually accompany the lung shadowing. In polyarteritis there is usually a leucocytosis in the peripheral blood in contrast to SLE in which there is usually a leucopenia. The leucocytosis is due to an increase in polymorphs unless there are asthmatic features in which case eosinophilia may contribute to the leucocytosis. Eosinophilia in the absence of asthmatic features is uncommon. Another presentation which should alert one is the presence of hypertension with a slight fever or non-specific abdominal pain which is occasionally severe enough to simulate an acute abdomen. The fever may be accompanied by a tachycardia which is out of all proportion to the height of the temperature. In the eye the usual changes of hypertension may be seen affecting the arteries; in addition nodes are occasionally seen in relation to the arteries. Unlike arteriosclerotic changes the arterial narrowing and irregularity which occurs in polyarteritis may be patchy and involve only one eye. Involvement of the central retinal artery may cause unilateral blindness.

Two other features occur more commonly in polyarteritis than in the other collagen diseases, the first is Raynaud's phenomenon and the second is peripheral neuropathy. The neuropathy tends to be mainly motor and involve individual peripheral nerves unlike rheumatoid arthritis which is predominantly sensory and has a "glove and stocking" distribution. Like all the collagen disorders there may be myositis and arthritis. The most suitable sites for biopsy are skin, muscle, artery, testis, liver and kidney. An EMG may be useful in detecting involved muscle and thus indicating the most suitable muscle to biopsy. Renal involvement tends to be of two main types: one in which the larger renal arteries are involved in common with arteries elsewhere in the body, this type of involvement producing systemic hypertension; the other type of renal involvement affects the smaller intrarenal vessels leading to a clinical picture similar to acute nephritis—in this type of renal involvement the blood pressure may be normal.

Polyarteritis usually runs a course of about a year; at the end of this time the disease either remits or the patient dies usually from hypertension or chronic renal failure. There is some evidence that steroids promote arterial thrombosis and precipitate malignant hypertension in polyarteritis (Fernandez-Herlihy, 1960). There is also some evidence that early treatment with steroids in pulmonary involvement will prevent the renal complications (Rose and Spencer, 1957). In the established case steroids should be given in sufficient doses to abolish symptoms; they probably need not be given in doses which completely suppress the disease as this does not improve the long-term prognosis (Medical Research Council, 1960). It is essential to note that before the advent of steroids over half the patients with polyarteritis recovered (Grant, 1940).

There are four conditions which are believed to be variants of polyarteritis:

1. Giant-cell or temporal arteritis.
2. Wegener's[99] granulomatosis.
3. Senile arteritis (polymyalgia rheumatica).
4. Takayasu's [100] disease.

The term temporal arteritis is of course a complete misnomer as the larger medium-sized artery in any organ may be involved particularly coronary, renal and mesenteric; none the less, the temporal arteries are the most frequently involved. When the temporal artery is inflamed, tender and non-pulsatile the diagnosis is easy but it is important to note that by the time the patient is seen the severe acute signs may have subsided and all that is left is headache and an elevated ESR. A recent study indicates that intensive treatment with steroids does seem to improve the 5-year survival in patients with polyarteritis nodosa (Frohnert and Sheps, 1967). Immunosuppressive drugs are justified in critical cases. It is essential to palpate the whole course of both terminal arteries comparing each side. Pulsation may only be diminished and not abolished; loss of pulsation may only be segmental and may only affect the terminal part of each artery. There may be other systemic manifestations such as fever, anaemia and weight loss. The intracranial arteries may be involved leading to hemiplegia and blindness. Temporal arteritis is a medical emergency and treatment should begin immediately with high doses of corticosteroids until the pain has subsided and steroids should be continued in moderate doses for six months as blindness may occur after the acute symptoms have subsided (Richardson, 1963).

Wegener's granulomatosis consists of a vasculitis affecting arteries and veins leading to granuloma formation in the upper air passages, lungs and kidneys.

Takayasu's disease ("pulseless" disease) consists of granuloma formation and narrowing of elastic arteries leaving the arch of the aorta and descending aorta with abnormal vessels in relation to the optic disc which are probably arteriovenous anastomoses. It used to be said that the disease only occurred in young girls but cases have been described in middle-aged men.

When confronted with a lesion which is due to arterial disease it is worthwhile considering whether the affected artery is large, medium or small. Certain conditions have a predilection for arteries of a certain size; in practice this is not rigid but may be useful (Table IV).

Buerger's Disease (Thrombo-angiitis Obliterans)

The evidence is now strong that this condition is not a distinct disease. The disease was variously considered to be a combination of peripheral

99. FRIEDRICH RUDOLF GEORG WEGENER (1843–1917). Berlin pathologist.
100. U. TAKAYASU. Japanese ophthalmologist.

TABLE IV

Size of artery	Main lesions
Large	Arteriosclerosis
	Syphilis
	Embolism (due to clots, or rarely to tumour or fungus emboli)
	Takayasu's disease
Medium	Polyarteritis nodosa
	Monckeberg's sclerosis
	Giant-cell arteritis
	Buerger's[101] disease
	Arteritis of severe infection and malignancy
	Embolism
	Arteriosclerosis
Small arteries and arterioles	Hypertension
	Dermatomyositis
	Scleroderma
	Raynaud's phenomena
	Rheumatoid arthritis
	Ergotism

arterial gangrene accompanied by thrombophlebitis, commoner in the lower limbs of young men who smoked heavily. Specific histological features were claimed. The evidence against Buerger's disease as a distinct entity has been reviewed by Wessler and his colleagues (Wessler *et al.*, 1960). Their conclusions underline a useful working rule in medicine—that unusual manifestations of common diseases are more common than rare diseases. Their evidence against the disease as a distinct entity is:

1. The histological changes in the veins thought to be specific for the disease occur in otherwise uncomplicated phlebothrombosis.

2. Histological changes in the arteries thought to be specific for the disease occur in otherwise uncomplicated arteriosclerotic gangrene.

3. All cases in which the diagnosis can be considered clinically have evidence of arteriosclerosis. Buerger himself said that for the diagnosis to be considered, evidence of arteriosclerosis should be absent.

4. In severe atherosclerosis perivascular fibrosis occurs and is often severe enough to involve venae comitantes causing venous thrombosis.

Scleroderma (Systemic Sclerosis)

There are two aspects of the pathology of scleroderma which are important: the first is that like polyarteritis there is an arteritis although it tends to affect smaller arteries, and the second is that unlike other

101. LEO BUERGER (1879–1943). New York surgeon.

collagen diseases there is first an increase and then a degeneration in collagen tissue. This occurs in sites related to the skin and mucous membranes of the gastro-intestinal tract and results in thickening and oedema of the dermis. The skin lesions consist of a combination of ischaemic atrophy due to the vasculitis and infiltration and hardening of the skin due to mucinous degeneration of the excess collagen tissue. The degenerating collagen tissue may calcify and the vasculitis result in telangiectasia and Raynaud's phenomena. The combination of calcinosis of fingers with telangiectasia or purpura around the mouth is known as the Thibierge-Weissenbach syndrome.

As a result of the thickened skin and ischaemia there will be disuse of the affected part and consequent osteoporosis and muscular atrophy. Subcutaneous fibrosis will cause contractures and deformity of joints. This deformity may resemble arthritis but unlike rheumatoid arthritis there is no joint swelling. Thrombosis of affected vessels may cause gangrene.

The changes of scleroderma may be localised particularly to the neck and the condition is then called morphoea, occasionally it is localised to the fingers and toes and is then known as acrosclerosis. In both these conditions there is usually no evidence of extension or visceral involvement with scleroderma. Acrosclerosis is by far the commonest clinical manifestation of scleroderma. A condition which is rare but may appear similar to the skin manifestation of scleroderma is scleroedema. This is a condition which almost always follows a streptococcal infection and is accompanied by oedema, fibrosis and induration of the skin which may closely resemble scleroderma, however, in scleroedema the hands and feet are spared and the condition is much worse over the face and trunk. It is not accompanied by vasculitis so that there is no atrophy of the skin or overlying telangiectasia.

In scleroderma visceral involvement may occur in the complete absence of any skin lesions. The commonest is involvement of the lower end of the oesophagus which may cause dysphagia, peptic oesophagitis, oesophageal dilatation and aspiration pneumonia. Loss of proper peristalsis may be demonstrated, before there is demonstrable narrowing of the oesophagus, if a barium swallow is taken with the patient lying down. Any part of the gastro-intestinal tract may be involved and if the small intestine is affected there may be malabsorption.

The respiratory system can be involved in four main ways:

1. Aspiration pneumonia.
2. Vasculitis affecting pulmonary arterioles leading to pulmonary hypertension.
3. Fibrosis and degeneration of collagen tissue causes interstitial fibrosis and a diffusing defect which involves mainly the lower zones.

4. Involvement of skin and diaphragm leads to diminished ventilation of the lungs.

The kidneys and heart are usually involved fairly late in the disease. The renal lesions resemble those of SLE and the main cardiac lesion is a cardiomyopathy possibly complicated by pulmonary hypertension, systemic hypertension and endocardial thickening causing mitral and tricuspid incompetence.

Treatment of scleroderma consists of corticosteroids if the disease is progressing rapidly or is causing discomfort as it often does. Low-molecular weight dextran (Rheomacrodex) is indicated if arterial lesions are severe. It is given intermittently every 4–6 weeks; it is required more often during the cold weather (Holti, 1965). There is some evidence that penicillamine prevents excessive formation of collagen and it may be beneficial in scleroderma (Harris and Sjoerdsma, 1966).

Dermatomyositis and Polymyositis

From a practical point of view there is no point in distinguishing between these two conditions provided it is appreciated that the skin is not invariable involved—the muscles alone may be affected. The affected muscles are those of the limb girdles and proximal limb muscles, those of the face and distal limbs are commonly not affected. The affected muscles become weak, atrophic and tender at rest and on palpation. The skin lesions consist of erythema which usually involves the face, chest and arms—involvement of the dorsum of the fingers is very suggestive. The rash is light-sensitive and may closely resemble SLE; however, visceral involvement, arthritis and LE cells are rarely seen in dermatomyositis. In patients over the age of 50 the majority will have an accompanying neoplasm, the common sites being the stomach, breast and ovary. The dermatomyositis may antedate the appearance of the carcinoma or rarely it may develop after the neoplasm has been cured. The response of established dermatomyositis to removal of the tumour is variable but it may be complete. Muscle and skin biopsy are important in diagnosis and estimation of muscle enzymes (phospho-creatine kinase, aldolase and transaminases) are useful indicators of progress. The disease does not usually relapse and remit; the most usual outcome is death after about six months or a slowly progressive downward course. Corticosteroids are usually given in large doses and it is justifiable to continue them for a long time; a careful search should always be made for a primary neoplasm, especially of the lung, ovaries and stomach.

Systemic Lupus Erythematosus

This is the most common and the most catholic of the collagen disorders. Multisystem involvement is the rule rather than the exception.

The commonest features are fever, arthritis, skin and renal involvement. Unlike the skin lesions of dermatomyositis and scleroderma, calcinosis does not occur. The disease is rare in men; a high clinical index of suspicion for SLE is important in a female patient who has a fever and raised ESR who is being investigated for otherwise unexplained:

Thrombocytopenia and purpura.
Haemolytic anaemia.
Lymphadenopathy and splenomegaly.
False positive WR.
Nephrotic syndrome.
Peripheral neuropathy.
Recent onset of psychosis or epilepsy.
Pleural effusions or pericarditis.
Patchy shadowing in the lung fields.
Hepatitis.

Discoid lupus refers to the occurrence of the skin lesions of SLE when they occur in the absence of any systemic manifestations. It is now accepted that many cases of discoid lupus eventually develop SLE.

Mild cases of SLE and most cases of discoid lupus can be treated symptomatically or with antimalarials. Hydroxychloroquine is more suitable than chloroquine. Both drugs may cause corneal deposits, retinopathy or a reversible neuromyopathy. The retinopathy may appear years after the drug has been stopped. Chloroquine characteristically causes a large scotoma for red. In acute and more severe chronic cases corticosteroids are given in doses large enough to control the disease (as judged by disappearance of fever, anaemia, thrombocytopenia, arthritis and skin lesions). Two factors are important in the practical management of SLE, the first is that the height of ESR is not a good guide to the dose of steroids and the second is that for some entirely unknown reason patients with SLE who are treated with steroids are much less prone to develop side-effects of steroid administration (Medical Research Council, 1961). The absence of side-effects has even been suggested as a method of distinguishing SLE from rheumatoid arthritis. The single most important factor in assessing the prognosis of SLE is the presence or absence of renal involvement.

The diagnosis can be confirmed by:

(a) LE cell factor
(b) Antinuclear factor
(c) Anti-DNA antibodies

If all of these are negative then a diagnosis of SLE is unlikely. Complement levels may be reduced if the disease is in an active phase. There is a strong correlation between lowered haemolytic complement levels and the presence of renal disease. This finding alone in the presence of known SLE justifies treatment because of the adverse prognosis of renal lesions.

Current opinion favours the combined use of azathioprine and prednisone sometimes with heparin if there is known renal or severe vascular involvement. If there is no renal involvement prednisone should be used in the minimum dose—if this fails then azathioprine should be added (Hughes, 1974).

Drugs and SLE

The commonest drugs known to cause the SLE syndrome are hydrallazine, isoniazid, phenytoin and procainamide. The syndrome is usually reversible when the offending drug is stopped; renal involvement and myocarditis are less common than with the spontaneously occurring form of SLE.

Serum Sickness

This has many features in common with the collagen disorders, and the arterial lesions which occur are indistinguishable from those of polyarteritis nodosa. The most important clinical features are fever, urticarial and erythematous skin reactions, arthralgia, lymphadenopathy, angioneurotic oedema which may involve the larynx, albuminuria and an eosinophilia. The condition is nearly always self-limiting and only occasionally requires steroids. Two unusual but diagnostically confusing features are the occurrence of a positive Paul[102]-Bunnell[103] test and the neurological lesions which consist of a peripheral neuropathy usually involving the arms and which may result in severe, permanent wasting of the muscles; rarely retrobulbar neuritis and optic atrophy occur.

Serum sickness generally comes on several days after an injection of serum or drug—there has to be time for the production of antibodies by the body and for the subsequent antibody-antigen reaction which results in the clinical features. If the patient already has antibodies to the injected serum then there may be an immediate anaphylactic reaction which is much more commonly fatal than serum sickness that develops after a few days. It is important to note that serum sickness can occasionally complicate blood transfusion.

Polymyalgia Rheumatica

Most rheumatologists regard this as a disease entity although it is uncommon and its existence is disputed by some. It has been precisely defined as pain and stiffness in the muscles with evidence of systemic

102. JOHN RODMAN PAUL (b. 1893). New Haven physician.
103. WALLS WILLARD BUNNELL (b. 1902). Framington, Connecticut, physician.

involvement (Andrews, 1966). It is virtually confined to the elderly and the muscular pains are always accompanied by a high ESR but not other evidence of rheumatoid arthritis. The muscle pain and stiffness are nearly always worse in the early morning and by mid-morning the patient is better. Depression and weight loss are almost inevitable. It is thought to be due to an arteritis similar to giant-cell arteritis. Following the acute onset of muscular pains there is often wasting of the muscles, particularly the proximal groups. Synonyms are anarthritic rheumatoid disease and senile arteritis. The most difficult differential diagnosis of severe cases is from polymyositis.

Weber[104] Christian Disease (relapsing, febrile, nodular, non-suppurative paniculitis)

The nodules are subcutaneous, the overlying skin is slightly erythematous; the nodules disappear, leaving areas of depressed skin due to underlying fat necrosis. There is sometimes systemic involvement with anaemia, a high ESR and fat necrosis of the viscera and omentum. Occasionally corticosteroids are necessary.

Other Forms of Fat Necrosis

1. *Intestinal lipodystrophy* (Whipple's disease).
2. *Insulin lipodystrophy* in which fat necrosis occurs at the site of insulin injections.
3. *Progressive lipodystrophy* in which there is loss of subcutaneous fat over some areas. A similar condition occurs in diabetes but in this case the loss of subcutaneous fat involves the whole of the body.
4. *Disseminated fat necrosis.*—This occurs in acute pancreatitis; there is necrosis of fat in parts of the body remote from the abdomen.
5. *Bazin's[105] disease* (*erythema induratum*), which is one of the tuberculids and affects the calves of young women.

Non-articular Rheumatism

Pain, stiffness and local tenderness occur when muscles, ligaments and tendons are used excessively or if a sudden unaccustomed strain causes rupture of a few fibres, leading to local confined oedema, stimulation of local nerve endings and muscle spasm. This much at least is uncontroversial. Considerable controversy, however, surrounds the three conditions, fibrositis, psychogenic rheumatism and paniculitis or fatty herniae. Most rheumatologists accept the condition "fibrositis", which is best defined as a condition characterised by local tenderness or referred pain which arises from palpable fibrous nodules or from "trigger points" which are constantly localised but non-palpable areas.

104. FREDERICK PARKES WEBER (b. 1863). London physician.
105. ANTOINE PIERRE ERNEST BAZIN (1807–1878). French dermatologist.

The pathology of the tender palpable nodules suggests that they are either due to a few muscle fibres which are in intense spasm (Elliot, 1944) or that they are due to herniation of fat through a tear in the surrounding fibrous envelopes (Copeman and Ackerman, 1944). Paniculitis refers to the occurrence of widespread fat herniae or excessive accumulation of fluid within fat contained in non-expanding fibrous envelopes so that the capsule surrounding the fat lobule is excessively stretched. Treatment consists of rest, analgesics, local heat, in an attempt to cause vasodilatation and reduction of oedema as well as discouraging muscle spasm. Local massage may also disperse nodules and "trigger areas" although injection of local anaesthetic into the tender points is often necessary.

The exact cause of non-articular rheumatism is not known, nevertheless, there are a number of factors which cause muscle tenderness which is similar to non-articular rheumatism, viz. some virus infections such as influenza and Bornholm[106] disease, any of the conventional collagen diseases, and excessive strain.

"Psychogenic rheumatism" refers to pain of musculo-skeletal origin that is due to psychogenic factors only and which does not have an organic basis. It is probably reasonable to regard non-articular rheumatism as quite distinct from psychogenic rheumatism.

GOUT (*L.* Gutta: a drop)

Uric acid and sodium biurate are the end products of purine metabolism. Clinical gout is caused by an increase in the body uric acid pool due to increased purine synthesis and decreased excretion. The arthritis is due to deposition of biurate crystals in the articular cartilages. The first attack of gout occurs in the big toe in 70 per cent of patients but the ankles or wrists are occasionally the site of the first attack. Hyperuricaemia at some time is a prerequisite for the development of gout, although the serum uric acid is often normal at the time of the acute attack; the level of uric acid at which gout occurs varies even in the same patient. A useful clinical rule is that acute gout always affects one joint at a time.

Nearly all patients who have several attacks of gout will develop tophi (*Gk:* volcanic rock), which consists of deposits of urates and an accompanying inflammatory reaction in the soft tissues particularly cartilages, tendons and ligaments. Tophi do not usually calcify and they are responsible for the soft tissue swelling seen in relation to joints affected by gout.

Chronic gouty arthritis refers to joint deformities which develop after frequent acute attacks of gout in those joints; it is usually painless

106. BORNHOLM—an island in the Baltic Sea.

and almost invariably accompanied by tophi. As a general rule gout never occurs in women before the menopause.

Alcohol, salicylates, guanethidine and thiazide diuretics impair the excretion of uric acid by the distal renal tubules; when a factor which diminishes uric acid excretion is combined with increased purine metabolism, which may be familial or racial (as in the Maoris of New Zealand), clinical gout will be produced.

The acute attack of gout is treated with colchicine 0·5 mg two-hourly for four doses or with phenylbutazone 200 mg six-hourly or a combination of both. Following the acute attack there are two ways in which the uric acid pool may be reduced; one is to promote increased excretion of uric acid and the other is to limit its production. The most widely used uricosuric agent is probenecid 100 mg t.d.s.; early in treatment uricosuric agents may precipitate an acute attack of gout, therefore, some physicians advocate prophylactic colchicine 0·5 mg b.d. for the first few months of treatment with uricosuric drugs.

In long-standing gout renal impairment may occur, and starts with deposition of urate crystals near the collecting ducts. This leads to tubular damage which manifests itself by inability to concentrate the urine, later glomerular damage occurs and the blood urea becomes elevated. Urate calculi are common in long-standing gout; they can be prevented and dissolved by a high fluid intake and alkalinising the urine which increases the solubility of the urates. Uricosuric drugs increase urinary excretion of uric acid and are contra-indicated in gouty nephropathy. Purines are metabolised via xanthine to uric acid; allopurinol is a drug which inhibits the enzyme xanthine oxidase thus preventing the breakdown of xanthine to uric acid. Allopurinol represents a major advance in the treatment of hyperuricaemia because it can be safely used in the presence of renal failure and, because it diminishes the excretion of uric acid, it may also be used to prevent the formation or recurrence of urate calculi. Allopurinol is indicated in secondary hyperuricaemia due to haematological disorders and to malignant disease treated with cytotoxic drugs or radiotherapy. In the absence of renal impairment gouty tophi can be dissolved by a combination of allopurinol and uricosuric drugs. Sometimes an acute attack of gout may be produced when allopurinol is first used.

Chondrocalcinosis or Pseudo-gout

This recently recognised condition is also called calcium gout, and crystal gout. It is characterised by deposition of crystals of calcium pyrophosphate in the articular cartilages, ligaments and tendons. The joints most commonly affected are the knees, hips and wrists, hence these joints are the most suitable for x-raying if the disease is suspected. The disease occurs in acute attacks which are less severe and less sudden in onset than true gout. The condition is more common in women, it may give rise to chronic arthritis which is punctuated by acute attacks. Like gout the overlying skin may be red and tender to touch, and the diagnosis can be confirmed by finding characteristic crystals in the joint fluid or in the synovial membrane. The disease appears to be more common in the presence of diabetes and hyperparathyroidism.

REFERENCES

American Rheumatism Association (1959). *Ann. rheum. Dis.*, **18**, 49.
ANDREWS, F. M. (1966). In *Modern Trends in Rheumatology*. Ed. Hill, A. G. London: Butterworth & Co.
British Medical Journal (1968). **1**, 460.
COPEMAN, W. S., and ACKERMAN, W. L. (1944). *Quart. J. Med.*, **13**, 37.
ELLIOT, F. A. (1944). *Ann. rheum. Dis.*, **4**, 22.
Empire Rheumatism Council (1950). *Ann. rheum. Dis.*, Suppl. 9.
Empire Rheumatism Council (1962). *Reports on Rheumatic Diseases*, No. 5.
FERNANDEZ-HERLIHY, L. (1960). *Med. Clin. N. Amer.*, **44**, 457.
FROHNERT, P. P., and SHEPS, S. G. (1967). *Amer. J. Med.*, **43**, 8.
GELL, P. G., and COOMBS, R. R. (1968). *Clinical Aspects of Immunology*. Oxford: Blackwell Scientific.
GRANT, R. J. (1940). *Clin. Sci.*, **4**, 245.
HÄLLÉN, J. (1966). *Acta. med. scand.*, Suppl. 462.
HARRIS, E. D., and SJOERDSMA, A. (1966). *Lancet*, **2**, 996.
HOBBS, J. (1968). *Proc. roy. Soc. Med.*, **61**, 884.
HOBBS, J. (1969). *Proc. roy. Soc. Med.*, **68**, 773.
HOLTI, G. (1965). *Brit. J. Derm.*, **77**, 560.
HUGHES, G. R. (1974). *Brit. J. hosp. Med.*, **12**, 309.
Medical Research Council Report (1960). *Brit. med. J.*, **1**, 1399.
Medical Research Council Report (1961). *Brit. med. J.*, **2**, 915.
MORGAN, B., and FOURMAN, P. (1969). *Brit. J. hosp. Med.*, **2**, 910.
RICHARDSON, J. (1963). *Connective Tissue Disorders*. Philadelphia: F. A. Davis Co.
ROSE, G. A., and SPENCER, H. (1957). *Quart. J. Med.*, **26**, 43.
WAKSMAN, B. H. (1962). *Medicine (Baltimore)*, **41**, 93.
WESSLER, S., SI CHUN MING, GUREWICH, V., and FREIMAN, D. G. (1960). *New Engl. J. Med.*, **262**, 1149.
WILLIAMS, R. C., and KUNKEL, H. G. (1962). *J. clin. Invest.*, **41**, 666.
YOUNG, V H. (1969). *Proc. roy. Soc. Med.*, **62**, 778.

6

NEUROLOGY

In neurology as in the other specialised branches of medicine there are clinical concepts which are reasonably straightforward and simple. These clear concepts are the cornerstone of more detailed knowledge and expertise. In neurology, the situation tends to become confused for the non-expert because of the rarity with which he has to apply the simple concepts and because the complicated anatomy can vary the clinical features so much. Nevertheless, it is possible to define, understand and remember enough of the essential concepts for practical purposes.

Internal Capsule

All motor and sensory fibres which begin or end in the cerebral cortex pass through the internal capsule. The internal capsule is part of the cerebral hemispheres; its middle part is occupied by motor fibres, behind these are sensory, visual and auditory fibres. As a working rule all motor and sensory fibres in one internal capsule serve the opposite side of the body; the exception is a collection of motor fibres that do not cross which supply muscles innervated bilaterally from both cerebral cortices. These muscles are mainly those of the trunk, neck and limb girdles. As well as motor and sensory fibres, the internal capsule also transmits autonomic and extrapyramidal fibres. Internal capsular lesions often involve the autonomic fibres leading to vasomotor and sweating disturbances in the weak limbs. Involvement of the extrapyramidal fibres accounts for the increased tone and spasticity of the weak muscles; this increased tone affects the extensor muscles of the limbs much more than the flexor muscles. In contrast in hemiplegias or paraplegias due to lesions in the spinal cord, the tone is increased in the flexor muscles, leading to paraplegia-in-flexion and painful flexor spasms. The fibres subserving movements of the head and eyes lie close together, and both are usually involved together. Lesions of the internal capsule cause weakness of muscles *of* the opposite (contralateral) side and weakness of movements *to* the contralateral side. Thus, following a lesion in one internal capsule, there is weakness of the opposite side of the body, and deviation of the head and eyes away from the weak (contralateral) side. In many cases this effect is transitory because many of the trunk, neck and eye muscles have bilateral innervation.

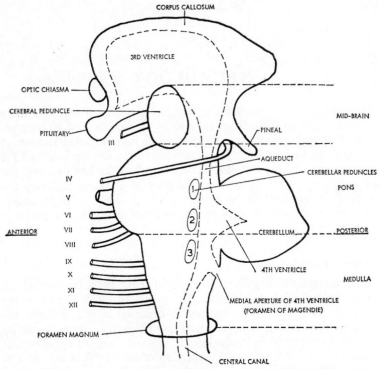

FIG. 11.—The brain stem showing the midbrain, pons and medulla and the origin of the cranial nerves.

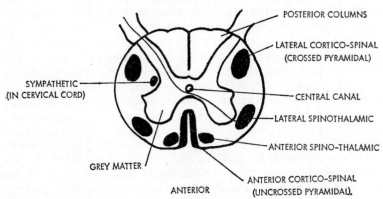

FIG. 12.—Cross-section of the spinal cord showing the position of the important tracts.

The Brain Stem (Fig. 11)

From the internal capsule all the fibres pass to the cerebral peduncle and thence to the brain stem. A simple concept that is often confused is that the brain stem is that part which joins the cerebral peduncles to the spinal cord. The brain stem consists of three principal parts:

1. Midbrain.
2. Pons.
3. Medulla.

The pons is so-called because there is a thick band of fibres passing anterior to it which "bridges" between the two cerebellar hemispheres. As well as transmitting nerve fibres from cerebral peduncles to spinal cord, the brain stem contains the nuclei of the cranial nerves and their interconnections.

The Spinal Cord

The overall structure of the spinal cord is similar throughout its length (Fig. 12), and there are only minor modifications due to increase in number of nerve fibres. Most motor and sensory nerve fibres decussate at some point in the nervous system. The main exceptions to this are a small number of motor fibres carried in the anterior corticospinal tract which generally serve bilaterally innervated muscles.

Nerve fibres subserving the various sensory modalities are carried in tracts which decussate at different levels and have a different destination in the brain stem. The principal sensory tracts, their site of decussation and the sensory impulses which they convey are shown in Table V. All sensory impulses enter the spinal cord by the posterior nerve roots and are, therefore, situated posteriorly for at least part of their journey to the brain. Hence, any posteriorly situated lesion in the spinal cord will generally affect some form of sensation first.

The signs of damage to the posterior columns are:

1. Loss of proprioception and vibration sense, leading to ataxia (because increased movements have to be performed in order to produce proprioceptive impulses and wrong movements are not appreciated and corrected quickly).
2. Loss of "deep" pain (loss of tenderness of the tendo Achillis).
3. Positive Rombergism.[107] Ataxia occurs with the eyes closed but not when they are open because lack of proprioception may be corrected by looking at the position the limbs are in.
4. Hypotonicity due to the fact that many spinocerebellar fibres travel in the posterior columns before entering the spinocerebellar tract.

107. MORITZ HEINRICH ROMBERG (1795–1853). Berlin physician.

TABLE V

Tract	Sensory Impulses	Site of Decussation
Posterior columns	Proprioception Vibration Deep pain Some light touch	In the medulla, after forming medial lemniscus
Anterior spinothalamic	Light touch	In the spinal cord several segments above their entry
Lateral spinothalamic	Superficial pain. Temperature Tickle	In the spinal cord immediately above entry
Spinocerebellar	Concerned with muscle tone and co-ordination	Probably do not cross

5. Diminished tendon reflexes—the sensory stimulus for the deep reflexes is a stretch (hence proprioceptive) reflex, hence diminished proprioception will diminish the tendon reflexes.

It is important to note that not all the above signs need be present to diagnose a posterior column lesion, the two most important causes of which are tabes dorsalis and subacute combined degeneration of the cord.

Loss of proprioception can be quickly tested by the examiner's placing the limbs and fingers of one side of the patient in a certain position and then getting the patient with his eyes closed to place the limbs and fingers of the other side in the same position.

Detailed Consideration of the Brain Stem (Fig. 11)

The motor and sensory fibres of the cranial nerves join their counterparts from the spinal cord. *It is essential to note that all the motor fibres of the cranial nerves are derived from the opposite cerebral cortex in the same way as are the motor fibres of the spinal nerves.* The motor fibres of the spinal nerves (corticospinal or pyramidal fibres) decussate in the upper part of the medulla just below the pons. They continue on the opposite side to the spinal cord where they become the pyramidal or lateral corticospinal tract. Most of the cranial nerves leave the brain stem higher than the decussation of the pyramids, hence the motor fibres of the cranial nerves must cross higher in the brain stem—they do not form distinct recognisable pathways before they reach their nuclei from which the lower motor neurones are derived.

The fact that the upper motor neurones of the cranial nerves decussate at a higher level than the decussation of the pyramids explains the phenomenon of crossed hemiplegia, i.e. weakness of the opposite side of the body with weakness of the cranial nerve muscles on the same side. A lesion which damages the cranial nerve *after* it has decussated, which also damages the pyramidal tract *before* it has decussated, will cause a crossed hemiplegia. The best known examples of crossed hemiplegias are:

1. Weber's [108] syndrome: ipsilateral lower motor neurone lesion of the oculomotor nerve with contralateral hemiplegia.
2. Millard[109]-Gubler[110] syndrome: lower motor neurone lesion of the abducens nerve which supplies the lateral rectus and contralateral hemiplegia.
3. Foville's[111] syndrome in which there is a hemiplegia with paralysis of conjugate deviation towards the side of the lesion, i.e. the eyes are fixed *towards* the weak side; in a hemiplegia due to a lesion in the internal capsule, the eyes tend to be fixed *away* from the weak side.
4. Hemiplegia on one side with weakness of muscles supplied by the lower cranial nerves (IX–XII) on the opposite side.

Most sensory fibres end in the thalamus, cerebellum or cerebral cortex. Like the motor fibres, all the sensory fibres decussate at various levels (except those going to the cerebellum via the spinocerebellar tracts). The thalamus is the main destination of sensory impulses; from it, selected impulses are relayed to the cerebral cortex on the same side. The cerebral cortex is concerned with discriminatory functions at a conscious level. The main ways of testing this clinically are:

1. Two-point discrimination.
2. Assessment of size, weight, texture and purpose of objects (stereognosis), e.g. naming the value of a coin.
3. Ability to recognise symbols written on the skin (graphaesthaesia).
4. Naming correctly which part of the body the examiner is touching.
5. Position sense (provided, of course, that the posterior columns are intact).

In the brain stem, the tracts of the spinal cord end as follows (Fig. 13):

1. The posterior columns, which contain uncrossed fibres, form the medial lemnisci which decussate in the medulla.

108. Sir Herman Weber (1823–1918). London physician.
109. Auguste Louis Jules Millard (1830–1915). Paris physician.
110. Adolphe Marie Gubler (1821–1879). Paris physician.
111. Achille Louis François Foville (1799–1878). Paris neurologist.

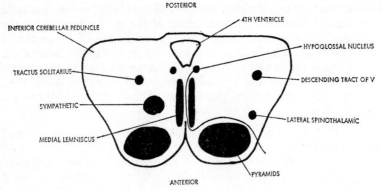

FIG. 13.—Cross-section of the medulla showing the position of the important tracts.

2. The anterior spinothalamic (light touch) which forms the reticular substance in the medulla, and then joins the medial lemniscus in the pons.

3. The lateral spinothalamic (pain and temperature), which continues through the medulla as the lateral spinothalamic tract and then also joins the medial lemniscus in the pons.

The medial lemniscus terminates in the thalamus.

Other clinically important structures which are seen in the brain stem are:

1. Medial longitudinal bundle which interconnects the nuclei of the cranial nerves and is concerned with co-ordination of face and eye movements.

2. Ascending tract of the trigeminal nerve which contains proprioceptive and touch fibres, corresponding to the posterior columns. The fibres immediately cross the midline and join the medial lemniscus.

3. Descending tract of the trigeminal nerve which carries pain and temperature impulses corresponding to the lateral spinothalamic tract. This tract descends to the level of C.2 on the same side as it enters, and then crosses the midline and joins the lateral spinothalamic tract.

4. Tractus solitarius, which contains fibres conveying taste.

5. Corticospinal tracts.

6. Nuclei of the cranial nerves. These occur as follows: Midbrain: oculomotor and trochlear. The oculomotor nerve emerges from the midbrain close to the cerebral peduncle so that a lesion in this area gives rise to a lower motor neurone oculomotor palsy on the same side and a hemiplegia on the opposite side (Weber's syndrome). Pons: abducens, trigeminal, facial and auditory. Medulla: glossopharyngeal, vagus, accessory and hypoglossal.

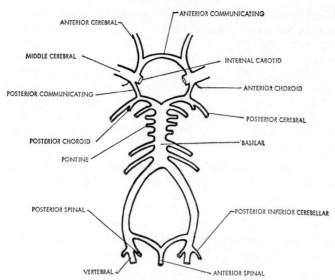

FIG. 14.—The arteries at the base of the brain and the circle of Willis.

The basilar artery runs along the anterior surface of the brain stem as far as the upper border of the pons, and is its main blood supply (Fig. 14). The three portions of the brain stem are also supplied by various other arteries. The most important are the posterior cerebral, supplying the midbrain (including the cerebral peduncles), the anterior inferior cerebellar artery, supplying the pons and posterior inferior cerebellar artery supplying the medulla. The posterior inferior cerebellar arteries are derived from the vertebrals and in practice, narrowing of one vertebral artery may result in ischaemia of the medulla. Ischaemia of the midbrain, if severe and bilateral, will result in a quadriplegia, because both cerebral peduncles are involved. The nuclei of the cranial nerves and their connections in this region of the midbrain will be involved (III and IV), resulting in lower motor neurone oculomotor and trochlear palsies and impairment of conjugate eye movements, as the nuclei subserving conjugate movements are in the same region. In lesser degrees of unilateral midbrain ischaemia, there will be a crossed hemiplegia caused by involvement of the corticospinal tract and third nerve. Particular features of midbrain ischaemia which are sometimes present are:

1. Hemiballismus due to involvement of part of the thalamus.
2. Thalamic syndrome.
3. Akinetic mutism (coma vigil) in which the patient appears to be almost awake, with the eyes open, and yet in a coma.

4. Lesions near the pineal result in impairment of upward movement of the eyes, due to the proximity of the nucleus concerned with upward conjugate deviation.

From a consideration of the structures of the pons, the probable consequences of partial ischaemia can be deduced. The important considerations are firstly the cranial nerve nuclei dealing with the conjugate lateral deviation and secondly the fact that in the pons the medial lemniscus is joined by the lateral spinothalamic tracts and the anterior spinothalamic fibres via the reticular formation; thus, the possible consequences are:

1. Lower motor neurone lesions of the cranial nerves arising from the area, i.e. abducent, trigeminal, facial and auditory nerves.

2. Impairment of lateral conjugate deviation.

3. Variable loss of sensation of one side of the body, depending on whether the medial lemniscus is involved before or after it has been joined by fibres from the anterior and lateral spinothalamic tracts.

4. Contralateral hemiplegia due to involvement of the corticospinal tracts.

Other considerations are the presence of fibres of the sympathetic nervous system which, if affected, will give rise to Horner's syndrome and the cerebellar tracts which, if affected, may cause cerebellar signs. Particular features of pontine lesions include pin-point pupils and hyperventilation.

Ischaemic lesions of the medulla are commoner than either midbrain or pontine lesions. From Fig. 13, the possible consequences of lesions in the medulla can be deduced. They are:

1. Involvement of the cranial nerves of the area: the glossopharyngeal and vagus, leading to dysarthria, dysphagia, and vocal cord paralysis (bulbar palsy). Involvement of the vestibular branches of the eighth nerve causes vertigo and nausea.

2. Involvement of the corticospinal tract leads to a contralateral hemiplegia.

3. Involvement of the medial lemniscus leads to loss of proprioception and vibration sense on the opposite side of the body.

4. Involvement of the cerebellar peduncle may lead to unilateral cerebellar signs.

From Fig. 13, it will be seen that if the lesion is mainly of the lateral side of the medulla, the descending tract of the trigeminal, the lateral spinothalamic and the sympathetic tract will be involved. This leads to contralateral loss of pain and temperature over the body and an ipsilateral loss over the face because the descending tract of the trigeminal is involved before it has decussated (which it does in the cervical spine), whereas the lateral spinothalamic fibres decussate soon after they enter the cord; in addition there will be an ipsilateral Horner's syndrome (lateral medullary syndrome). If the medial part of the medulla is mainly involved the above will be absent, but instead the medial lemniscus and the hypoglossal nucleus will be involved and there will be unilateral atrophy of the tongue which will be absent in the lateral medullary syndrome.

LOCALISING FEATURES OF MOTOR LESIONS

Site

Cerebral cortex
Flaccid weakness. Flexors and extensors equally affected ("global weakness").
Cortical sensory loss may be present.

Internal capsule
Spastic weakness.
Extensors more affected than flexors.
Distal limb muscles more affected than proximal muscles.
Paralysis of head and eye movements so that patient looks away from the weak *limbs*.

Brain stem
Crossed hemiplegia, i.e. ipsilateral cranial nerve palsy with contralateral limb palsy.

Cord lesion
Flaccid.
Flexors more affected than extensors.

Root and peripheral nerve
Lower motor neurone lesion.
Peripheral nerve lesions usually affect both motor and sensory function in muscles and skin supplied by the nerve. The following is a *rough* guide to the muscles supplied by clinically important motor nerve roots:

C 5 & 6	Biceps and deltoid	L 2 & 3	Adductors
C 7 & 8	Triceps	L 3 & 4	Quadriceps
C 7	Finger extensors	L 4 & 5	Dorsi flexors
C 8	Finger flexors	L 5 & S 1	Hamstrings
T 1	Small muscles of the hand	S 1 & 2	Plantar flexors and small muscles of the feet

The Plantar Reflex

One of the perennial discussions in which non-neurologists indulge is the significance of the plantar response and the correct means of eliciting it. It is now generally accepted that the "extensor" response is part of the general *flexor* response of the limbs reacting to injury and that the extensor hallicus longus is in fact physiologically a flexor muscle because its contraction results in shortening of the limb.

The reflex is best elicited by firm, slightly painful stroking of the lateral border of the sole. The normal response when the nervous system is intact is a downward movement of the big toe and slight downward movement of the remaining toes, as if the foot were relaxing itself to receive a painful stimulus. When the plantar response is elicited the important movement of the big toe is the early movement; the later movements particularly when the ball of the foot is stroked may develop into a general "flexor" movement of the limb (i.e. dorsiflexion) as part of the withdrawal reaction.

It is helpful to consider the movements of the foot and leg which occur in normal people when different parts of the foot are stimulated. All the reflex movements of the limb are "designed" to reduce the effects of harmful stimuli affecting the sole of the foot, bearing in mind that the human foot has been modified for the erect posture. It has been shown that all the movements are co-ordinated (i.e. there is reflex inhibition of opposing muscles). Stimulation of the ball of the foot *in normals* results in dorsiflexion of the toes, flexion of ankle and knee. Stimulation of the hollow of the foot results in plantar flexion of the toes, flexion of the ankle, etc. Stimulation of the plantar surface of the heel results in plantar flexion of the toes and extension of the heel, flexion of the knees, *extension* of the hips (i.e. the heel is raised off the ground). Thus the ball of the foot is the only area of the sole where *dorsiflexion* is the *normal* response.

The distinction between a normal response and patients with upper motor neurone lesions is that the pathological "extensor" plantar response (dorsiflexion) can be elicited from a much wider receptive field, i.e. the area from which dorsiflexion can normally be elicited (the balls of the feet) extends over a wider area of the sole. The reason why the outside of the foot is stimulated is that it is a *less* sensitive area than the inside of the sole—stimulation of the inside of the sole with a minor pyramidal lesion may still produce a normal plantar flexor downward response.

CEREBRAL CORTEX

The surfaces of the cerebral hemispheres are divided by certain fissures which are constant. These are the lateral fissure (Sylvian[112] fissure) and the central sulcus (Rolandic[113] fissure). In front of the

112. FRANCISCUS SYLVIUS (1614–1672). Dutch anatomist.
113. LUIGI ROLANDO (1773–1831). Turin anatomist.

central sulcus is the motor area and behind it is the sensory area. The lobes of the cerebral cortex are not clearly defined by any internal arrangement, but are merely areas of the surface of the cortex which are in contact with the bones of the skull of the same name. However, it is usually convenient to consider the functions of the different areas of the cortex in terms of the named lobes (Fig. 15).

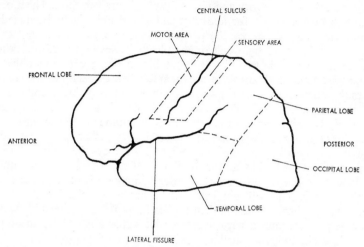

FIG. 15.—The cerebral cortex showing the position of the lobes and the motor and sensory areas.

The area in front of the central sulcus (known as the pre-central gyrus) is concerned with motor functions of the opposite side of the body. The part of the motor area concerned with movements of the feet is at the top and the part concerned with movements of the head is at the bottom, i.e. the body image is represented upside down. The area behind the central sulcus (the post-central gyrus) is concerned with appreciation of sensation and this is represented in precisely the same way as in the motor area, i.e. feet at the top and head at the bottom.

The Speech Centres

The centre concerned with the reception of information which will lead to speech is situated in the sensory cortex; and the centre concerned with the motor side of speaking is situated in the motor area. As a rule, only the dominant cerebral hemisphere contains the speech centre. In a right-handed person, this is the left cerebral hemisphere. Lesions of one or other of the two speech centres give rise to motor or sensory dysphasia. In motor dysphasia, the patient knows what he wants to say, but cannot say it. It is best tested for by asking the patient to obey a command (such as "close your eyes" or "open your mouth"), to write down his reply to a question or to ask him to nod when you supply him with the correct answer to a question you have given him.

The two ways in which the sensory speech area is stimulated are either by the patient reading or hearing a question or command. Thus, sensory dysphasia can be due to inability to comprehend the spoken word (auditory dysphasia) or the written word (visual dysphasia). In their pure forms, auditory and visual dysphasia are very rare. The more common occurrence is for auditory and visual aphasia to be mixed; under these circumstances, the patient may be able to speak, but the words are often unrecognisable or completely irrelevant to the question. Although he is able to talk, he is unable to name common objects although he may still be able to use them for their correct purposes (e.g. a comb or a glass of water). Thus, a rough way of assessing dysphasia is to ask the patient a simple question and, if he is unable to reply, he probably has either motor aphasia or has not understood the question (auditory sensory aphasia). In order to establish whether he understands he is asked to perform a simple movement. If he obeys the command this will confirm that he has motor dysphasia. If he does not do a simple movement in response to a verbal order he may do it in response to a written order. This will confirm that he has a combined motor and auditory dysphasia. If the patient replies in an incomprehensible way, then he probably has a sensory dysphasia. Aphasia is usually accompanied by an inability to calculate (acalculia) or to write (agraphia).

Dysarthria refers to difficulty with the mechanical act of producing spoken words and is due to disorder of the muscles of articulation, which include the tongue, facial and laryngeal muscles. Various phrases are traditionally used when testing for dysarthria—these particular phrases are used because they test all the groups of muscles involved in speaking (labials, linguals, palatal and laryngeal). The traditional phrases are: "British constitution", "baby hippopotamus", "West Register Street" and "Methodist Episcopal Church".

The important causes of dysarthria are:

1. Lesions of the cranial nerves serving the muscles of articulation, which include the facial, glossopharyngeal, vagus and hypoglossal nerves. A lower motor neurone lesion of the nerves gives rise to a "bulbar palsy".

2. Disorders of the co-ordination of movement, seen particularly in cerebellar lesions.

3. The muscles of articulation are innervated from both cerebral cortices, hence a lesion of one internal capsule will not produce dysarthria, but if both internal capsules are affected, dysarthria will follow —"pseudo-bulbar palsy".

4. Disease or weakness of the muscles of articulation, e.g. myopathies and myasthenia gravis.

The Visual Pathways

The visual areas of the cerebral cortices are in the posterior part of the occipital lobes. The macular region of each eye is represented in both occipital lobes, furthermore, the macular area of each occipital lobe has a dual blood supply via the middle and posterior cerebral arteries. Figure 16 shows the visual pathways. Defects of vision of one-half of the visual field are hemianopias; because of the effects of the lens of the

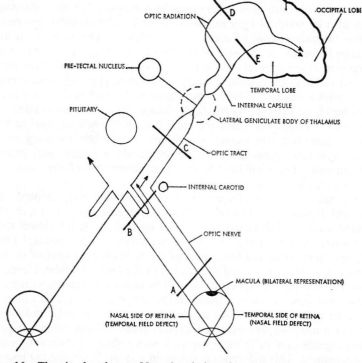

PARIETAL LOBE
OPTIC RADIATION
D
OCCIPITAL LOBE
PRE-TECTAL NUCLEUS
E
TEMPORAL LOBE
INTERNAL CAPSULE
PITUITARY
LATERAL GENICULATE BODY OF THALAMUS
C
OPTIC TRACT
INTERNAL CAROTID
B
OPTIC NERVE
MACULA (BILATERAL REPRESENTATION)
A
NASAL SIDE OF RETINA
(TEMPORAL FIELD DEFECT)
TEMPORAL SIDE OF RETINA
(NASAL FIELD DEFECT)

Fig. 16.—The visual pathways. Note the pituitary in relation to nasal fibres from both retinae, the optic radiation, the internal carotid artery and the muscular fibres passing to both optic tracts.

eye a temporal hemianopia is due to a lesion of the nerve fibres supplying the nasal side of the retina, and vice versa. A field defect which affects the corresponding field of vision of both eyes, i.e. the nasal field of one eye and the temporal field of the other is a homonymous hemianopia. If only a quarter of the visual field is involved it is a quadrantanopia, and if only a small portion of the field is involved, it is a scotoma. The macula is concerned with fixation of vision and is the area of maximum visual acuity.

From Fig. 16 it will be seen that a lesion of the optic nerve (A) will lead to complete blindness in one eye. A lesion at (B) will lead to complete blindness in one eye and a temporal hemianopia in the other eye, due to the fact that fibres from the nasal side of the retina loop into the optic nerve of the opposite eye. Enlargement of the pituitary from below is almost always asymmetrical, it compresses fibres from the lower nasal side of one eye first and hence causes an upper temporal field defect. Later, the defect may involve the lower temporal field and become equal in both eyes (bitemporal hemianopia). The optic chiasma may also be involved by a meningioma or by fibrosis following meningitis (meningococcal, tuberculous or syphilitic). The internal carotid arteries lie on the lateral side of the chiasm; excessive atheroma or an aneurysm of the internal carotid may press on the temporal fibres from the eye on that side, causing a nasal hemianopia. The optic tract carries fibres backwards to the lateral geniculate body, and in the optic tract the fibres from each eye remain fairly distinct, hence any lesion affecting the tract (C) does not affect the congruous fields of both eyes to the same extent; the hemianopia or scotoma is therefore not congruous. The commonest lesions affecting the optic tracts are meningitis, pituitary tumours, temporal lobe lesions and aneurysms of the posterior communicating or internal carotid arteries.

The optic fibres pass from the lateral geniculate body through the internal capsule, and fan out, before converging again to reach the occipital cortex. Fibres from the upper part of the retina (lower field of vision) pursue a long course and are related to the parietal lobe, whereas fibres from the lower part of the retina (upper field of vision) pursue a shorter course and are related to the temporal lobe. Hence, a lesion of the parietal lobe (at D) will produce a lower homonymous quadrantanopia, whereas a lesion of the temporal lobe (at E) will produce an upper homonymous quadrantanopia. In the optic radiation, fibres from both eyes serving congruous areas of both retinae lie very close together, unlike in the optic tract where fibres of congruous areas are separated. This difference is the main way of distinguishing lesions of the optic tract from those of the optic radiation. Tract lesions will cause non-congruous hemianopias or scotomata, but radiation lesions will produce congruous hemianopias or scotomata.

Damage to one occipital lobe will produce a homonymous hemianopia but the macula will be spared because it has bilateral representation. Damage to both occipital cortices occurs if both posterior cerebral arteries are damaged or if the basilar artery is occluded because both the posterior cerebral arteries arise from the basilar. Bilateral occipital cortical infarction leads to cortical blindness, in which the patient is totally blind but the pupillary light and accommodation reflexes remain intact. In all other forms of neurological bilateral blindness, either the optic nerves or tracts have to be involved and the afferent fibres for the pupillary light reflex will be damaged, leading to loss of the pupillary light reflex. In cortical blindness the optic nerves and tracts are intact and the damage is distal to the point where the pupillary afferent fibres leave the visual fibres to go to the pretectal nucleus of the midbrain.

DISTURBANCES OF FUNCTION OF THE LOBES OF THE CEREBRAL CORTEX

Frontal Lobes

The frontal lobes are concerned with intellectual functions as well as containing the motor area within the precentral gyrus. Damage to the frontal lobes leads to forgetfulness, dementia and incontinence with indifference. If the lesion involves the motor area, there may be Jacksonian[114] focal epilepsy and weakness of the corresponding area of the body. Motor aphasia will occur if the dominant hemisphere is involved. The frontal lobes lie directly over the olfactory tracts, which may be compressed, leading to anosmia; alternatively, a meningioma, arising from the olfactory groove, may compress the frontal lobes. A parasagittal meningioma (one occurring in the midline in the sagittal or antero-posterior plane) above the cerebral hemisphere will press on the top of the frontal lobes, leading to loss of motor function at the top of the motor area (i.e. affecting the legs). The frontal lobe may press on the optic nerves, giving rise to optic atrophy on that side, if the tumour enlarges and causes a raised intracranial pressure there may be papilloedema in the opposite eye. The occurrence of papilloedema in one eye and optic atrophy in the other is known as the Foster Kennedy[115] syndrome. A physical sign believed to be pathognomonic of frontal lobe tumours is the "grasp" reflex, which affects the limbs of the opposite side of the body and is similar to the physiological grasp reflex of babies.

Parietal Lobes

The parietal lobes are mainly concerned with sensory recognition and orientation of the body image. Lesions which involve the post-central gyrus will cause cortical sensory loss in the corresponding part of the body. The important tests of cortical sensation are stereognosis, two point discrimination, localisation of a stimulus to the correct part of the body, and recognition of letters or figures drawn on the skin. Parietal lobe lesions may cause a lower homonymous quadrantanopia. If the dominant lobe is involved, there will be sensory aphasia ac-

114. JOHN HUGHLINGS JACKSON (1835–1911). London neurologist.
115. FOSTER KENNEDY (b. 1884). New York neurologist.

companied by inability to calculate (acalculia), inability to read (alexia) and inability to write (agraphia). Lesions of the non-dominant parietal lobe (usually the right lobe) cause inattention and inability to recognise the left half of the body. This can be tested by touching both sides of the body at the same time, the patient will always say that the right side only has been touched. The combination of confusion of right and left, inability to identify the fingers and acalculia, is known as Gerstmann's[116] syndrome. A curious feature of parietal lobe lesions is that the signs vary from day to day.

Temporal Lobe

The upper homonymous quadrantanopia of temporal lobe lesions has already been mentioned; other features are hallucinations of taste and smell, often accompanied by excessive lip smacking. Patients who have temporal lobe epilepsy often have auditory hallucinations and a dazed look. The best known temporal lobe symptom is an excessive number of déjà-vu phenomena (a feeling of having been in the same situation before).

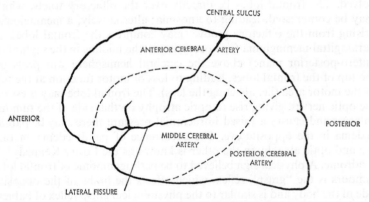

FIG. 17.—The cerebral cortex showing the distribution of the cerebral arteries.

Blood Supply of the Cerebral Cortex (Fig. 17)

Anterior cerebral artery.—This artery supplies the frontal lobes and the superior portion of the cerebral cortex (leg area). A large branch of the anterior cerebral, Heubner's[117] artery (medial striate artery) supplies the anterior portion of the internal capsule which carries fibres supplying the upper part of the body. Occlusion of the artery beyond the origin of Heubner's artery gives rise to:

116. JOSEF GERSTMANN (b. 1887). Vienna neurologist.
117. JOHANN OTTO LEONHARD HEUBNER (1843–1926). Leipzig and Berlin paediatrician.

1. Motor dysphasia (on dominant side) because of involvement of precental gyrus of the frontal lobe.

2. Cortical (flaccid) weakness of opposite leg.

3. Cortical sensory loss in opposite leg because of involvement of superior surface of cerebral cortex.

4. Frontal lobe involvement may cause a grasp reflex, incontinence and intellectual deterioration.

Occlusion of Heubner's artery affecting the anterior limb of the internal capsule and extrapyramidal nuclei leads to contralateral weakness in the upper body—the weakness is accompanied by spasticity.

Middle cerebral artery.—This artery supplies the majority of the internal capsule (via the lateral striate arteries), the cortical speech areas, and the part of the motor and sensory cortex concerned with the upper part of the body as well as the larger part of frontal, temporal and parietal lobes. Obstruction of the lateral striate branches of the middle cerebral artery results in:

1. Contralateral spastic weakness.

2. Hemianopia (involvement of visual fibres in internal capsule).

3. Obstruction of frontal branches leads to flaccid (cortical) weakness and cortical sensory loss of the upper part of the body. Interruption of branches to the parietal and temporal lobes result in parietal and temporal lobe signs (see pp. 267 and 268).

Posterior cerebral artery.—This supplies the occipital lobe and a branch to the thalamus and midbrain. Occlusion distal to the thalamic branch produces an homonymous hemianopia with sparing of the macula; occlusion proximal to the thalamic branch will produce the thalamic syndrome in addition. The thalamic syndrome consists of increased sensitivity to stimuli from one-half of the body with a feeling of severe pain in various parts.

If both posterior cerebral arteries are occluded "cortical blindness" results. The patient is blind but all the pupillary reflexes are intact; the patient is completely unaware when a light is shone into the eyes. The fundal appearances are normal. In other forms of blindness due to lesions of the retina, optic nerve or optic tracts, the pupillary reflexes are usually affected, there are changes seen in the fundus and the patient is usually aware of the fact that a light is being shone into the eyes. A curious feature of "cortical blindness" is that the patient may be unaware of or deny his inability to see.

Transient Ischaemic Attacks

These are brief episodes of neurological symptoms and signs which recur and are thought to be due to temporary arterial insufficiency. The intervals between recurrences vary widely from a few minutes to several months. Their occurrence almost invariably means that there is *wide-spread* although not necessarily *severe* cerebral arteriosclerosis. They are precipitated by a variety of causes:

1. Haemodynamic disturbances—hypotension and fall in cardiac output, or dysrhythmias which are often transient.
2. Anaemia and polycythaemia.
3. Emboli—from any stenotic or atheromatous lesion within the arteries supplying the circle of Willis, from the left atrium, left ventricle or aortic valve.
4. Temporary obstruction to arteries supplying the circle of Willis, particularly compression of the vertebral arteries in cervical spondylosis. The carotid arteries may occasionally be compressed by the transverse process of the atlas when the head is rotated.
5. Subclavian steal syndrome in which blood flows from one sub-clavian artery to the other via the vertebrals and basilar artery because of occlusion of one subclavian artery at its origin; this diverts blood from the circle of Willis.
6. Hypertensive crises.
7. Rarely cerebral tumour and cerebral aneurysms.

Spasm of the cerebral vessels has largely been discontinued as a cause of these transient neurological disturbances (Pickering, 1948; Marshall, 1968).

The clinical features of transient ischaemic attacks vary widely but they can be roughly grouped into ischaemia of the carotid and middle cerebral artery territories and ischaemia in the region supplied by the basilar artery—this includes the posterior cerebral arteries into which the basilar artery drains.

Carotid and middle cerebral features are:

Transient monocular blindness due to interruption of flow in one retinal artery.
Confusion due to frontal lobe ischaemia.
Hemiplegia
Hemianopia ⎫ due to internal capsular ischaemia.
Horner's syndrome.
Stuttering hemiplegia.

Basilar and posterior cerebral features are:

Vertigo
Dysarthria
Dysphagia ⎫ Pontine and medullary signs.
Facial pain
Hemiplegia

Altitudinal or hemianopic visual field disturbances due to ischaemia of optic radiation or occipital lobe (posterior cerebral artery).

Drop attacks believed to be due to ischaemia of the reticular formation.

Rarely, temporal lobe symptoms.

Management.—The known aetiological factors should be excluded or treated (e.g. anaemia, polycythaemia, hypertension, emboli arising from the heart).

Carotid and vertebral artery angiography (four-vessel angiography) should probably be performed:

1. In young patients (say those under 55).

2. If the clinical features suggest carotid artery or middle cerebral ischaemia.

3. If there is a carotid artery bruit or diminished pulsation on one side. (It is important to try and palpate the internal carotid artery in the tonsillar fossa.)

4. If signs and symptoms are unequivocally related to moving the head and neck.

5. To exclude a tumour or cerebral aneurysm as the cause.

6. If the patient is normotensive.

If a definite stenosis of the extracranial vessels is found surgery (disobliteration) should be considered together with anticoagulants.

If no stenotic lesion is found anticoagulants alone are used if the usual contra-indications are absent—they are usually given empirically *for one year* and then gradually withdrawn *provided* symptoms do not recur.

Apart from transient ischaemic attacks and extracranial artery stenosis the main indications for anticoagulants for vascular disorders affecting the brain are:

1. Cerebral embolism.

2. "Stroke in evolution."

Features suggesting embolic infarction are:

1. Signs are complete at the onset.

2. The signs are usually attributable to occlusion of a single artery.

3. Headache is often present due to compensatory vasodilatation.

The prognosis is poor if recovery is not rapid because there is usually no pre-existing atherosclerosis of the cerebral arteries to encourage collaterals.

The main indication for carotid and cerebral angiography following a completed stroke are (Marshall, 1968):

1. Young patients.
2. Cardiovascular accident preceded by transient ischaemic attacks suggesting a lesion in one of the extracranial vessels.
3. Skull or arterial bruit.
4. Possibility of preceding trauma.
5. Possibility of a cerebral tumour.

One difficult problem particularly for the non-expert is the decision about further radiology in the management of patients with transient ischaemic attacks. This subject has recently been reviewed (Kendall and Marshall, 1974). They suggest that practically all normotensive patients with carotid transient ischaemic attacks should be investigated because these attacks are ten times more likely to progress to a completed stroke than vertebro-basilar ischaemic attacks. In these patients angiography is indicated to answer two questions:

1. Has the patient a lesion relevant to his symptoms?
2. If so, is it surgically correctable?

In the case of vertebro-basilar transient ischaemic attacks the situation is different because they are much less likely to progress to a completed stroke and secondly the scope of surgery is much more limited. There are two main situations in which angiography is indicated; firstly when there is a supraclavicular bruit or inequality of brachial blood pressures, indicating a subclavian steal situation, and secondly when the attacks are clearly related to neck movements in which case simple surgery may be effective in removing an offending osteophyte.

CRANIAL NERVES

OPTIC NERVES

The optic nerve is surrounded by the meninges and the subarachnoid space. The dura fuses with the sclera and the optic nerve pierces the sclera through a series of holes known as the lamina cribrosa. The central artery and vein of the retina also pierce the lamina cribrosa and travel in the optic nerve for a short distance before leaving it, crossing the subarachnoid space and joining the ophthalmic vessels. The practical importance of this crossing of the subarachnoid space by the vein is that any change in pressure in the subarachnoid space can easily compress the vein, leading to congestion of the veins in the retina.

The fibres from the macular area occupy the central portion of the optic nerve, they are not so vulnerable to changes of pressure in the subarachnoid space surrounding the optic nerves, but are more prone to damage by inflammatory lesions of the optic nerves. Hence, retro-

bulbar neuritis gives rise at an early stage to severe disturbance of vision
with a central scotoma, involving the blind spot and fixation spot
(macula), whereas in papilloedema, due to raised intracranial pressure,
vision is little disturbed until the papilloedema has been present for
some time. When visual disturbances do occur in papilloedema, they
consist of some enlargement of the blind spot, which is due to oedema
increasing the size of the nerve head in the eye, and constriction of
peripheral fields of vision. The fixation point is not affected. This
difference in visual disturbance is the main distinguishing feature between papilloedema and retrobulbar neuritis.

The optic disc consists of the fibres of the optic nerve entering the
back of the eye, turning at right angles and being distributed to the
retina. Because all the fibres turn outwards and individual fibres are
transparent, there will be a funnel-shaped hole in the centre of the disc
(the optic cup); in the bottom of the hole a few fibres of the nerve pierce
the sclera, and although the nerve fibres cannot be seen, the holes in the
sclera through which they travel are seen as the lamina cribrosa. It is
sometimes helpful in understanding the anatomy of the optic disc to
use an analogy—imagine a hollow pipe opening flush onto a flat surface; emerging from the pipe are many pieces of string which are distributed in all directions over the flat surface. Provided there are many
pieces of string they will obviously have to be heaped on top of each
other as they turn at right angles after leaving the pipe. Furthermore, as
they all turn outwards there will be a funnel-shaped hole in the
centre.

The contour of the optic disc is sharply defined: it consists of the
layers of the retina coming to an end as the optic nerve emerges through
the sclera. As the fibres of the optic nerve turn outwards, over the inside of the eye, they tend to become heaped up between the optic cup
and the edge of the disc. In the normal, the optic nerve protrudes about
2 mm above the surface of the retina. The optic disc is normally slightly
paler on the temporal than on the nasal side—it is important to be aware
of this normal temporal pallor because increased temporal pallor is a
sign of disseminated sclerosis, but it takes considerable experience to
say whether the temporal pallor is more than normal. Another important normal feature of the optic disc is blurring of its nasal margins. The
contour of the disc should normally only be blurred on the nasal side:
similar blurring of the contour elsewhere indicates papilloedema.

Papilloedema

The earliest sign of papilloedema is swelling of the veins, which
normally are approximately twice the thickness of the arteries: they are
swollen if they are more than twice the thickness. The next step in the
development of papilloedema is blurring of the disc margins and then

the disc becomes more red than usual. Normally, the optic disc is much paler than the surrounding retina, and one which is the same colour as the retina is almost certainly abnormal. The oedema of the optic nerve causes the funnel-shaped hole in the centre of the nerve (the optic cup) to become filled with fluid, so that the lamina cribrosa cannot be seen. As oedema and congestion continue, small veins rupture, leading to haemorrhages in the layers of the retina. All the nerve fibres in the retina radiate outwards from the optic disc, so that haemorrhage between the nerve fibres will tend to be linear (or sometimes flame-shaped). This radial arrangement of the nerve fibres also applies to the macular area, so that any oedema which collects near the macula appears to radiate from it—this is called the "macular star", and it occurs in severe papilloedema.

If the raised intracranial pressure is not relieved, the congestion of the disc remains. The continued pressure on the optic nerve causes the fibres to atrophy, and when they do so they become white. This causes the optic disc to appear very pale. The increased pressure tends to involve the central retinal artery, which may become narrowed causing attenuation of the arteries of the retina, and the veins usually remain congested. Because of the accompanying oedema, the disc margin remains blurred, the optic cup remains filled with fluid and, therefore, indistinct and the lamina cribrosa cannot be seen. This is the appearance of secondary optic atrophy because it occurs secondary to papilloedema. Primary optic atrophy is atrophy of the optic nerve, due to external pressure or inflammation—there is no interference with the venous drainage or arterial supply of the eye. The disc in primary optic atrophy will appear paler than usual but because there is no oedema, the contour, the optic cup, and the lamina cribrosa will be easily seen. The arteries and veins of the retina are normal. Consecutive optic atrophy refers to atrophy of the optic nerve due to disease within the eye, damaging the nerves of the retina after they have left the optic nerve. The appearances of the optic nerve are the same as those of primary optic atrophy, but in addition, the cause of the optic atrophy can also be seen within the eye. The two commonest causes are glaucoma and choroiditis. When the optic disc is inspected, the following should be noted: circulation (arteries and veins), colour, contour, cup, cribriform plate and the complete retina.

Some conditions cause inflammation of the optic nerve: if the nerve is only affected behind the eyeball the condition is called retrobulbar neuritis. In the early stages of retrobulbar neuritis there are no abnormalities to be seen in the optic disc, although vision may be severely affected. Later primary optic atrophy follows. Optic neuritis refers to inflammation of the optic nerve where the nerve can be seen with the ophthalmoscope within the eye, the appearances are those of papilloedema. The causes of optic neuritis and retrobulbar neuritis are the same, namely:

1. Disseminated sclerosis.
2. Tabes dorsalis.
3. Vitamin B_1 and B_{12} deficiency.
4. Toxic causes (such as tobacco, alcohol particularly methyl alcohol, quinine and lead).

The pupillary reaction in retrobulbar neuritis may be helpful: the pupil reacts briskly to accommodation and consensual light reaction, but slowly to the direct light reaction because the afferent light pathway has been interrupted by the damage to the optic nerve. Conditions which may be associated with papilloedema are:

1. Intracranial tumours; papilloedema is usually more severe with tumours arising in the posterior fossa.
2. Malignant hypertension; probably causes papilloedema by raising the intracranial pressure, although local spasm of arterioles may lead to local ischaemia and oedema and thickened arteries may press on veins, causing venous congestion.
3. Venous obstruction affecting the central vein of the retina. Causes include: orbital neoplasms, cavernous sinus thrombosis, superior vena cava obstruction and thrombosis of the central retinal vein.
4. Unusual causes of papilloedema, such as severe anaemia, polycythaemia and raised blood CO_2.

Once primary optic atrophy has occurred, the changes are permanent, so that, should raised intracranial pressure arise later, papilloedema will not occur. In a tumour of a frontal lobe which presses on one optic nerve, optic atrophy occurs on that side; later as the tumour grows, the intracranial pressure rises, leading to papilloedema in the opposite eye—this is known as the Foster Kennedy syndrome.

Thrombosis of the central artery of the retina results in extreme pallor of the retina, with narrowing of the retinal arteries and a "cherry-red" spot at the macula. There is, of course, sudden complete blindness. Thrombosis of the central vein of the retina results in papilloedema and oedema of the rest of the retina with grossly congested veins and numerous haemorrhages. Unlike papilloedema the condition is usually unilateral, the retinal oedema extends to the periphery of the retina and visual acuity is affected. In papilloedema visual acuity usually remains normal until the late stages. Following retinal vein thrombosis anastomotic vessels may develop or the retinal appearances may return to normal. Vision may be severely affected even though the retinal appearances have returned to normal.

Following subarachnoid haemorrhage, a subhyaloid haemorrhage may be seen in the eye, situated between the retina and the vitreous humour. In this position it takes up the shape of the eye and has a curved lower margin, its upper border is horizontal. The exact cause is not known, as the subarachnoid space is not in continuity with the subhyaloid space in the eye; it may result from a sudden increase in venous pressure in the central retinal vein due to a sudden outpouring of blood into the subarachnoid space.

The appearances of choroiditis are of white, opaque areas of any size, surrounded by a black, pigmented margin. The retinal vessels are always seen superficial to an area of choroiditis. In glaucoma, the increased intra-ocular pressure causes an increase in size of the optic cup which is the weakest part of the sclera. The cup may become so large that its base is wider than its apex, so that it shelves under the emerging fibres of the optic nerve. Continued pressure may lead to atrophy of the nerve fibres and a pale disc. If a small vessel is followed from the retina onto the disc it suddenly disappears as it enters the optic cup, whose walls are sloping outwards towards its base. The small vessel will reappear again as it crosses the floor of the optic cup to enter the lamina cribrosa.

At the optic disc, two physiological conditions may cause confusion. The first is the myopic crescent which occurs in severe myopia; it merely consists of an opaque crescent lying against one margin of the disc, and the other is opaque medullated nerve fibres, which radiate out from the disc; these are white and may simulate optic atrophy.

The walls of the retinal arteries are normally not visible. All that is seen is the column of blood within the artery and the reflection of light from the curved surface of the artery. Normally this light reflex is of constant thickness along the length of the vessel; when atheromatous plaques are deposited on the intima, the visible column of blood appears indented, and, therefore, the artery appears to have increased in tortuosity. Deposition of atheroma in the intima of the arteries leads to a smaller lumen and a thinner column of blood which appears as arterial narrowing. The thickening and infiltration of the wall of the artery with atheroma leads to the wall becoming white and visible, the artery will now appear as a column of blood on either side of which is a white margin. This is known as "silver wiring". Because the arterial wall is thickened and irregular, the light reflex will vary in thickness and appear interrupted. At the stage of "silver wiring" veins will be compressed by the thickened arterial wall, leading to the appearance of arterio-venous nipping. All the changes mentioned may be seen in severe atheroma in the absence of hypertension. However, in the presence of long-standing hypertension, the same changes may be seen—they are due to atheroma which has been accelerated by the hypertension. Hypertension alone will produce a change in the retinal arteries: this consists of irregular spasm of the arteries, and consequently an irregularity of the light reflex in narrowed arteries. The retinal artery appearances of hypertension may, of course, be superimposed on those due to accelerated atheroma.

Accelerated hypertension may go on to produce haemorrhages and "soft" exudates—these are poorly demarcated and are probably caused by resolving small retinal infarcts as a result of the arterial narrowing. "Hard" exudates have a well-defined border and are due to degeneration of part of the retina. They are also seen in hypertension but are more common in diabetes. In malignant hypertension there is always papilloedema. These changes in the retinal arteries and retina form the basis for a graded classification of the severity of the retinal changes in hypertension.

Grade I Indicates mild changes in the retinal arteries.
Grade II Indicates arteriovenous nipping.
Grade III Indicates haemorrhages and exudates.
Grade IV Indicates papilloedema.

From the previous discussion it will be seen that Grades I and II may indicate atheroma and not always hypertension. For this reason it is probably better to qualify the grades by a description of the changes in the retinal arteries.

Movements of the Eye

Voluntary eye movements in all directions are controlled bilaterally by centres in the frontal cortices. In the midbrain, there are the nuclei for oculomotor and trochlear nerves and nuclei dealing with conjugate deviation of the eyes upwards and downwards. In the pons, there is the nucleus of the sixth nerve and a centre dealing with lateral conjugate deviation. All the nuclei are interconnected by the medial longitudinal bundle.

The abducens nerve (VI) supplies the lateral rectus, the trochlear (IV) supplies the superior oblique and the oculomotor nerve (III) supplies the remainder of the ocular muscles. The lateral and medial recti move the eye outwards and inwards, the superior and inferior recti elevate and depress the eyes when they are turned outwards, and the superior and inferior obliques depress and elevate respectively when the eye is turned inwards.

The third nerve emerges from the midbrain close to the cerebral peduncles, passes between the posterior cerebral and superior cerebellar arteries and then passes through the cavernous sinus where it is very close to the fourth and sixth nerves and the ophthalmic division of the fifth nerve.

The third nerve also supplies the levator palpebrae superioris and the constrictor muscle of the pupils. If the nerve is paralysed there is ptosis due to drooping of the levator palpebrae superioris, a dilated pupil due to the unopposed action of the sympathetic impulses, and paralysis of all eye muscles except the lateral rectus and superior oblique. Thus, the eye is rotated outwards (by the lateral rectus) and downwards (by the superior oblique).

The fourth nerve arises from the dorsum of the midbrain, passes between the posterior cerebral and superior cerebellar arteries and enters the cavernous sinus.

The sixth nerve arises from the pons and its nucleus is very close to that of the seventh nerve. It has a very long intracranial course before entering the cavernous sinus. It passes with the seventh nerve through the cerebello-pontine angle over the petrous bone where it lies close to the fifth nerve. Because of their long intracranial course, the third, fourth and sixth nerves are subject to a large number of lesions, some of which are common to them all. The three nerves have their origins in the brain stem; midbrain lesions will affect the third and fourth, while pontine lesions will affect the sixth. Within the brain stem, they are subject to:

1. Vascular lesions.
2. Neoplasms.
3. Encephalitis.
4. Disseminated sclerosis.

They all lie on the meninges and are, therefore, prone to damage in:

Meningitis.
Syphilis.
Meningioma.
Carcinoma of meninges.

They have a common pathway in the cavernous sinus and through the superior orbital fissure and can be damaged in:

Cavernous sinus thrombosis.
Aneurysm of the internal carotid artery.
Lesions within the orbit.

Like all nerves they may be victims to polyneuritis and myasthenia gravis.

The third nerve passes near the posterior cerebral and posterior communicating arteries, and may be pressed by aneurysms of these arteries. It may also be damaged by a raised intracranial pressure: the nerve is fixed where it pierces the dura to enter the cavernous sinus, but the brain stem is pushed downwards by cerebral tumours towards the foramen magnum, causing excessive stretching of the nerve. The same applies to the sixth nerve but the fourth nerve is not usually affected.

The only lesion which usually damages the fourth nerve alone is an aneurysm of the posterior cerebral artery. The sixth nerve is more vulnerable than the third to a rise in intracranial pressure and may be damaged by the transient rise of intracranial pressure which occurs following a subarachnoid haemorrhage.

The sixth nerve crosses the cerebello-pontine angle where it may be involved in an acoustic neuroma (in which the eighth, seventh and fifth nerves may also be affected). As the nerve passes forwards, it crosses the apex of the petrous temporal bone, and lies near the fifth nerve: in this situation it may be involved in periostitis of the petrous temporal bone which results from otitis media, usually in childhood. The combination of sixth nerve palsy with pain in the distribution of the trigeminal nerve is known as Gradenigo's[118] syndrome.

The main symptom from any ocular palsy is diplopia and the main signs are strabismus (or squint) and inability to move the eyes in certain directions. The eyes should be tested one at a time by moving the finger in all directions to see in which directions the eye will not move. There are three basic rules with regard to the assessment of diplopias:

1. Diplopia is present when the eye is moving in the direction of the paralysed muscle.

2. Diplopia is maximal when the eye is looking in the direction of pull of the paralysed muscle.

3. The most peripheral image of the two is from the eye with the weak muscle so that covering one eye at a time will distinguish which eye has the weak muscle.

Strabismus

Some conditions cause deviation in the direction of the optical axis of each eye which remains constant irrespective of which direction the eyes are looking: this is known as concomitant strabismus. It occurs if there is slight asymmetry of strength of corresponding muscles of each eye—it is a common occurrence in children and often follows an attack of measles. A paralytic or divergent strabismus is a squint due to paralysis of ocular muscles and it will only be present when an attempt is made to move the eye in the direction of the paralysed muscles; in other positions the optical axes of both eyes will be parallel.

In a concomitant strabismus, the range of movements of each eye is normal, and the deviation in the direction in which both eyes are look-ing is constant in all positions; furthermore, it is present at rest. In a paralytic strabismus the squint is not usually present at rest and is worse on looking in the direction of pull of the paralysed muscle. A fundamental difference between paralytic and concomitant strabismus

118. GIUSEPPE GRADENIGO (1859–1926). Naples otologist.

is that there is no diplopia in a concomitant strabismus because the image from one eye is suppressed. It is usually found that one eye has a severe refractive error and the image from this eye is the one that is usually suppressed, although the eye can be used if the other is covered.

The centres concerned with voluntary conjugate movement of the eyes are situated in the frontal lobes; however, in addition, there are, in the brain stem, the centres concerned with involuntary conjugate movements: the centres in the brain stem are near the nuclei of the corresponding cranial nerves. It is possible to have lesions between the voluntary centre and the reflex centres for conjugate movements. Such lesions will abolish conjugate eye movements when the patient is asked to look in a particular direction or to follow a moving finger; however, conjugate movements will be intact if the patient is asked to look at a fixed object and his head is slowly rotated. The lesions responsible for such supranuclear ocular palsies are always bilateral.

The Pupils

The constrictor pupillary muscle is controlled by parasympathetic fibres, travelling via the third nerve and ciliary ganglion. The dilator pupillary muscle is supplied by fibres from the cervical sympathetic chain, the fibres travelling both via ciliary ganglion and via the ophthalmic division of the trigeminal nerve. The pupillary light reflex is stimulated by afferents travelling in the optic nerve to the lateral geniculate body and thence to the bilateral nuclei in the midbrain concerned with pupillary constriction: this nucleus lies very close to that of the third nerve, through which the motor side of the reflex is mediated.

The reaction to accommodation is complex: it involves convergence of the eyes, using both medial recti, contraction of ciliary muscle rendering the lens of the eye more globular and constriction of the pupils. The afferent side of the reflex probably arises from the frontal cortex; the motor side is mediated by the third nerve; however, there is some evidence that the fibres concerned with the accommodation reaction do not pass through the ciliary ganglion, unlike those concerned with the pupillary light reflex.

The essential features of the Argyll Robertson[119] pupil is that it reacts to accommodation but not to light. The most likely position for a lesion which interferes with the light but not the accommodation reflex is in the ciliary ganglion because it is believed that the fibres of the oculomotor nerve carrying accommodation reflex impulses do not pass through the ganglion. The other possible position for such a lesion is in the midbrain near the aqueduct where the light-reflex fibres decussate on their way to the third nerve nuclei of the two sides. Other features of

119. DOUGLAS MORAY COOPER LAMB ARGYLL ROBERTSON (1837–1909). Scottish physician.

the Argyll Robertson pupil are that the pupil is irregular, that it is con-tracted and that there is depigmentation of the iris. The fact that con-traction is a cardinal feature of the Argyll Robertson pupil means that the lesion does not only involve the oculomotor nerve fibres, otherwise the pupil would be dilated. This suggests that the sympathetic innerva-tion is also impaired, which is added evidence for the lesion being in the ciliary ganglion, because some sympathetic pupillary fibres travel to the eye via the ciliary ganglion. The Argyll Robertson pupil occurs with conditions other than syphilis, including diabetes, post-encephalitic Parkinsonism, polyneuritis, as well as vascular and neoplastic lesions involving the midbrain.

The Holmes[120]-Adie[121] pupil is quite distinct from the Argyll Robertson pupil. It is larger than normal, does not react to light, but may react to accommodation very slowly. The condition is virtually always unilateral, confined to women and associated with diminished tendon jerks.

Ptosis

The upper lid is elevated by the levator palpebrae superioris, which is supplied by the sympathetic and by the third nerve. The sympathetic supply is mainly responsible for maintaining the tone of the muscle at rest; if the sympathetic supply is interrupted but the third nerve is intact, the upper lid will appear ptosed at rest, but can be raised norm-ally when the patient is asked to look upwards: this is the situation in Horner's syndrome. In ptosis due to paralysis of the third nerve, the levator palpebrae superioris is paralysed and the upper lid can only be raised by overaction of the frontalis muscle which is seen as excessive wrinkling of the forehead. Despite the overaction of the frontalis, the upper lid cannot be raised as much as normally when the patient looks upwards.

The important causes of ptosis are:

Horner's syndrome due to interruption of the sympathetic system anywhere from the upper thorax to the ciliary ganglion. The main condi-tions causing this are enlarged cervical lymph glands, syringobulbia and syringomyelia, and vascular lesions of the medulla.

Tabes dorsalis and lesions of the third nerve.

Mild bilateral congenital ptosis.

Hysteria, in which case the ptosis is always unilateral.

TRIGEMINAL NERVE

The motor and sensory divisions arise from nuclei in the pons. When the sensory division enters the brain stem the fibres subserving pain and

120. SIR GORDON MORGAN HOLMES (1876). London neurologist.
121. WILLIAM JOHN ADIE (1886–1935). London physician.

temperature descend on the same side to the level of the third cervical segment, cross the midline and ascend in the lateral spinothalamic tract. The fibres of this descending tract which reach the lowest level are those derived from the upper part of the face. This explains why syringomyelia which affects the middle of the cervical cord may cause loss of pain and temperature of the upper part of the face. The sensory fibres of the trigeminal nerve carrying touch and proprioceptive impulses cross the midline as soon as they enter the brain stem and ascend to the thalamus and cerebral cortex by way of the medial lemniscus.

The sensory and motor roots leave the pons and cross the cerebello-pontine angle; the sensory root relays in a large ganglion which lies near the sixth nerve at the apex of the petrous temporal bone, where it may be involved in spread of infection from otitis media. From this ganglion the ophthalmic division travels in the cavernous sinus with the three ophthalmic nerves; hence, any lesion within the cavernous sinus (internal carotid artery aneurysm or thrombosis of the cavernous sinus) generally involves the three ophthalmic nerves and the ophthalmic division of the fifth nerve.

The ophthalmic division conveys sensation from the cornea and remainder of the eye; it is the afferent part of the corneal reflex, the motor part being the facial nerve which innervates the orbicularis oculi. Stimulation of the cornea of one eye results in bilateral contraction of the orbicularis oculi, so that even in the presence of a lower motor neurone facial nerve weakness on one side the corneal reflex can still be tested. Loss of the corneal reflex is an early sign of a tumour in the cerebello-pontine angle.

The ophthalmic division of the trigeminal nerve is more frequently affected by herpes zoster than the other two sensory branches. Involvement of the ophthalmic division may lead to anaesthesia of the cornea and subsequent ulceration, keratitis and blindness. The fifth nerve supplies sensation to the whole of the face, pharynx and nose except for taste sensation. Taste sensation from the anterior two-thirds of the tongue is carried for a short distance in the lingual nerve which is a branch of the mandibular division of the fifth nerve; taste fibres then leave the lingual nerve to join the chorda tympani of the facial nerve in the facial canal. Thus, a peripheral lesion of the mandibular nerve may affect taste over the anterior two-thirds of the tongue, although such lesions are very rare.

Because of the extensive distribution of branches of the trigeminal nerve, pain may be referred to an area remote from its origin. The most important examples of this clinically are pain in the ear and temples in the case of an apical tooth abscess or carcinoma of the maxillary antrum. Pain from the eye (as in glaucoma) may be referred to the temples or to the dura mater (causing severe headache). The exclusion of referred pain is important in the diagnosis of trigeminal neuralgia. The drug carbamazepine (Tegretol) has considerably improved the treatment of trigeminal neuralgia; it does not relieve referred pain. The motor branch of the fifth nerve supplies the muscles of mastication.

SEVENTH NERVE

The facial nerve is purely motor, its nucleus is situated in the pons and as the nerve emerges from the brain stem it is closely associated with the nucleus of the sixth nerve. It crosses the cerebello-pontine angle, passes into the internal auditory meatus and then into its own bony canal. In the bony canal it gives off a branch to the stapedius muscle, then forms the geniculate ganglion which receives taste fibres via the chorda tympani from the anterior two-thirds of the tongue. The facial nerve emerges from the skull via the stylomastoid foramen and is then distributed to the facial muscles which include the platysma of the neck.

Lower motor neurone lesions beyond the nucleus of the facial nerve cause complete paralysis of all the facial muscles on one side. The nucleus of the facial nerve in the pons receives two sets of upper motor neurone fibres which run together; one set derived only from the opposite cerebral cortex is concerned with movements of the lower facial muscles and the other set derived from both cerebral cortices is concerned with movements of the upper facial muscles. Thus, an upper motor neurone lesion of the facial nerve will cause total paralysis of the lower facial muscles, but the upper facial muscles can still be moved because the part of the facial nucleus on each side concerned with the upper facial muscles is supplied by both cerebral cortices. An internal capsular lesion which causes a facial weakness will only affect the lower face on one side whereas a Bell's palsy will affect the whole of the face on one side. The principal sites of damage to the facial nerve are:

1. *Pons.*—Lesions here will be associated with a lateral rectus palsy, damage to the fifth nerve (both descending and immediately decussating parts), spinothalamic tract and pyramids (before they have decussated).

2. *Cerebello-pontine angle.*—The commonest tumour is an acoustic neuroma. If the facial nerve is damaged in this situation there will be loss of taste over the anterior two-thirds of the tongue and hyperacusis because the nerve to the stapedius muscle will be paralysed. In the cerebello-pontine angle the fifth, sixth and eighth nerves are also affected.

3. *The facial canal.*—The nerves will be affected by suppuration from the middle ear; taste from the anterior two-thirds of the tongue will be lost.

4. *In the face* the commonest lesion is Bell's[122] palsy, although it may also be affected in neoplasms of the parotid gland.

Although loss of taste and hyperacusis are unusual in a Bell's palsy they do sometimes occur, indicating that the lesion is sometimes within the facial canal. The cause of the condition is not known. There are several controlled trials which show that prednisolone given soon after the onset of Bell's palsy accelerates recovery which is also more complete than in untreated cases. It is worth giving corticosteroid therapy up to 7 days after the onset of palsy. The usual dose regimen is prednisolone 80 mg daily for 5 days followed by 60, 40, 20, 10 mg for one day each (Taverner *et al.*, 1971).

As a rule if there is some *recovery* of voluntary function after one week, full functional recovery of the nerve will occur. Ideally the management of cases of Bell's palsy should include nerve excitability tests; these are extremely simple to perform and involve no discomfort for the patient. Small electric currents are passed via electrodes applied to the skin over the stylomastoid foramen, the lowest current which stimulates the facial nerve producing a twitch of the corner of the mouth is recorded. Nerve excitability tests should be done 7, 14 and 21 days after the facial palsy has developed; by 14 days electrical recovery should have started (i.e. the current needed to excite the nerve should be less than on day 7). If recovery has not started by day 21 decompression of the facial nerve *may* be indicated although the results of decompression of the nerve are difficult to evaluate.

EIGHTH NERVE

The cochlear portion of the nerve is concerned with hearing and the vestibular part with balance and position sense. Both parts arise from the pons, cross the cerebello-pontine angle close to the seventh, fifth and sixth nerves, enter the internal auditory meatus and terminate in the cochlear and vestibular apparatus in the inner ear. In the pons the cochlear fibres pass up both lateral lemnisci to the temporal cortices. Whereas vestibular fibres join the medial longitudinal bundle which co-ordinates the nuclei of the cranial nerves concerned with movements of the face and eyes, some vestibular fibres terminate in the cerebral cortex, and these are concerned with the appreciation of vertigo.

Deafness

Deafness is caused by lesions of the middle ear, cochlea, auditory nerve or its central connections. Damage to the middle ear leads to conduction deafness; this can be distinguished from "nerve" deafness

122. SIR CHARLES BELL (1774–1842). Scottish surgeon.

by Weber's[123] and Rinne's[124] tests: bone conduction of sounds is better than air conduction if there is middle-ear disease, i.e. a conduction deafness.

The important causes of middle-ear deafness are otitis media and otosclerosis; the important causes of cochlear destruction are mumps, Ménière's disease and idiosyncrasy or overdose of quinine, salicylates and streptomycin; the important causes of auditory nerve deafness are acoustic neuroma, Paget's disease and meningitis (usually syphilitic). Cochlear deafness can be distinguished from nerve deafness by audiometric tests by the fact that in cochlear deafness once a sound can be heard at all it appears louder than it should ("loudness recruitment").

Nystagmus

Nystagmus generally consists of two phases, one rapid and the other slow. There are three groups of causes of nystagmus each of which has distinguishing features. They are:

1. Lesions of the eye in which the nystagmus is associated with defective vision and consists of two phases which are equal in speed.

2. Lesions of the vestibular system (labyrinth and vestibular nerve). These are usually accompanied by damage to the auditory apparatus or auditory branch of the eighth nerve, with frequently coexisting deafness and tinnitus. Vestibular nystagmus is always accompanied by vertigo and usually lasts only a few weeks because central compensation occurs.

The direction in which nystagmus is greatest is sometimes helpful in establishing its cause. The simple rule is that in vestibular nystagmus the slow phase is towards the diseased side and the excursions are greatest when looking in the direction of the quick phase. This means that vestibular nystagmus is constant in the direction of its slow and fast phases and is maximum in its excursion when the patient is looking *away* from the affected labyrinth or nerve. The commonest causes of vestibular nystagmus are Ménière's[125] disease and middle ear infections.

3. Central lesions (usually brain stem and cerebellum). There is usually no vertigo, deafness or tinnitus, unlike vestibular nystagmus. The slow phase is always directed to the rest position of the eyes so that the direction of the slow and fast phases changes with full excursion of the eyes. The commonest causes of central nystagmus are disseminated sclerosis, cerebellar lesions, hereditary ataxias and syringomyelia.

Caloric tests are of limited value in elucidating the cause of nystagmus and vertigo. The principle on which they are based is simple but their interpretation is often difficult. The principle is that when hot and then

123. FRIEDRICH EUGEN WEBER-LIEL (1832–1891). Berlin and Jena otologist.
124. HEINRICH ADOLF RINNE (1819–1868). Hildesheim otologist.
125. PROSPER MÉNIÈRE (1799–1862). Paris physician.

cold water is run into one ear each induces nystagmus in opposite directions; normally the nystagmus lasts for about two minutes. In disease of the vestibular apparatus or vestibular nerve (e.g. Ménière's disease or acoustic neuroma) the nystagmus in both directions from the affected ear is shorter than normal ("canal paresis"). In disease of the central connections the nystagmus in one direction from stimulation of both ears (hot in one and cold in the other) is increased ("directional preponderance").

NINTH NERVE (Glossopharyngeal)

This supplies the muscles of the pharynx, taste from the posterior third of the tongue and sensation from the inside of the mouth.

TENTH NERVE (Vagus)

The motor branch supplies the soft palate in addition to the muscles of the pharynx and larynx.

ELEVENTH NERVE (Accessory)

This is entirely motor and is joined by a branch from the upper cervical spine; together they supply the trapezius and sternomastoid muscles.

TWELFTH NERVE (Hypoglossal)

This is the motor nerve of the tongue. A lower motor neurone lesion causes atrophy of one-half of the tongue—this is a very dramatic physical sign, it occurs within days and is always severe and unmistakable; the tongue deviates from the weak side as it lies in the mouth but protrudes from the mouth *towards* the weak side. In bulbar palsy there is bilateral wasting of the tongue; in pseudobulbar palsy the tongue is not wasted but it can only be protruded with difficulty because it is stiff and spastic (in keeping with the fact that pseudobulbar palsy is due to bilateral upper motor neurone lesions).

The ninth, tenth, eleventh and twelfth cranial nerves are usually involved together in lesions within the posterior fossa (syndrome of the jugular foramen).

Raised Intracranial Pressure

The cerebrospinal fluid is produced by the choroid plexuses of the lateral ventricles deep in the cerebral hemispheres, it passes to the third ventricle of the midbrain, through the narrow aqueduct into the fourth

126. HUBERT VON LUSCHKA (1820–1875). Tübingen anatomist.
127. FRANÇOIS MAGENDIE (1783–1855). Paris physician and physiologist.

ventricle of the medulla (Fig. 11). Note that so far the fluid has been *inside* the substance of the brain and brain stem. It leaves the fourth ventricle by three holes, the two foramina of Luschka[126] laterally and the median foramen of Magendie,[127] and for the first time the fluid finds itself in the subarachnoid space surrounding brain and spinal cord. The fluid is absorbed by the arachnoid granulations on the surface of the brain. A point often overlooked is that wherever the obstruction to flow of the CSE occurs there is *always* enlargement of the ventricular system of the brain and it is the increased pressure in the ventricular system which causes enlargement of the cerebral hemispheres. It is this enlargement of the cerebral hemispheres which gives rise to the increased pressure in the subarachnoid space. Another factor which contributes to the later increase in pressure of CSF is that a small rise in intracranial pressure causes obstruction of the venous drainage of the arachnoid granulations leading to decreased absorption of CSF. A cerebral tumour causes back pressure dilatation of the ventricular system by pushing the cerebral hemispheres downward and blocking the hole between the free edges of the tentorium. Meningitis causes enlargement of the ventricular system by obstructing the flow in the subarachnoid space over the surface of the cerebral hemispheres.

Classification of hydrocephalus into communicating and obstructive is of no value clinically because the pathogenesis of the increased pressure in both cases is the same, namely increase in size of the ventricular system causing swelling of the cerebral hemispheres. Obstructive hydrocephalus refers to obstruction to the flow of CSF before it has left the ventricular system—it will occur in ependymomas of the third ventricle, pineal and midbrain tumours, congenital stenosis of the aqueduct between third and fourth ventricles and obstruction to outflow from the fourth ventricle such as may occur in the Arnold-Chiari malformation or basilar impression. Communicating hydrocephalus refers only to the fact that there is free communication between the ventricular system and subarachnoid space—in the case of a communicating hydrocephalus the block is within the subarachnoid space usually at the hiatus of the tentorium. Raised intracranial pressure develops much more quickly with tumours in the posterior fossa than in other sites because they readily obstruct the openings in the roof of the fourth ventricle.

The clinical features of raised intracranial pressure are:

1. Papilloedema due to obstruction to retinal veins.
2. Headache, vomiting and epilepsy.
3. Mental changes.
4. Pressure-cone features and false localising signs.

There are two positions where the brain and brain stem can attempt to expand if there is a rise in intracranial pressure. The midbrain passes between the two free edges of the tentorium; increased pressure above the tentorium, as in cerebral tumours, will force part of the temporal lobes through the hiatus compressing any structures in contact with the tentorium—these are the midbrain, the cerebral peduncles, the third and sixth nerves and the posterior cerebral arteries. The features of a tentorial pressure cone are therefore:

1. Contralateral hemiplegia due to pressure on the cerebral peduncle on the side of the tumour. Occasionally the brain is displaced laterally, compressing the opposite cerebral peduncle, in which case the hemiplegia is on the side of the lesion—hence the description "false localising sign".

2. Ipsilateral third nerve palsy leading to a fixed dilated pupil.

3. Ipsilateral lateral rectus palsy (sixth nerve).

4. Occlusion of one posterior cerebral artery leading to homonymous hemianopia.

5. Midbrain infarction.

If the increased pressure occurs in the posterior fossa, part of the cerebellum is forced through the foramen magnum and the medulla will be compressed at its anterior and posterior parts as well as being pushed downwards. This is the foramen magnum pressure cone. It leads to:

1. Compression of the nuclei of the posterior columns leading to loss of proprioception.

2. Compression of pyramidal tracts anteriorly.

3. Acute angulation of the lower cranial nerves leading to a bulbar palsy. The nerves are fixed by the foramina through which they emerge from the skull, hence if the medulla is pushed downwards the nerves will be unduly stretched.

4. Severe pain in the occipital region and the neck.

5. Occasionally there are cerebellar signs.

The same clinical features as in the foramen magnum pressure cone may be seen in abnormalities of the base of the skull. The most important of these are:

1. Arnold[128]-Chiari malformation in which herniation through the foramen magnum occurs as a congenital anomaly. The condition may present as hydrocephalus if the outflow of the CSF from the fourth ventricle is obstructed. The condition is often associated with syringomyelia and meningocele.

2. Congenital fusion of cervical vertebrae (Klippel[129]-Feil[130] deformity).

128. JULIUS ARNOLD (1835–1915). Heidelberg pathologist.
129. MAURIC KLIPPEL (1858–1942). Paris neurologist.
130. ANDRÉ FEIL (b. 1884). Paris neurologist.

3. Basilar impression and platybasia in which the upper cervical spine is invaginated into the base of the skull. It may occur as a congenital anomaly or be due to bone disease such as Paget's disease or osteomalacia.

Benign intracranial hypertension.—This is a rare condition in which the intracranial pressure is raised in the absence of a tumour but the ventricles are often normal in size. Papilloedema and a sixth-nerve palsy may occur; the condition is usually self-limiting but the papilloedema may damage vision permanently. The exact cause of the raised intracranial pressure is not known but certain conditions are commonly associated with it.

1. Sudden reduction or increase in corticosteroid dosage.
2. Addison's disease.
3. Hypoparathyroidism.
4. Pregnancy, obesity and the menarche.
5. Previous head injury.
6. Chlortetracycline administration.
7. Sagittal sinus thrombosis (otitic hydrocephalus).
8. Anaemia.
9. Polycythaemia.
10. Nalidixic acid.
11. Oral contraceptives.

Normal Pressure Hydrocephalus

Another relatively common condition is normal pressure hydrocephalus in which there is enlargement of the ventricles associated with cerebral atrophy and neuropsychiatric manifestations, particularly unsteadiness of gait and urinary incontinence, but in which the CSF pressure is normal. It is believed that flow of CSF from the ventricles is disturbed possibly by arachnoid adhesions over the surface of the brain preventing absorption of CSF by the arachnoid granulations in the superior longitudinal sinus. Adhesions may follow previous meningitis or subarachnoid haemorrhage. It is an important condition to pick up because pneumoencephalography nearly always causes a deterioration and secondly, good results are obtained from drainage procedures of the ventricles. The condition can be diagnosed by injecting radioactive labelled albumin into the CSF and noting by brain scan its abnormally prolonged retention in the cerebral ventricles.

Blood Supply of the Brain and Spinal Cord

Figure 14 shows the principal arteries supplying the brain. The basilar artery runs on the under surface of the brain stem supplying branches to the medulla and pons. The midbrain is supplied by the posterior cerebral arteries. Occlusion of one of the vessels feeding the circle of Willis[131] may give rise to symptoms even though the remainder of the circle of Willis is patent. The converse is also true, namely that ischaemic symptoms may not be present even if there is total occlusion of one, two or even three of the main vessels feeding the circle of Willis. It is important to remember that all the cerebral arteries leaving the circle are end-arteries and there is no collateral circulation.

The middle cerebral artery is more or less a continuation of the internal carotid artery, hence occlusion of the internal carotid will usually cause the features of middle cerebral artery occlusion. However, an aneurysm of the internal carotid may involve the optic chiasma or optic tracts leading to a nasal or homonymous hemianopia respectively; or an aneurysm of the internal carotid may occur in the cavernous sinus leading to damage to the third, fourth, sixth or ophthalmic division of the fifth nerve. Obstruction of the internal carotid may involve a small branch of the artery before it joins the circle of Willis; this is the anterior choroidal artery which supplies part of the optic radiation near the internal capsule leading to a homonymous congruous scotoma or hemianopia.

As it leaves the midbrain the third nerve lies close to the posterior cerebral and posterior communicating arteries so that an aneurysm on either may lead to an isolated third-nerve palsy. The posterior cerebral artery supplies the occipital visual cortex so that complete occlusion causes a complete homonymous hemianopia but the macula is spared. However, small branches of the posterior cerebral supply the lower part of the optic radiation (which contains fibres from the lower part of the retinae), hence partial occlusion or a transient fall in blood flow in the posterior cerebral will cause an upper homonymous quadrantanopia. This explains why patients with vertebro-basilar insufficiency may complain of a defect of vision which is "like a curtain coming down".

The upper part of the optic radiation is supplied by the middle cerebral artery, hence ischaemia due to narrowing of the middle cerebral (or internal carotid) may cause a field defect in the lower part of the visual fields.

Aneurysms on the anterior cerebral or anterior communicating artery may compress the optic nerves leading to optic atrophy or they may compress the frontal lobes leading to frontal lobe symptoms.

Subarachnoid Haemorrhage

The commonest cause of blood in the subarachnoid space is rupture of any aneurysm of one of the cerebral arteries; however, blood may occur in the CSF in a number of other conditions which it is important

131. THOMAS WILLIS (1621–1675). English anatomist and physician.

to recognise. Bleeding may not necessarily be arterial, and in severe encephalitis capillaries may be damaged and lead to oozing of blood into the CSF; severe meningitis and pyaemias may cause venous damage and venous bleeding. Other causes of blood in the CSF include:

Intracerebral haemorrhage.
Bleeding into cerebral tumours.
Haemorrhagic diathesis (including anticoagulants).
Bleeding from angiomas.
Bleeding from anteriovenous malformations.

Arterial aneurysms always occur at the junction of two blood vessels, and are probably due to congenital weakness of the wall of the blood vessels which becomes critical when associated hypertensive or arteriosclerotic changes are present. At least two-thirds of ruptured aneurysms occur in women and half these are hypertensive. Anterior and middle cerebral aneurysms are considerably more common than posterior cerebral or posterior communicating aneurysms.

The diagnosis of a ruptured cerebral aneurysm is confirmed by finding blood in the CSF, but one very important practical point is that lumbar puncture should be delayed at least six hours after the ictus as it may take this time for blood to pass down into the spinal subarachnoid space; occasionally, it takes very much longer.

The mortality from rupture of a cerebral aneurysm is about 50 per cent. About one-third of those that die will do so within 48 hours from the effects of the first haemorrhage. Of the other two-thirds that die, most will succumb within six weeks from a second bleed—the greatest risk is in the second week after the first bleed. Of the patients who survive one-fifth will have severe neurological damage. Broken down the approximate percentages are:

	Per cent
Survival without severe impairment	40
Survival but with severe impairment	10
Die within 48 hours	15
Die within 6 weeks having survived 48 hours	25
Die after 6 weeks	10

Management of Subarachnoid Haemorrhage

Patients who are comatose are managed conservatively once the diagnosis has been made, but virtually all will die. This somewhat nihilistic view is accepted by the majority of neurosurgeons and it may be the only practical policy; however, some neurosurgeons believe that early cerebral angiography is indicated in younger patients in case the intracerebral haematoma is readily accessible and removable. Patients who do not have evidence of severe neurological damage or severe coincidental disease have bilateral carotid and vertebral angiography as soon as practicable. If no aneurysm is found the prognosis is considerably better; if an aneurysm is found the type of treatment depends on several factors. The statistical survival and morbidity figures are available for series of aneurysms at given sites treated medically and surgically. Aneurysms of the middle cerebral arteries have a better prognosis if treated surgically in men but conservatively in women (McKissock *et al.*, 1962). Aneurysms of the anterior cerebral and anterior communicating arteries have the same prognosis whether treated medically or surgically (McKissock *et al.*, 1965). However, aneurysms arising from the posterior cerebral or posterior communicating arteries have a much better prognosis when treated surgically both from the point of view of subsequent mortality and quality of survival (McKissock *et al.*, 1960). The main snag with the figures is that they show the outcome of series of patients treated in a particular way, but they do not help in deciding which form of treatment to adopt in an individual patient. Although one form of treatment may give larger survival figures in a series, an individual patient with certain characteristics may do better with the form of treatment which would not benefit the series as a whole. An attempt has been made to get over this problem by considering as many facets of the patient as possible. It is possible to draw up a list of factors to be considered as indicating benefit from surgical treatment of aneurysms at different sites. An example is given in Table VI; + indicates that the factor correlates with benefit from surgery, − indicates

TABLE VI

Factor	Aneurysm of anterior cerebral	Aneurysm of posterior cerebral
Increased age	+	−
Sex of patient	+	+
Hypertension	+	−
Conscious level when first seen	+	−
Presence of vascular spasm in the angiogram	−	+
Presence of a haematoma	−	+
Size of the aneurysm	−	+
Shape of the aneurysm	+	−
Direction of the aneurysm	+	−

that the factor is not important in considering surgery (Richardson *et al.*, 1966).

Subarachnoid haemorrhage due to leakage of blood directly into the spinal subarachnoid space is almost invariably due to an angioma. At the time of the bleed the patient has severe pain in the back which comes on so suddenly that it feels as if he has just been kicked in the back.

Thrombosis in the venous sinuses of the brain is rare, but when it occurs it is usually as a result of sepsis or trauma. Thrombosis in the cavernous sinus will cause damage to the third, fourth, sixth and ophthalmic division of the fifth nerve as well as exophthalmos and papilloedema due to congestion of the veins behind the eye. The other important sinus which may be affected is the sagittal sinus which runs antero-posteriorly in the midline. It runs over the frontal and parietal lobes of both cerebral cortices in the top of the falx cerebri. Thrombosis of the sagittal sinus will cause damage to the top of both cerebral cortices and, therefore, produces loss of sensation and movement in the legs—"crural dominance". Other conditions which cause crural dominance are thrombosis of the anterior cerebral arteries, para-sagittal meningioma or a subdural haematoma.

Blood Supply of the Spinal Cord

The anterior spinal artery (Fig. 14) arises from both vertebral arteries at the level of the medulla and passes down the anterior border of the spinal cord, and it sends branches to the lower medulla; occlusion of the anterior spinal artery at its origin will give rise to the medial medullary syndrome (involvement of corticospinal tracts, medial lemniscus and hypoglossal nerve). There are two small posterior spinal arteries which also arise from the vertebral arteries. The spinal arteries receive additional blood from the segmental arteries, although the extent to which segmental arteries contribute to the arterial supply of the cord varies. There are two very important and fairly constant segmental arteries: one arises from the costocervical trunk and enters the lower cervical cord and the other arises from one of the lower thoracic or upper lumbar segmental arteries usually on the left side and is known as the artery of Adamkiewicz.[132] It is believed that blood from the artery entering the lower cervical region flows mainly downwards and that the cervical cord above this region is supplied either by the anterior spinal or segmental arteries. Blood entering via the artery of Adamkiewicz flows both up and down the cord. The amount of anastomosis between the segmental arteries and the longitudinal spinal arteries is variable. If the anastomosis is poor it is easy to see how localised disease in one segment which occludes a vital artery can damage the tract of the spinal cord, even though the blood supply of the remainder of the cord is adequate. From the site and distribution of the main segmental boosters to the arterial supply it will be appreciated that there are two zones of the spinal cord which are particularly

132. ALBERT ADAMKIEWICZ (1850–1921). Cracow and Vienna pathologist.

vulnerable to ischaemia; the first is the lower cervical region just above the segment that the artery from the costocervical branch enters, as blood from the artery is believed to flow mainly downwards. The second zone vulnerable to ischaemia is the mid-thoracic region between the area of the cord supplied by the costocervical booster and that supplied by upward flow from the artery of Adamkiewicz.

Damage to the blood supply of the cord is particularly likely to occur due to damage to the artery of Adamkiewicz as in dissection of the aorta, left lower thoracotomies and lower left intercostal nerve blocks. The distribution of the blood supply to the spinal cord explains some of the anomalies of severe neurological damage with relatively minor lesions in certain areas, such as mild cervical spondylosis in the absence of evidence of cord compression. Damage to the arterial supply of the cord may occur following neck injuries, particularly "whip-lash" injuries.

Meningitis

The cardinal signs of inflammation of the meninges are neck stiffness due to reflex spasm of extensors of the neck when the head is flexed and Kernig's[133] sign which is spasm of the hamstring muscles when the knee is extended with the hips fully flexed. Meningism is the occurrence of neck stiffness in the absence of meningeal infection, it occurs particularly in subarachnoid haemorrhage and acute febrile illness in children. In meningism the pressure in the CSF is usually increased, the chloride is low but the protein and cell content are normal. Fibrosis of the meninges may occur following meningitis, resulting in isolated cranial nerve palsies, hydrocephalus or epilepsy. Meningococcal meningitis is the commonest form of meningitis in children and young adults and usually occurs as a result of overcrowding. Asymptomatic carriers may carry the organism in their throats for 2–3 weeks, but widespread treatment with sulphonamides of a population at risk will eliminate organisms carried by these asymptomatic carriers and will usually bring an epidemic to an end. There is often an erythematous or purpuric skin rash; another notorious feature is the syndrome of acute adrenal insufficiency or the Waterhouse[134]-Friderichsen[135] syndrome. The meningococcus is always sensitive to the sulphonamides in this country although resistant strains have been reported from the United States. Sulphonamides are usually combined with penicillin in case the pneumococcus is responsible for the meningitis. The most suitable sulphonamide is probably sulphadiazine rather than sulphadimidine.

133. Vladimir Mikhailovich Kernig (1840–1917). St. Petersburg physician.
134. Rupert Waterhouse (b. 1873). Bath physician.
135. Carl Friderichsen (b. 1886). Copenhagen physician.

Sulphadiazine is not as strongly bound to the plasma proteins and reaches the CSF in higher concentrations than sulphadimidine, however sulphadiazine is more likely to produce crystalluria.

In cases of meningitis in which the infecting organism is not known many physicians use a combination of sulphonamide, penicillin and chloramphenicol to cover the meningococcus, the pneumococcus and *H. influenzae*. Pneumococcal meningitis usually occurs as a result of spread from the nose or sinuses which harbour the organisms—this type of meningitis is particularly liable to occur following fractures of the skull which involve the nasal sinuses.

Meningitis due to *Haemophilus influenzae* is fairly common and may present in an interesting way: the meningitis may not be acute and it may cause a localised collection of fluid which behaves in the same way as subdural haematoma. Chloramphenicol is the drug of choice in treatment.

As a rule all forms of meningitis are accompanied by some inflammation of the brain and spinal cord (encephalitis and myelitis) and conversely all forms of encephalitis have some degree of meningeal irritation and meningism—this is particularly true of the viral infections of the nervous system. Non-viral causes of meningo-encephalitis are:

Tuberculosis.
Syphilis.
Malaria.
Trypanosomiasis.
Brucellosis.
Leptospirosis (Weil's disease and canicola fever).
Toxoplasmosis.
Behçet's disease (possibly due to a virus).
Sarcoidosis.
Torulosis (cryptococcosis).
Typhoid and typhus (*Gk*. typhos, mist; referring to mental and visual mistiness).
Carcinomatosis.

Viral Causes of Meningo-encephalitis

The diagnosis of virus infection can be substantiated by:

1. Clinical features.
2. Leucopenia and lymphocytosis.
3. Demonstration of the virus by electron microscopy.
4. Circumstantial evidence by observing a particular cytopathogenic effect of the virus on certain cells in the laboratory or producing an illness in animals which previous experience has shown to be due to a known virus.

5. Demonstration of serum antibodies. There are two main ways of demonstrating antibodies:

Complement fixation tests.—When antibody-antigen reactions take place complement (which is a globulin) is used up. Various dilutions of sera are incubated with a known quantity of virus antigen. In those dilutions in which an antibody reaction has taken place complement will be used up (or fixed). Any complement remaining means that not enough antibody from the patient is present to react with the known amount of virus antigen. Complement is detected by observing haemolysis of red cells when they are mixed with haemolysin. Haemolysis of the cells will not occur unless complement is present.

Neutralisation tests.—Serial dilutions of the patient's serum (containing antibody) are mixed with a known quantity of virus and inoculated into tissue cultures, the viruses not neutralised by antibody will grow. The dilution from which no growth on the tissue culture occurs indicates the titre of viral antibody present.

Complement fixation tests are better for the diagnosis of acute infections because the rise in antibody occurs quickly and subsides quickly and the test is quicker and easier to perform. Neutralisation tests are more time-consuming and the antibody titre may not fall even years after an infection. The main snag of serological tests for virus infections is that in many cases the virus has to be available for the tests to be performed. In the case of Coxsackie and ECHO viruses there are so many groups that may cause infection that it is not practicable to test for antibodies against the 30 odd members of each group. In order to perform the serological tests the virus has to be grown from the patient, usually from the stools but sometimes from throat swabs or CSF. The antibody titre against any virus grown is tested and if the titre is rising then this is presumptive evidence that the infection has been recently acquired. In some infections the virus has never been grown so that it is impossible to test for an antibody against it, e.g. infective hepatitis.

The main virus infections of the nervous system are:

1. Acute lymphocytic meningitis.
2. Acute aseptic meningitis. (Both of these may be due to Coxsackie and ECHO viruses.)
3. Poliomyelitis.
4. Arbor virus encephalitides.
5. Nervous system secondarily involved, as in:
   Mumps.
   Glandular fever.
   Herpes simplex.

Herpes zoster.
Exanthemata.
Psittacosis.
Infective hepatitis.
Rickettsial diseases.
Royal Free disease.
Epidemic vomiting, vertigo and cervical myalgia.

Acute lymphocytic and aseptic meningitis refer to the occurrence of meningeal irritation with a predominance of lymphocytes in the one case and a normal cell count in the other. The commonest causes of these two forms of meningitis are Coxsackie and ECHO virus infections; however, both forms of meningitis may occur in any of the other virus infections of the nervous system. When due to Coxsackie and ECHO virus infections the disease has a good prognosis. The diagnosis can be confirmed by growing the virus from the faeces or CSF, demonstrating a rising titre of neutralising antibodies and excluding other causes of lymphocytes in the CSF such as tuberculosis, poliomyelitis, glandular fever and herpes infections.

The arbor viruses are a group that are always spread by insect vectors and which cause three main types of illness:

Short, prostrating fevers, e.g. dengue and sandfly fever.
Haemorrhagic tendencies, e.g. yellow fever and various haemorrhagic fevers.
Encephalitis, e.g. St. Louis encephalitis, Japanese B encephalitis and Russian Spring fever.

Diseases caused by arbor viruses should not be confused with those caused by rickettsiae which are organisms larger than viruses, but can exist free from animal cells. There is, however, one important similarity between arbor viruses and rickettsiae—they are both exclusively spread by insect vectors. The main rickettsial diseases are typhus, Q fever and scrub typhus (tsutsugamushi disease).

SYPHILIS

The primary chancre usually occurs within 2–3 weeks of infection, it is associated with regional lymphadenopathy and always with blood dissemination of spirochetes. The primary chancre usually heals within six weeks. Secondary syphilis consists of the visible manifestations of blood-borne spread of the spirochetes. The most important manifestations of secondary syphilis are mucous and cutaneous; it is vitally important to realise that the lesions of secondary syphilis may recur in crops and that the lesions are highly infectious. It has been found by experience that after a period of 2–4 years the lesions of secondary syphilis no longer recur. However, despite the fact that skin and mucous lesions will not recur the spirochetes may still persist in the nervous and cardiovascular systems and can cause structural damage. Any stage of syphilis following the primary chancre, in which there is no evidence of structural damage, is known as latent syphilis. The stage of secondary syphilis before the mucocutaneous crops stop recurring is known as early latent syphilis and after the period 2–4 years when crops of lesions will no longer occur, is known as late latent syphilis. It is worth emphasising that latent syphilis can only be diagnosed if syphilitic infection can be proved to have occurred by positive serology, but there must be no evidence whatsoever of any structural lesion in the nervous or cardiovascular systems. Should the CSF in anyway be abnormal then structural change in the nervous system must have occurred and the syphilis cannot be latent even if the structural lesion cannot be found— this state is called asymptomatic neurosyphilis. The changes in the CSF which indicate neurosyphilis are an increase in lymphocytes, the presence of a positive WR in the CSF, the presence of globulin (normally globulin does not occur in the CSF; it is tested for by Pandy's[136] test) and alteration of the Lange[137] colloidal gold test. It is worth noting at this point that if the patient has received anti-syphilitic treatment, the blood WR may be negative even though asymptomatic neurosyphilis is present.

Beside the mucocutaneous manifestations of secondary (or early latent) syphilis there may be an iritis, retinitis or alopecia areata. Following early latent syphilis or late latent syphilis, structural changes may occur and the two parts of the nervous system involved are the meninges and the blood vessels—this is the stage of meningovascular neurosyphilis or tertiary syphilis. Later the spirochetes may directly involve parenchymatous nerve tissue leading to so-called quaternary syphilis: the manifestations of this are general paresis of the insane (GPI), in which the parenchymatous tissue of the cerebral hemispheres is affected, and tabes dorsalis in which the posterior nerve roots are involved.

The Serological Tests of Syphilis

There are two main types. The reagin tests that detect the presence of a non-specific antibody which develops after syphilis, yaws and leprosy; this is tested for either by a complement fixation test such as the Wassermann[138] reaction (WR) or by flocculation tests such as the Kahn[139]

136. KALMAN PANDY (b. 1868). Budapest psychiatrist.
137. CARL FRIEDRICH AUGUST LANGE (b. 1883). Berlin physician.
138. AUGUST PAUL VON WASSERMANN (1866–1925). Berlin bacteriologist.
139. REUBEN LEON KAHN (b. 1887). Lansing, Michigan, serologist.

and VDRL tests (Venereal Disease Reference Laboratory). The other type of serological tests are the treponema immobilisation test (TPI) and the Reiter protein complement fixation test (RPCF) which is almost specific for syphilis. The TPI tests for the presence of an antibody against the treponemes.

Following the primary chancre the reagin tests become positive after about two weeks while the TPI usually becomes positive after about two months. As a general rule the RPCF test remains positive for life even following adequate treatment. In untreated patients the reagin tests will become negative in about a quarter of the patients—"biological cures". Following adequate treatment of primary or secondary (early latent) syphilis the reagin tests will become negative after about six months in 90 per cent of the patients. In the remainder, the titre of reagin may drop but not reach zero, it may remain low or it may later rise again (sero relapse). Rarely, following adequate treatment, the reagin titre does not fall at all. Sero relapse is generally followed by clinical relapse—it is impossible to establish whether relapse has really occurred or whether there has been a fresh infection. It is very important to detect sero relapse because there is evidence that the clinical manifestations will be more severe than those of relapse in the untreated patient.

Neurosyphilis may develop with a negative blood WR, hence it is essential to examine the CSF one year after a primary lesion has been treated even if the blood WR is negative; if the CSF is normal the patient is followed for a further year or two to ensure that there is no sero relapse. If the patient presents with late latent syphilis, i.e. more than 2–4 years after the primary chancre, positive blood WR, no clinical features and a normal CSF, he should be treated because in the absence of previous treatment it is possible that he may develop the cardiovascular complications even though his CSF is normal. The patient who presents in the stage of early latent syphilis, i.e. less than 2–4 years following the primary infection, positive WR, no clinical features and negative CSF, is also treated and provided the CSF is normal after one year he is followed for a further year or so to ensure that sero relapse does not occur. It is important to note that a patient is only discharged if his blood WR is negative or if the titre is very low; normally patients should be followed for 2–5 years after treatment.

The treatment at the primary stage consists of ten days penicillin to which *Treponema pallidum* is always sensitive. The type of penicillin used varies; the main ones are:

1. Procaine penicillin daily injection of 2 ml (600,000 units).
2. Delayed released procaine penicillin combined with aluminium monostearate (PAM) every second or third day.
3. Benzathine penicillin one injection only.

Following the first dose of penicillin there may be adverse effects from a sudden release of toxic material from killed organisms— Jarisch[140]-Herxheimer[141] reaction. This may be important if there is a lesion situated near the opening of the coronary arteries or the origin of one of the spinal arteries. It is important to note that this type of reaction will only occur following the first dose of penicillin; any reactions which occur after the first dose of penicillin are likely to be due to hypersensitivity to penicillin in which case tetracycline is usually used instead. These reactions are common and usually consist only of pyrexia and malaise which lasts a few hours. The patient should be warned to expect it otherwise he may cease to attend. These reactions do not occur following bismuth injections, hence bismuth is often given first when late untreated syphilis is being treated for the first time. In patients who have cardiovascular or nervous system involvement a Jarisch-Herxheimer reaction could be serious if it involved a spinal, cerebral or coronary artery.

In the treatment of late latent syphilis, or neuro- or cardiovascular syphilis, 2–3 weeks of penicillin are given. Sometimes bismuth injections are administered at weekly intervals of four weeks before penicillin treatment of neuro- or cardiovascular syphilis to diminish the risk from Jarisch-Herxheimer reactions. The CSF should be examined before and after treatment; further treatment is indicated if the CSF continues to be abnormal after six months or if there is a progression of signs.

Neurological Manifestations of Syphilis

It cannot be emphasised enough that syphilis may simulate any known lesion in the nervous system by the following mechanisms:

1. Syphilitic endarteritis may affect any blood vessel, e.g. cerebral arteries, anterior spinal artery and branches.
2. Meningeal involvement may cause meningitis.
3. Cerebral tumours may be simulated by gummata.
4. Meningioma may be simulated by local collections of fluid as a result of local meningitis—meningitis serosa cirumscripta. These may also simulate a subdural haematoma and if very localised may be responsible for individual cranial or spinal nerve palsies and epilepsy.
5. Posterior column lesions occur in tabes dorsalis.
6. Parenchymatous involvement of the nervous system occurs in GPI.

Tabes Dorsalis (*L*. tabes: wasting)

The name refers to the wasting of the posterior columns; the old

140. ADOLF JARISCH (1850–1902). Vienna and Innsbruck dermatologist.
141. KARL HERXHEIMER (1861–1944). Frankfurt dermatologist.

name of locomotor ataxia reflected the predominant symptom of ataxia as a result of loss of proprioception. The reason why only the posterior columns are affected is not known; the explanation that the posterior nerve roots are constricted by local thickening of the arachnoid is probably untrue because the sensory loss is selective. Optic atrophy occurs almost always and is due to:

1. Constriction of the optic nerves by arachnoiditis.
2. Degeneration of the retina due to a retinitis during the secondary stage.
3. Direct damage to the fibres of the optic nerves by the organisms —this is, therefore, one form of retrobulbar neuritis.

Tabes dorsalis is very rare in women. The main features of tabes are:

Argyll Robertson pupils and ptosis.
Optic atrophy.
Charcot[142] joints.
Loss of ankle and knee jerks.
Loss of deep pain sensation.
Posterior column loss leading to lack of position sense, ataxia and positive Romberg's test and loss of vibration sense.
Delayed appreciation of pinprick.
Perforating ulcers of the feet and painful tabetic crises.

The WR in the blood and CSF are positive in about 60 per cent of patients, but is negative in about 20 per cent; following treatment the CSF abnormalities and blood WR may revert to normal.

SYRINGOMYELIA

The syrinx (*Gk.:* pipe) is situated in the cervical region of the cord or brain stem (syringobulbia). It occurs anterior to the central canal in relation to the decussation of the fibres of the lateral spinothalamic tracts. It is also near the anterior horn of the grey matter, through which the motor root enters the cord, and it is near the pyramidal tracts. Thus, the characteristic features of syringomyelia in a segment of the cervical cord are:

1. Loss of pain and temperature sensation in skin supplied by that segment or the one below.
2. Lower motor neurone lesions in the motor nerve of that segment due to involvement of the anterior horn of the grey matter.
3. Upper motor neurone lesions below the affected segments due to involvement of the pyramidal tracts.

142. JEAN MARTIN CHARCOT (1825–1893). Paris neurologist.

The commonest segment to be affected initially is the first thoracic, hence wasting of the small muscles of the hand with loss of pain and temperature sensation in the hands is the characteristic presenting feature. If the gliosis surrounding the syrinx or the syrinx itself spreads then the lateral spinothalamic tracts as well as the decussation of some lateral spinothalamic fibres may be compressed, leading to loss of pain and temperature in dermatomes below the lesion. Syringobulbia produces similar changes in relation to the medulla.

Three signs which occur in the cranial nerves when the disease is still limited to the cervical cord are Horner's syndrome, nystagmus and loss of pain and temperature in the lower part of the face. The Horner's syndrome is due to involvement of the sympathetic pathway in the cervical cord, the nystagmus is due to involvement of fibres of the vestibulospinal tracts and the loss of pain and temperature in the lower face is due to involvement of the descending tract of the trigeminal nerve as it descends into the cervical cord.

MOTOR NEURONE DISEASE

The pathological changes in motor neurone diseases are situated in the anterior horn cells, the pyramidal tracts and the motor cranial nerve nuclei in the medulla and pons. The position of the lesions causes the three dominant clinical features, namely: progressive muscular atrophy (lower motor neurone), amyotrophic lateral sclerosis (pyramidal tracts) and progressive bulbar palsy (motor cranial nerve nuclei). Certain clinical features of the disease are characteristic: it never begins before the age of 40, there are never any sensory disturbances or pain, the sphincters are never affected and the course of the disease is never more than seven years.

The disease most frequently starts with lower motor neurone lesions in the hands with wasting and fasciculation of muscles and diminished reflexes. Later, there are pyramidal signs which also begin in the cervical spine, and these lead to upper motor neurone signs in the legs with weakness, no wasting, extensor plantar responses and exaggerated reflexes. The upper motor neurone signs may then affect the arms leading to further weakness but no further wasting, thus the weakness of the arms may be more severe than the wasting would suggest. Eventually lower motor neurone signs may develop in the legs leading to abolition of the reflexes. The effect of the disease on the reflexes is variable depending on whether lower or upper motor neurone signs predominate.

Lower motor neurone lesions affecting the lower cranial nerves lead to progressive bulbar palsy. Upper motor neurone signs may be present in the lower cranial nerves leading to pseudobulbar palsy which is associated with spasticity of the muscles, stiffness but not wasting of the tongue and an exaggerated jaw jerk.

The main differential diagnosis is myelopathy due to cervical spondylosis, syringomyelia and bilateral cervical ribs; however, sensory changes are present in all these and the presence of a bulbar or pseudobulbar palsy will exclude lesions in the cervical spine.

PERONEAL MUSCULAR ATROPHY

This misnamed condition is not all that uncommon and has a very characteristic appearance. Muscle wasting occurs in the legs but the wasting has a definite upper margin above which all the muscles are normal—thus the wasting may affect the leg below the mid-thigh or below the mid-calf. There are sometimes mild posterior column signs. The disease is familial and usually begins in the teens. The arms are only rarely affected.

ABNORMAL INVOLUNTARY MOVEMENTS

The three important types of abnormal involuntary movements are:

1. **Tremor**—in which one single movement is continually repeated rapidly.

2. **Athetosis**—in which the movements are writhing in nature and are completely purposeless.

3. **Chorea**—in which the movements are often semi-purposeful, like continually clutching for the bed-clothes or more complicated like continually opening and closing the eyes.

The common causes of each are:

Tremor: old age, Parkinsonism, cerebellar disease, thyrotoxicosis, familial tremor, hysteria and alcoholism (delirium tremens).

Athetosis: familial, psychogenic and vascular lesion of the basal ganglia.

Chorea: pregnancy (chorea gravidarum), rheumatic fever (Sydenham's chorea), old age, psychogenic causes and Huntington's[143] chorea.

4. **Myoclonus.**—Sudden quick contractions of whole muscles.

5. **Tic.**—Repeated complicated movements.

6. **Tonic-clonic contractions** (convulsions).

7. **Jacksonian epilepsy.**

Parkinsonism[144].—It is essential to realise that nowadays Parkinsonism is regarded as a collection of common clinical features which have a variety of causes:

143. GEORGE SUMNER HUNTINGTON (1851–1916). New York physician.
144. JAMES PARKINSON (1755–1824). English physician.

1. Idiopathic degeneration of the basal ganglia—paralysis agitans or Parkinson's disease.
2. Arteriosclerotic degeneration of the basal ganglia.
3. Encephalitis lethargica.
4. Toxic, e.g. phenothiazines, manganese and carbon monoxide poisoning.

There are some helpful distinguishing features: Parkinson's disease usually comes on earlier than arteriosclerotic Parkinsonism. In Parkinson's disease the mental state is normal and there are no upper motor neurone signs. Arteriosclerotic Parkinsonism comes on at a later age, is often associated with a history of transient weakness of the limbs, there are usually bilateral upper motor neurone signs due to ischaemia of the internal capsules so that the reflexes are increased and the plantar responses are extensor; the reflexes in Parkinson's disease are normal. There may be evidence of a pseudobulbar palsy if there is bilateral softening of the internal capsules in arteriosclerosis; other arteriosclerotic manifestations such as dementia or epilepsy may occur. Post-encephalitic Parkinsonism comes at an earlier age than Parkinson's disease and like Parkinsonism associated with phenothiazine administration is usually accompanied by oculogyric crises.

The two important features of Parkinsonism are tremor and rigidity, and it is worth emphasising that each feature may occur alone; it is easy to miss mild Parkinsonism in an old person in whom the only feature is slowness of facial expression.

The main pathological feature of idopathic Parkinsonism is loss of pigmentation in the substantia nigra. There is loss of the neurotransmitter dopamine which is normally antagonised by acetylcholine leading to an alteration in the relative amounts of each.

The tremor affects the distal muscles first and is worse at rest. The rigidity is accompanied by increased tone—this can often be demonstrated by passively flexing the other arm. Hypokinesia is often the most difficult of the features to recognise. Parkinsonism can present in unusual ways; for example, unexpected falling or ankle oedema due to relative immobility of the feet. There are two main approaches to pharmacological treatment, the first is to attempt to increase the concentration of dopamine in the brain and the second is to inhibit the action of acetylcholine with anticholinergic drugs. The concentration of dopamine can be increased by giving levodopa which is a precursor of dopamine. Unfortunately levodopa does not cross the blood-brain barrier in high concentrations. The concentrations of levodopa can be increased by giving a drug, carbidopa, which prevents outside the CNS the breakdown of levodopa to dopamine. However, although carbidopa does not cross the blood-brain barrier the increased concentrations of levodopa which do cross the barrier in small amounts will be available to the brain to be converted into dopamine.

When confronted with a patient whose face appears slightly abnormal there are five common conditions which should be considered:

Parkinsonism.
Myoxedema.
Mild pseudobulbar palsy.
Acromegaly.
Paget's disease.

Entrapment Syndromes

This rather graphic name refers to those conditions caused by mechanical constriction of nerve roots or spinal cord. The commonest causes of entrapment are cervical spondylosis, herniation of a lumbar intervertebral disc and cervical ribs.

A number of simple anatomical points are worth making. The intervertebral discs are anterior to the spinal cord. Herniation of the discs occurs laterally compressing the nerve roots as they leave the spinal canal between the vertebrae. Herniation and osteophyte formation can occur on the posterior part of the disc compressing the cord from before backwards. For some reason, in the cervical region compression of the nerves in the intervertebral foramen affects the sensory root more than the motor. Sensory disturbances are, therefore, much commoner than motor disturbances in cervical spondylosis. In the cervical region, as the disc protrudes backwards, the anterior part of the cord will be compressed first; this is the part where the pyramidal tracts are located, hence cervical spondylosis severe enough to compress the cord as well as nerve roots may lead to upper motor neurone signs in the legs. The anterior spinal artery may be directly compressed in this situation leading to more extensive damage to the anterior part of the cord, particularly the pyramidal tracts.

An interesting sign of spinal cord compression in the cervical region is inversion of the biceps and triceps reflexes—tapping the biceps tendon leads to contraction of the triceps. The biceps muscle is supplied by C5 and 6 and the triceps by C6 and 7; if there is compression at the level of C6 there will be upper motor neurone signs below this level which will include C7, the main nerve supply of the triceps muscle. Thus, there will be a lower motor neurone lesion of the biceps muscle and an upper motor neurone lesion of the triceps; because they have one nerve in common which can carry the afferent impulse from stimulation of the biceps tendon, the triceps will contract in the manner of an upper motor neurone lesion, i.e. briskly. Disc protrusion and calcification, osteophyte formation and osteoarthritis all contribute to the pathogenesis of spondylosis. The osteophyte formation will cause narrowing of the canal carrying the vertebral artery possibly leading to vertebro-basilar insufficiency.

Prolapsed Intervertebral Disc

Approximately 60 per cent of disc protrusions affect the L5–S1 disc (S1 nerve root), 30 per cent affect the L4–L5 disc (L5 nerve root) and combined lesions occur in about 10 per cent. The lumbar pain which occurs in acute disc protrusion is probably related to tearing of the annulus fibrosis and protrusion of the nucleus pulposus. The *lumbar* pain of long-standing disc protrusion is probably due to stretching of the posterior longitudinal ligament of the spine and reflex protective spasm of the erector spinae muscle. Disc protrusion which results in pressure on the nerve root results in pain along the course of the nerve root, tenderness of the nerve and pain of myotome distribution, i.e. in the *muscles* supplied by the nerve. This accounts for the well-known symptom of pain radiating down the back of the thigh (in the course of the sciatic nerve and in the region of the biceps femoris), and down the back of the lower leg in the region of gastrocnemius (S1) or anterolateral part of the leg in the region of the tibialis anterior (L5).

Note that the *pain* does not radiate in the cutaneous distribution of the affected nerve root, i.e. lateral part of the lower leg and medial side of the foot (L5) and sole and lateral side of the foot (S1). However, compression of the nerve root may result in *paraesthesiae* and/or *numbness* in the appropriate *cutaneous* distribution. Further nerve root compression will result in a lower motor neurone palsy of the muscles by the affected nerve root. These are:

L5 and S1: (1) Glutei (extension of thigh—G. maximus; abductors —G. medius and minimus).
(2) Biceps femoris (flexion of the knee).
(3) Peronei (eversion of the foot).

L5 (with L4): Dorsiflexors of the foot ("extensor" muscles and tibialis anterior).

S1 (with S2): (1) Plantar flexors of the foot (gastrocnemius and soleus).
(2) Small muscles of the foot (patient is asked to "make the sole of the foot into a cup").

Note that the dorsiflexors of the foot are supplied by the lateral popliteal nerve. Lesions of this nerve may result in foot drop—this may also occur with lesions affecting the nerve roots; however, if the lateral popliteal nerve is involved peripherally there is no involvement of the glutei. Gluteus medius is best tested by asking the patient to abduct the thigh against resistance. Gluteus maximus extends the thigh; this can be tested either with the patient lying prone or in the supine position by passing one's arm behind the lower end of the thigh, raising the leg 3–4 inches off the bed and then asking the patient to "push my arm into the bed".

Other evidence of lower motor neurone weakness will be loss of diminution of deep reflexes (loss of ankle jerk in lesions of S1; note that L5 lesions do not affect either the knee or the ankle jerk—the knee jerk is mediated through roots L3 and L4). Other signs of prolapsed intervertebral disc which should be carefully sought are:

1. Restricted movements of the lumbar spine.
2. Loss of normal lumbar lordosis.
3. Lumbar scoliosis (the direction of the scoliosis is no guide to the side of the disc protrusion).
4. Tenderness on palpation of the lumbar spine.
5. "Sagging" of the glutei on one side.
6. Tenderness with "percussion" over the sciatic nerve.
7. Restriction of straight leg raising.

Occasionally lumbar disc protrusion may be painless or a disc other than L4—L5 and L5—S1 may protrude. L3—L4 disc lesions result in loss of the knee jerk. It is usually the posterolateral part of the intervertebral disc which is the site of herniation of the nucleus pulposus, rarely the posterior part of the disc is the site of herniation. This central protrusion may cause bilateral symptoms and signs and may compress the cauda equina. The cauda equinal consists of all the nerve roots below L2 at which level the spinal cord ends; for this reason prolapse of the L4–L5 or L5—S1 discs can never produce *upper* motor neurone signs. Compression of the cauda equina whether by central disc protrusion or tumour produces a flaccid paraplegia with numbness and sphincter disturbance which in the case of the bladder causes hesitancy, urgency and then retention of urine. Space-occupying lesions in the cauda equina are more likely to produce compression of the lower sacral nerves because these nerves travel the whole distance of the lumbar sac from the point where the cord ends to their emergence from the spinal column—the lowest sacral nerves, therefore, have a longer course than the other nerve roots which constitute the cauda equina. Nerve roots which occur in the upper part of the cauda equina will not, of course, be compressed by tumours arising below their points of exit from the spine. Muscles supplied by the affected nerve roots are always weak and wasted, there is usually pain of sciatic distribution; pain is nearly always an early symptom of cauda equina lesions. Impotence, urinary symptoms, numbness and lower motor neurone weakness occur later. Rectal examination is mandatory particularly as it may reveal a patulous anal sphincter which is sometimes an early sign of cauda equina compression.

Sacral, anal and perianal anaesthesia are nearly always present.

Evidence of cauda equinal compression is a medical emergency: unless the pressure of the nerve roots is relieved permanent paralysis will result; the nerves of the bladder are particularly sensitive in this respect. A myelogram is generally performed before proceeding to a laminectomy.

Claudication of the cauda equina.—In 1961 Blau and Logue described a syndrome which most clinicians have been able to confirm. The syndrome consists of bilateral pain and paraesthesiae brought on by exercise and relieved by rest, the peripheral arterial pulses are normal and neurological examination may show weakness of the foot dorsiflexors and reflex changes. It is suggested that the cause of the syndrome is intermittent claudication of the cauda equina.

It is important to note that lumbar disc protrusion may cause a marked elevation of the protein in the cerebrospinal fluid.

Cervical rib (scalenus anterior) syndrome.—The syndrome is caused by the subclavian artery and first thoracic nerve being damaged either by acute angulation over a cervical rib (or radio-translucent fibrous band representing the cervical rib) or compression between first rib and insertion of scalenus anterior (on the first rib). Symptoms usually begin in middle age and may be precipitated by carrying heavy loads, shoulder bags or anything which causes the shoulder to sag. The syndrome is commoner in women than men. Vascular symptoms are much commoner than nerve pressure symptoms and consist of pallor, coldness and cyanosis of the fingers. The radial pulse may be weak especially if palpated with the arm held downwards; if narrowing of the artery occurs there may be post-stenotic dilatation, thrombus formation and recurrent peripheral emboli. A murmur may be heard over the narrowed artery, the radial pulse may become weaker if the patient turns his head towards the side of the lesion and takes a deep inspiration—this will tense the scalenus anterior which is one of the accessory muscles of respiration. The costoclavicular syndrome is much rarer than the cervical rib syndrome. The subclavian artery and rarely the first thoracic nerve are compressed between the first rib and clavicle. The radial pulse will become obliterated if the patient pulls his shoulders (and clavicles) backwards as in standing to attention. Both the cervical rib and costoclavicular syndromes may closely resemble Raynaud's disease.

PERIPHERAL NEUROPATHY

Peripheral neuropathy is defined as bilateral symmetrical muscle weakness usually accompanied by sensory disturbances due to dysfunction of several peripheral nerves simultaneously. The principal causes are:

1. Toxins, e.g. alcohol, lead, arsenic, isoniazid, nitrofurantoin, gold, aniline, and benzene derivatives.
2. Deficiency of vitamins B_1 and B_{12}.
3. Metabolic disorders, e.g. diabetes, uraemia, porphyria and amyloid disease.
4. Carcinoma.
5. Collagen disorders: polyarteritis, SLE, rheumatoid arthritis.
6. Allergy, e.g. serum sickness.
7. Infections: almost any infection from typhoid to tubercle may be complicated by a peripheral neuropathy.
8. Acute infective polyneuropathy or Guillain-Barré syndrome.

The cause of polyneuropathy in an individual case is often not found. Occasionally, an industrial, geographical, dietary, social or family history is helpful. One rather surprising problem in clinical practice is to distinguish between a polyneuropathy and myopathy. The presence of sensory impairment will indicate neuropathy, but if sensation is normal it may be difficult, because in both there is muscle wasting and tenderness, with diminished reflexes. In some cases of peripheral neuropathy both the nerves and the myoneural junction may be involved, as in many cases of carcinoma—hence the use of the term carcinomatous neuromyopathy.

An electromyogram will indicate reduced interference pattern in a myopathy and nerve conduction times will be slowed in a polyneuropathy. In a difficult case, nerve biopsy is performed.

As well as an aetiological classification the peripheral neuropathies can be classified on a pathological basis. This has a closer relationship to the natural history and physiological changes which occur in the peripheral neuropathies. As a very general rule neuropathies associated with loss of the nerve axon (or neurone) recover slowly while those associated with demyelination may recover rapidly; loss of the myelin sheath (and Schwann's cell) may be patchy but conduction time in the nerve is usually slow. Infiltrations and ischaemia of the peripheral nerves form separate groups.

Pathological Classification of Peripheral Neuropathies

Axonal or neuronal damage

Toxic causes —alcohol
　　　　　　　porphyria
　　　　　　　uraemia
　　　　　　　isoniazid
　　　　　　　lead
　　　　　　　acrylamide
Deficiences —vitamin

Hereditary   —peroneal muscular atrophy
             hereditary sensory neuropathy
Others   —carcinomatous sensory neuropathy

Proximal segmental demyelination

Guillain-Barré neuropathy
Diabetes

Distal segmental demyelination

Carcinomatous mixed neuropathy
Diabetes
Myeloma neuropathy

Ischaemia

Polyarteritis
Diabetes
Entrapment neuropathies

Infiltrations

Reticulosis
Amyloidosis
Sarcoidosis
Refsum's syndrome

Acute Infective Polyneuropathy

This usually starts with a fever, headache and sore throat, with gradual onset of weakness in the distal muscles of the legs some days later. The weakness gradually spreads upwards to the trunk, arms and sometimes the cranial nerves. The muscles are usually very tender. Severe paraesthesiae occur at this stage, even if there is no objective sensory loss. In severe cases, there is a bulbar palsy, paralysis of respiratory muscles, sphincter disturbances and an encephalitis.

The pathological changes are not restricted to the peripheral nerves. There may be a myelitis, arachnoiditis, encephalitis and occasionally inflammatory changes in the liver and kidneys. The cerebrospinal fluid usually shows a marked increase in protein with either a normal or only slightly increased cell count. This is often called the Guillain[145]-Barré[146] syndrome.

Some confusion exists about the eponyms Guillain-Barré syndrome, Froin's[147] syndrome and Landry's[148] paralysis. Guillain and Barré described cases of infective polyneuropathy with the "dissociation

145. GEORGES GUILLAIN (b. 1876). Paris neurologist.
146. JEAN ALEXANDER BARRÉ (b. 1880). Strasbourg neurologist.
147. GEORGES FROIN (b. 1874). Vienna physician.
148. JEAN BAPTISTE OCTAVE LANDRY (1826–1865). Paris physician.

albumino-cytologique". Froin described a high protein content in the CSF associated with xanthochromia due to obstruction of the spinal subarachnoid space. Since then Froin's syndrome has come to mean a high CSF protein content due to any cause, including meningitis, blockage of the subarachnoid space and acute infective polyneuropathy. Landry described a clinical syndrome consisting of weakness, beginning in the lower limbs and spreading upwards, called acute ascending paralysis, and it is now accepted that this is one way in which any of the polyneuropathies may present—Landry's paralysis is not a specific disease entity. One further important fact to note is that "dissociation albumino-cytologique" is not specific for acute infective polyneuropathy. It may occur with nearly all the causes of polyneuropathy. But in acute infective polyneuropathy the level of protein in the CSF is usually higher than that found in other types of neuropathy.

With regard to the diagnosis of acute infective polyneuropathy, it is obviously essential to exclude as far as possible the other causes of polyneuropathy. The most important ones being the metabolic causes, such as diabetes, uraemia and porphyria; it is important to note that the neurological complications of diabetes may appear before the diabetes causes other symptoms, so it is essential to exclude diabetes by a formal glucose tolerance test. A polyneuropathy may complicate any severe infection including septicaemia, and it will improve as the infection is controlled.

The prognosis of acute infective polyneuropathy is variable; as a general rule, sporadic cases have a favourable prognosis. In the epidemic form, some epidemics are associated with a mild disease, and others with a more severe form. The place of corticosteroids has not been clearly established; however, one thing is certain, severe cases may sometimes respond dramatically and unexpectedly to steroids (Miller, 1966). For this reason, high doses are usually given in the first week, and moderate doses given for a further month.

Autonomic Neuropathy

Many causes of peripheral neuropathy, particularly diabetes, may cause damage to the autonomic nervous system. The sites at which lesions may produce autonomic dysfunction are in the afferent, central and efferent part of the reflex. The afferent side is best demonstrated by testing the automatic compensatory changes in the cardiovascular system in response to alterations in cardiac output, and the two easiest ways of doing this are to observe the blood pressure in response to changes of posture or the Valsalva manoeuvre. The central pathways can be tested by observing the rise in blood pressure in response to mental arithmetic or in the ability of the patient to sweat in response to heat. The efferent autonomic pathways are rather easier to test, the parasympathetic efferents in the vagus can be tested by blocking the vagus with atropine and observing an increase in heart rate. If the vagus is already damaged there will be no response to atropine. The ability of the vagus to stimulate the production of gastric acid can be tested by an insulin test meal. Sympathetic efferent pathways can be tested by infusing noradrenaline, and demonstrating a rise in blood pressure indicating that the blood vessels are able to respond; or acetylcholine can be locally injected into the skin and if the post-ganglionic fibres of the sympathetic are intact, piloerection will follow. Symptoms which should suggest the possibility of an autonomic neuropathy are postural hypotension, diarrhoea, impotence and loss of sweating.

As well as peripheral neuropathies which may damage either the afferent or efferent pathways of the autonomic reflexes, some central lesions may impair autonomic function. The most important of these is damage to the sympathetic pathways in the spinal cord, or medulla, as a result of syringomyelia, vascular or neoplastic lesions. The hypothalamus is the co-ordinating centre of autonomic activity and damage to the hypothalamus results in disturbances of sleep rhythm, temperature regulation, appetite regulation, disturbance of glucose metabolism and diabetes insipidus.

Treatment of an autonomic neuropathy is often difficult; if postural hypotension is a problem, the patient should wear thick, tight elastic stockings on the legs and should only stand up slowly. It sometimes helps for patients to sleep feet-down so that blood is already pooled within the legs, therefore, when he stands up, postural hypotension is minimised. The sympathetic system may be stimulated by sympathomimetic drugs such as ephedrine or, if cardiovascular symptoms are severe, a salt-retaining drug which increases the plasma volume may help (e.g. fludrocortisone).

ORGANIC PSYCHOSES

It is of great practical importance to be aware of the organic causes of mental symptoms. Many causes of mental symptoms are reversible if treated promptly. As a working hypothesis it is convenient to divide the organic psychoses into those which present acutely with a short illness and those with a more long-standing illness. In general the acute mental symptoms are those of delirium and the chronic mental symptoms those of dementia. Delirium refers to a sudden onset of confusion, restlessness and disorientation. Dementia refers to a gradual onset of diminished intellect, memory, assimilation of new ideas, social awareness together with inattention and confusion. There is often no change of mood (called by the psychiatrists "affect") although this depends on the previous personality of the patient.

The main disorders of affect (mood) are depression, anxiety and mania; in a mild form depression and mania are called apathy and excitement. These disorders of affect may be part of well-recognised psychiatric disorders which are as well-defined as most organic disease. The four most important psychiatric diseases of affect are endogenous and reactive depression, involutional melancholia and manic-depressive psychosis.

The important causes of delirium are:

1. **Infection.**—The delirium resulting from infections remote from the nervous system may be surprisingly severe, sometimes necessitating admission to a mental hospital before the correct diagnosis is made. Infections of the nervous system such as malaria and meningitis may also present as delirium.

2. **Injury** either directly to the head or rarely to the long bones resulting in a fat embolus.

3. **Intoxications,** the most important of which are alcohol, barbiturates, cocaine and heroin. Withdrawal of addictive drugs may also cause delirium.

4. **Metabolic** such as hypoglycaemia, uraemia, hypocalcaemia, hypernatraemia, hypoxia and hepatic failure.

5. **Cerebrovascular accidents.**

6. **Miscellaneous** such as Korsakow's[149] psychosis, puerperal psychosis and post-epileptic confusional states.

The important causes of dementia are:

1. **Arteriosclerosis.**
2. **Cerebral tumours.**
3. **Cerebral degeneration.**
4. **Chronic intoxications** such as alcohol, bromides or corticosteroids.
5. **Vitamin deficiency** such as B_{12} and probably folic acid, B_1 and B_2.
6. **Endocrine abnormalities** such as myxoedema, Cushing's disease, hypo- and hyperparathyroidism.
7. **Inherited disorders** such as Huntington's chorea and Wilson's disease.
8. **Infectious diseases** are rarely responsible, the only exceptions being GPI and trypanosomiasis.
9. **Old brain injury.**
10. **Chronic epilepsy.**

Presenile dementias.—These are dementias which begin below the age of 60, and there is sometimes a family history. There are three main types, and although there is considerable difference in the pathology

149. SERGEI SERGEYEVICH KORSAKOW (b. 1874). Moscow physician.

between Alzheimer's[150] and Pick's[151] disease, clinically it is not easy to distinguish them. The pathological changes in Alzheimer's disease generally involve all layers of the cortex and involve most lobes whereas in Pick's disease only the outer layers of the frontal lobes are affected. In Alzheimer's disease there is a gradual onset of complete dementia which affects all intellectual and social functions. In Pick's disease, which is commoner in women, the onset is usually 5–10 years later than Alzheimer's disease and there is often only loss of some of the higher intellectual functions and removal of social inhibition. Jakob[152]-Creutzfeld[153] disease consists of premature dementia accompanied by degeneration of cerebellum, pyramidal and extrapyramidal systems. The disease is invariably fatal in 2–3 years unlike the other forms of pre-senile dementia which may survive for 10–15 years.

The important headings to remember when assessing dementia are:

1. Ability to reason and to form valid judgements.
2. Memory for recent events.
3. Alteration of affect and emotional reactions.
4. Presence of delusions.
5. Loss of personal care and hygiene.

Mild dementia is surprisingly common in general medical out-patients. If one does not detect four to five new and unsuspected cases a year one is probably missing a few. Besides the usual careful history, examination and routine investigations the following investigations should always be performed in a suspicious case:

Protein-bound iodine
Plasma B_{12}
Wassermann reaction
Blood urea
Liver function tests
Serum calcium
Skull x-ray
EEG.

DISORDERS OF MUSCLE

The two main groups of primary muscle disorders are the muscular dystrophies and the diseases characterised by myotonia or delay in

150. ALOIS ALZHEIMER (1864–1915). Breslau neurologist.
151. ARNOLD PICK (1851–1924). Prague psychiatrist.
152. ALFONS MARIA JAKOB (1884–1931). Hamburg neurologist.
153. HANS GERHARD CREUTZFELD (b. 1885). Kiel neurologist.

relaxation of the muscles. However, a number of other conditions may affect the muscles secondarily (Thomas, 1970).

Inflammatory causes:
Polymyositis and dermatomyosis
Carcinomatous polymyositis
Sarcoidosis
Polymyalgia rheumatica
Trichiniasis
Bornholm disease.

Metabolic and endocrine causes:
Hypo- and hyperkalaemia
Familial periodic paralysis
Congenital absence of
    myophosphorylase (McArdle's
    syndrome)
Metabolic bone disease
Steroids
Thyrotoxicosis.

Toxic causes:
Alcohol
Chloroquine
Paraquat
Clofibrate.

Miscellaneous:
Primary amyloidosis
Ischaemic myopathy
Myoglobinuria
Myasthenia gravis.

From a clinical point of view it is often necessary to distinguish muscle weakness due to a disease of the muscle itself from disease of the peripheral nerves. This can be done fairly simply by recording the electrical potentials of a muscle at rest and on contraction with a needle electrode placed in the muscle (electromyogram or EMG). In the normal there is no activity at rest, on voluntary contraction individual motor units will be recorded and on maximum contraction so many motor units are occurring at the same time that no individual motor unit potential will be seen (interference pattern). A motor unit consists of many muscle fibres supplied by one nerve fibre.

In a myopathy in which there is a patchy involvement of muscle fibres within one motor unit, the motor unit potentials recorded on slight exertion will be smaller than normal because there are less muscle fibres contracting, also the interference pattern will be a lower voltage than normal because of damage to some fibres of each motor unit. In complete denervation the degenerating nerve occasionally fires off impulses spontaneously and denervated muscle fibres also may contract spontaneously which results in occasional discharges at rest, some of which resemble normal motor unit potentials while others are of a lower voltage. There is no activity with attempted contraction of the muscle. In the normal muscle at rest there are never any spontaneous motor unit potentials. If the nerve is recovering, on voluntary contraction a few motor unit potentials will be seen but not as many as normal, hence there will be less of an interference pattern although the height of the interference pattern is normal in contrast to a myopathy in which the height of the interference pattern is reduced.

As well as the EMG the other important diagnostic procedures in suspected muscle disorder are muscle biopsy and estimation of the muscle enzymes.

DISEASES CHARACTERISED BY MYOTONIA

In these conditions the muscles contract and relax more slowly than normal, but this tends to improve with exercise and as the patient gets older. As a result of the slower muscular contraction there may be difficulty in balance and if the muscles are tapped a local dimple forms which lasts for several seconds. A curious feature is that the tendon reflexes are always normal.

Myotonia congenita (Thomsen's[154] disease). This is always present from birth and tends to improve as the patient gets older, the muscles are always well developed. Variants of the condition are myotonia paradoxa in which the myotonia gets worse after exercise and paramyotonia in which the myotonia is worse on exposure to cold.

Dystrophia myotonica.—As its name suggests, this is a combination of muscular dystrophy and myotonia and the combination is pathognomonic of the condition which usually begins in adult life, the dystrophic or wasted muscles are those of the face, neck and distal parts of the limbs. Other features which may be present are cataract, testicular and ovarian atrophy and frontal baldness.

Diphenyl hydantoin, procainamide and corticosteroid may each relieve the symptoms of myotonia but do not affect the progress of dystrophia myotonica.

MUSCULAR DYSTROPHIES

There is progressive weakness and atrophy of the affected muscles but never any sensory disturbance. There are three main clinical types:

1. *Pseudohypertrophic* which occurs exclusively in young boys—the muscles of the limb girdles are mainly affected. It is fatal by the age of 20; death is usually due to cardiac failure secondary to the myocardial involvement which always occurs.

2. *Facioscapulo humeral* which occurs in either sex. The upper limb girdle as well as the face and neck are involved, the prognosis is good. The disease is often found in a mild, non-progressive form in the relatives of affected cases.

154. ASMUS JULIUS THOMAS THOMSEN (1815–1896). Danish physician.

3. *Limb girdle.*—This type begins in either the upper or lower limb girdles. It begins in early adult life and affects the two sexes equally.

Two other variants which may occur are a distal limb dystrophy and a dystrophy affecting the external eye muscle in the absence of any other evidence of myopathy.

Muscular dystrophies are always painless, the reflexes are lost and there are no sensory disturbances. Motor neurone disease is about the most difficult differential diagnosis; helpful distinguishing features may be an onset below the age of 40, a positive family history and the absence of fasciculation of the muscles in muscular dystrophy. In peroneal muscular atrophy which may be confused with the distal limb type there is usually some sensory impairment. Polymyositis is usually painful and more widespread.

REFERENCES

BLAU, J. N., and LOGUE, V. (1961). *Lancet*, 1, 1081.
KENDALL, B. E., and MARSHALL, J. (1974). *J. roy. Coll. Phycns Lond.*, 9, 30.
McKISSOCK, W., RICHARDSON, A., and WALSH, L. (1960). *Lancet*, 1, 1203.
McKISSOCK, W., RICHARDSON, A., and WALSH, L. (1962). *Lancet*, 2, 417.
McKISSOCK, W., RICHARDSON, A., and WALSH, L. (1965). *Lancet*, 1, 873.
MARSHALL, J. (1968). *The Management of Cerebro-vascular Disease*. London: J. & A. Churchill.
MILLER, H. (1966). *Brit. med J.*, 2, 1219.
PICKERING, G. (1948). *J. Amer. med. Ass.*, 137, 423.
RICHARDSON, A. E., JANE, J. A., and YASHOU, D. (1966). *Arch. Neurol. (Chic.)*, 14, 172.
THOMAS, P. K. (1970). *Brit. med. J.*, 1, 413.

7

DERMATOLOGY

Skin disorders are estimated to constitute 15 per cent of all disorders seen in general practice. The number of common primary skin conditions is comparatively small; much of the confusion of dermatology results from the fact that nearly all primary skin conditions are complicated by secondary lesions of some sort. A clear description of a skin lesion will often be enough to suggest the diagnosis and differential diagnosis. The cutaneous manifestations of systemic diseases are common enough to warrant a working knowledge of dermatology.

The secondary lesions which may complicate primary skin disorders are:

1. Excessive scratching (excoriation).
2. Scaling (loss of epidermal cells).
3. Crusting (hardened, adherent skin exudates).
4. Lichenification (thickening and scaling through chronic irritation).
5. Infection.
6. Pigmentation.
7. Ulceration and fissures.
8. Over-treatment with dermatological preparations.

All skin lesions should be described in full including the following:

Size and colour.
Location.
Single or multiple.
Border (whether well circumscribed or irregular).
Whether complicated by one of the secondary lesions.
Whether lesions are occurring in crops.
Always look for evidence of previous skin lesions (e.g. scars, telangiectasia or altered pigmentation).
The important primary lesions are:

Macules: Up to 1 cm in size, well circumscribed, *flat*, discolourations of the skin, e.g. freckles, measles rash and vitiligo.
Papules: Up to 1 cm in size, circumscribed, *elevated*, e.g. warts, lichen planus and weals.
Plaques: Similar to macules but larger, e.g. mycosis fungoides.
Nodules: Up to 1 cm in size, solid, may penetrate the skin, e.g. epitheliomas and xanthomata.

Tumours: Nodules larger than 1 cm.

Bullae: Well circumscribed elevations, containing fluid, usually larger than 1 cm.

Vesicles: Bullae smaller than 1 cm.

Pustules: Similar to bullae, but may be smaller and contain purulent fluid, e.g. acne and impetigo.

Petechiae, purpura and *ecchymoses*—all refer to extravasation of blood. Petechiae are up to 1 cm in size. Purpura and ecchymoses are larger.

The location on the body of lesions is one of the most important clues which the dermatologist has, e.g. the differentiation of smallpox from chickenpox.

Psoriasis characteristically involves extensor surfaces and flexures. It is rare on the face but may involve the scalp.

Seborrhoeic dermatitis involves only the hair, face, front of the chest and the pubic area.

Pityriasis rosea involves only the trunk.

Lichen planus usually involves the anterior wrists and shins.

Secondary syphilis involves mainly the trunk, mucocutaneous junctions, soles and palms.

Eczema involves the flexures, including the neck and ankles.

Histology of the Skin

The skin consists of two main layers: the dermis which consists of connective tissue, blood vessels and sebaceous glands, and an outer layer—the epidermis. The purposes of the epidermis are to protect the tissues from mechanical trauma, loss of fluid and from damage by excessive sunlight. The epidermis consists of two main types of cells, the first are cells producing keratin which provides mechanical protection and is impermeable to water and the second are cells producing melanin pigment which prevents excessive ultra-violet light penetrating the skin and burning the tissues.

The outer layer of the epidermis is the horny layer (stratum corneum) and it consists of keratinised cells which are water repellent and are constantly being shed. The cells of the horny layer have migrated through several other layers of the epidermis from the basal or germinal layer which lies next to the dermis. The basal layer is the origin of all the cells in the epidermis (keratin- and melanin-producing). From the germinal layer cells migrate to the prickle layer—so-called because the cells are separated by fine fibrils or "prickles". The cells then acquire granules which are the precursors of keratin and form the granular layer. The granules enlarge until they come to occupy most of the cell and since the keratin granules are clear the next layer is relatively clear and is called the lucid layer. This eventually becomes the horny layer.

Melanin pigment is formed from an amino acid, tyrosine, the process is under the control of the melanin-stimulating hormone (MSH), produced by the intermediate part of the pituitary gland. The skin pigmentation of Addison's disease is due to excessive production of a closely related hormone that also stimulates the melanophores of the skin, this is the adrenocortical stimulating hormone (ACTH) which is produced by the anterior lobe of the pituitary.

The amino acid tyrosine is metabolised from another amino acid phenylalanine and disorders of tyrosine metabolism give rise to four inborn errors of metabolism. Inborn errors of metabolism are due to an inherited deficiency of an enzyme catalising a metabolic process.

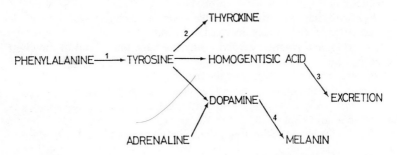

Absence of enzyme 1 leads to accumulation of phenylalanine and phenylketonuria. Absence of enzyme 2 results in a goitrous cretin. Absence of enzyme 3 results in accumulation of homogentisic acid and alkaptonuria in which the urine, ligaments and cartilages are stained black (ochronosis). Absence of enzyme 4 results in a complete absence of melanin (albinism).

Skin Biopsies

Even an experienced dermatologist may rely on a biopsy of the skin before making a definite diagnosis. The main descriptive terms of skin pathology are:

Acanthosis: thickening of the prickle cell layer of the epidermis.

Acantholysis: separation of the prickle layer, as in vesicular and bullous lesions.

Spongiosis: intercellular oedema of the epidermis, separating individual cells, occurs particularly in eczema.

Hyperkeratosis: thickening of the horny layer (stratum corneum) usually associated with thickening of other layers of the skin.

Parakeratosis: imperfect keratinisation with retention of nuclei in the horny layer and loss of the granular layer. It is seen in psoriasis and other scaling conditions.

The explanation and use of these terms will become clear in relation to specific skin diseases.

PSORIASIS (*Gk:* to itch)

This is one of the commonest skin disorders, it has a strong familial tendency. The disease is commoner in temperate climates and usually presents for the first time during the teens or early twenties; the first attack is often precipitated by some coincidental illness. Exacerbations of the disease may be precipitated by local skin trauma, anxiety, other skin disorders, drugs and local or systemic infections. There are usually changes in thermoregulation, and in the small bowel mucosa. There is a rise in metabolic activity even in apparently uninvolved skin.

The lesions tend to be symmetrical and occur in sites exposed to trauma and in the flexures; they are characterised by well circumscribed red macules which become covered with fine silvery scales. Despite its name the lesions of psoriasis only occasionally itch. The diagnosis may be confirmed by rubbing the lesions and allowing the scales to drop off (grattage): after the last scale has been removed the dermis is exposed and numerous small bleeding points are seen.

The pathological changes in the dermis consist of slight oedema (spongiosis)—a feature of almost all skin lesions—acanthosis and parakeratosis.

The nails are frequently involved, with minute pitting, by loss of translucency, thickening of the nail-bed and accumulation of keratin. Psoriasis may be accompanied by arthritis of the rheumatoid type in which case the nails are always involved. The arthritis differs from rheumatoid arthritis in that the distal interphalangeal joints are always involved, there are never rheumatoid nodules and the serological tests for rheumatoid arthritis are always negative. Areas of psoriasis may appear at sites previously damaged by trauma (Koebner's[155] phenomenon). This principle has been extended to other forms of skin damage, e.g. by other skin diseases. Thus, psoriasis may appear in an area previously involved with eczema or herpes zoster.

Treatment.—*Mild cases* usually require no treatment. *Chronic cases* require tar ointments and baths which tend to prevent parakeratosis. Keratolytics are useful in scaling conditions because they help to remove the horny scales, e.g. zinc oxide and salicylic acid paste (Lassar's[156] paste). Dithranol (Anthralin, USNF) is a keratolytic agent which has a specific action on psoriasis by cutting down the number of mitoses. It produces erythema after the scales have been removed and this may be followed by normal epithelialisation. Topical steroid

155. HEINRICH KOEBNER (1838–1904). Breslau dermatologist.
156. OSKAR LASSAR (1849–1907). Berlin dermatologist.

creams are used in intractible cases. Corticosteroids inhibit glycolysis and hence energy for mitosis. They nearly always produce a remission but the relapse rate is high and rapid. Dithranol, tar ointments and tar baths are slower to produce a remission but it usually lasts much longer. Occasionally psoriasis is complicated by pustulation and exfoliation; these are probably commoner when steroid ointments are used.

ECZEMA (*Gk:* to boil over)

This word is synonymous with dermatitis although strictly dermatitis should apply to any inflammation of the skin. By common usage, eczema applies to atopic or allergic eczema, and dermatitis to contact dermatitis.

Both eczema and dermatitis are characterised by erythema, oedema, vesical formation, exudation and weeping. The exudate becomes dry and crusted. Hence, eczema and dermatitis both go through two phases: wet and dry. Later, itching may lead to scratching and lichenification of the skin.

Atopic or infantile eczema (Atopy—*Gk:* out of place).—Atopy refers to a type of hypersensitivity unique to man. There is an inherited predisposition to asthma, hay-fever and eczema which may be mediated by antigens. The people who exhibit atopy are sensitive to many ubiquitous foreign proteins which are not normally antigenic, these proteins become antigenic by combining with a circulating reagin which acts as a hapten (*Gk:* to grasp). A hapten is a substance which is not antigenic in itself but when combined with another substance (in this case the foreign protein) causes it to become an antigen and stimulate antibody formation. The foreign proteins most frequently incriminated are pollens, dusts and certain foods.

Infantile eczema usually develops before puberty and it occurs particularly after recent vaccination, hence vaccination may have to be postponed if the infant has a family history or has recently had an attack of eczema. The erythema and vesicles usually begin on the face and spread to the trunk. Severe itching is an invariable accompaniment, this leads to excoriation and lichenification. Later, the eczema may decline but the lichenification may remain, particularly on flexor surfaces and the neck, as an itchy, dry, thickened area—this may wax and wane in severity and is known as Besnier's[157] prurigo. As the eczema subsides, asthma may develop.

Eczema may develop in adult life, the skin is usually dry (xeroderma) and frequently becomes secondarily infected. When the disease starts in adult life the lesions tend to be well-circumscribed—"discoid" or "nummular" lesions. (*L:* nummularius: of money, i.e. coin-like).

157. ERNEST BESNIER (1831–1909). Paris dermatologist.

Pathology.—Intra- and extracellular oedema occurs in the epidermis (spongiosis). Vesicles form in the prickle cell layer and are forced to the surface by proliferation of cells in the basal layers. The horny layer contains nucleated cells (parakeratosis). These cells stick to each other and form the scales.

Treatment.—Mild keratolytics help remove the scales and promote epithelialisation, e.g. zinc oxide and salicylic acid paste. (Zinc oxide is used as a "vehicle" for salicylic acid.) Tar compounds are also used to reverse the parakeratosis. Local application of steroids may be helpful.

Contact dermatitis.—This may be caused by irritants or substances to which the skin is "sensitive". The responsible agent may be detected by "patch" testing.

Other Forms of Dermatitis

Seborrhoeic dermatitis occurs in relation to hair-bearing skin. It may involve the eyelashes, leading to crusts forming on the lash, and red eyes from excessive rubbing. The neck, front of chest and pubic region may be affected.

Pompholyx causes intense irritation of palms (cheiropompholyx) or soles (podopompholyx) with numerous small blisters. The condition may be idiopathic or complicate blocked sweat ducts or fungus infections.

Hypostatic eczema is due to increased pressure in the veins of the lower limbs. They are frequently pigmented due to deposition of haemosiderin, sometimes there are pure white areas in the pigmentation. The area may become ulcerated and infected. Hypostatic ulcers should be distinguished from arteriosclerotic ulcers which are usually smaller, deeper and well-circumscribed; they are frequently painful when the limbs are in the dependent position.

PITYRIASIS (*Gk:* bran)

The term was originally used to describe any skin rash in which bran-like scales predominated. The main ones are:

1. Pityriasis rosea.
2. Pityriasis capitis (dandruff).
3. Pityriasis rubra (exfoliative dermatitis).
4. Pityriasis versicolor (tinea versicolor).

Pityriasis rosea.—This well-circumscribed erythematous maculo-papular rash is limited to the trunk. The lesions ("medallions") vary in size, from ½ to 3 cm and consist of a peripheral zone which is scaly and a central zone which is discoloured, smooth and soft. The generalised eruption is preceded by a "herald patch" which may be the only lesion for about two weeks. The disease is self-limiting.

Pityriasis versicolor.—This is a symptomless rash which appears most frequently on the back. It is very common and may be difficult to see. It is characterised by non-itching brownish-coloured scaling macules. Treatment is an aqueous solution of sodium thiosulphate or an anti-mycotic ointment such as Whitfield's[158] ointment.

NAEVI (PIGMENTED MOLES)

These are classified according to whether they arise from the dermis or the junction between the epidermis and dermis. If the junctional type is associated with an inflammatory reaction it is probably malignant. Any naevus occurring on the sole of the foot or palm of the hand is potentially malignant.

SEBORRHOEIC OR SENILE WARTS

These are seen very commonly in old people and consist of numerous pedunculated pigmented papillomata.

FUNGUS DISEASE OF THE SKIN

Ringworm or tinea are names given to the clinical manifestations of infections with fungi. Different fungi affect different parts of the body. They are treated either with systemic griseofulvin or with local applications of an antifungal agent such as Whitfield's ointment.

Candida albicans.—Is a yeast-like parasite which may involve the skin and mucous membranes particularly of diabetics. It is also responsible for systemic infections such as endocarditis, meningitis, gastro-enteritis, septicaemia and bronchitis.

PARASITIC DISEASES

The most important of these are lice (pediculosis) and scabies. Lice live and lay their eggs in hair or clothing. They cause intense irritation when they bite to obtain blood and the bites may become secondarily infected. Prolonged infestation results in generalised pigmentation (vagabond's disease) and may cause lymphadenopathy, particularly of the posterior cervical and occipital groups.

Scabies causes intense irritation and is found in "burrows" between the fingers. Generally all members of a family are infested.

BULLOUS LESIONS

Erythema multiforme.—This generally begins as erythema (redness of the skin due to dilatation of superficial blood vessels), and usually goes on to bulla formation. Usually no cause can be found, although some-

158. ARTHUR WHITFIELD (1868–1947). Dermatologist, King's College Hospital, London.

times it is associated with streptococcal infections and drug eruptions. The disease is generally self-limiting but sometimes the patient is very toxic and corticosteroids are necessary.

A variant of erythema multiforme is the Stevens[159]-Johnson syndrome in which the mucosa of mouth, genitalia and eyes may be involved. Blindness may ensue if there is conjunctival involvement.

Dermatitis herpetiformis.—This is a rare disease in which there are numerous urticarial and bullous lesions that resemble herpes zoster. It tends to run a very prolonged course and is often associated with a blood eosinophilia. "Pemphigoid" is the name given to dermatitis herpetiformis when it occurs in the elderly, when it may be associated with internal malignancy.

Pemphigus.—This is a disease of the elderly in which blisters appear on normal skin and mucous membranes. The blisters are often very large, become secondarily infected and are associated with toxaemia. Sometimes the disease is associated with generalised exfoliation. If the skin is rubbed firmly in a patient with pemphigus a thin-walled blister forms in the traumatised area (Nikolsky's[160] sign). In the other bullous diseases a similar blister may form but it has a thick wall because the plane of separation is the epidermo-dermal junction, whereas in pemphigus the plane of separation is between the stratum corneum and the remainder of the epidermis.

Cutaneous Vasculitis

This group of disorders has in common involvement of dermal blood vessels as its most impressive feature. In some forms the vasculitis may be generalised or accompanied by panniculitis (inflammation extending to the fat). Cutaneous vasculitis is conveniently classified (Borrie, 1967):

1. Allergic vasculitis (Henoch-Schoenlein or anaphylactoid purpura). It is important to note that the vesicles do not always contain blood, they may contain white degenerated lymphocyte and resemble small postules.
2. Nodular vasculitis (erythema induratum or Bazin's disease).
3. Livedo reticularis with nodulation (cutaneous polarteritis).
4. Livedo reticularis with ulceration.

Cutaneous Manifestation of Systemic Disease

Erythema nodosum.—The nodules are commoner in women and appear on the lower legs and extensor surfaces of the arms. They are

159. ALBERT MASON STEVENS (b. 1884). New York paediatrician.
160. PYOTR VASILYEVICH NIKOLSKY (b. 1855). Warsaw dermatologist.

painful and consist of bright red, rounded nodules, often up to 5 cm in diameter; they are usually accompanied by fever. They gradually fade, and never ulcerate. An accompanying arthralgia is common and may precede the skin lesions. The common causes are:

1. Streptococcal infections.
2. Rheumatic fever.
3. Drug sensitivity (commonly sulphonamides, aspirin, phenacetin and oral contraceptives).
4. Tuberculosis.
5. Sarcoidosis.
6. Unknown.

Lupus erythematosus.—The commonest cutaneous manifestation is the chronic, localised discoid variety which is not always associated with the systemic form of lupus. The characteristic rash consists of red, discoid macules which appear on the face and are worse when exposed to sunlight. The discs are painless and heal from the centre, they finally consist of thin, whitish scars.

Scleroderma.—This may exist in a purely localised form (morphoea) or may involve only hands, feet and face (acrosclerosis) or the skin may be involved in the systemic form of the disease, but this accounts for only about 5 per cent of cases of skin scleroderma. The involved skin is pale, tight and may be indurated. In acrosclerosis the finger may become stiff or fixed and claw-like. In the systemic form, the mucous membranes are involved together with the joints and lungs (diffuse interstitial fibrosis and honeycomb lung). Raynaud's phenomenon is also common.

Sarcoidosis.—There are three cutaneous manifestations of sarcoidosis:

1. Erythema nodosum.
2. Lupus pernio, in which chilblains form on the nose and face as well as the hands and feet.
3. Symmetrical, purplish macules, usually on the trunk.

Vitamin deficiency.—Vitamin A deficiency causes excessive dryness of the skin and may involve the eyes, causing xerophthalmia and permanent blindness as well as the reversible night blindness. Later the skin becomes hyperkeratotic. In cases of suspected deficiency the vitamin A level in the blood can be measured. Vitamin A may be toxic in large amounts, the main manifestations are fever, hepatomegaly and bone tenderness. Polar bear livers are toxic because they contain such large quantities of the vitamin.

Vitamin B_2 (riboflavin) deficiency causes pellagra. Early deficiency starts as glossitis with fissures at the corner of the mouth (cheilosis) and greasy, scaly skin which finally becomes pigmented. The nose is involved early—"pellagrinous nose"; other manifestations of pellagra include diarrhoea and dementia as well as dermatitis. The exact cause of the various clinical features of pellagra is not universally agreed—it so often happens that diets are deficient in several vitamins. Riboflavine (B_2) deficiency probably causes the dermatitis and gastro-intestinal disturbances of pellagra. Malabsorption and/or deficiency of B_{12} or folic acid accounts for the megaloblastic anaemia often seen in pellagra. The neurological features (encephalopathy and neuropathy) are attributable to deficiency of thiamine (B_1), pyridoxine (B_2), tryptophane or niacin. Pyridoxine is necessary for the conversion of tryptophane to niacin.

Vitamin C deficiency results in scurvy, the main skin manifestations of which are easy bruising, petechial haemorrhages, particularly perifollicular haemorrhages.

Biochemical screening tests which may be helpful in establishing nutritional deficiency are:

1. Vitamin A level in blood.
2. Increased blood pentose and pyruvate in vitamin B_1 deficiency.
3. High level in serum of methyl nicotinamide in niacin and pyridoxine deficiency.
4. Blood level or leucocyte level of ascorbic acid in scurvy (vitamin C deficiency).
5. Serum folate and B_{12} level.
6. Serum calcium, phosphorous and alkaline phosphatase.
7. Prothrombin time.

Syphilis.—The primary chancre occurs between 10 and 20 days after infection, usually in the genital area, and may be accompanied by adenitis. Secondary syphilis occurs 5 weeks to 2 years after the appearance of the primary chancre, and the skin lesions of secondary syphilis are macular, papular or pulstular. They are usually coppercoloured, bilateral and non-itching, they affect the palms and soles more frequently than other skin lesions. There is almost always mucous membrane involvement, which is unusual in other skin diseases, except pemphigus, erythema multiforme and occasionally lichen planus. The mucous membrane lesions consist of "mucous patches" which are painless, shallow ulcers (if long and thin they are known as "snail track" ulcers). Condylomata lata are moist, highly infectious papular lesions occurring in moist areas, e.g. around the anus or scrotum or between the toes. Other manifestations of secondary syphilis are: alopecia, leucoderma of the neck, anaemia, lymphadenopathy and atrophy of the skin.

Congenital syphilis may be associated with a generalised bullous eruption at birth. Later there may be a coppery maculo-papular rash which may become secondarily infected and scarred (rhagades).

Tuberculosis.—Cutaneous involvement is most frequently due to the bovine bacillus. Involvement of the skin occurs in two forms, one in which the lesions are due to the presence of tubercle bacilli in the skin and the other in which the skin is sensitised to tubercle bacilli which are present elsewhere in the body—the latter are called tuberculids and are atypical manifestations of the tuberculin reaction.

Lupus vulgaris.—This is the commonest cutaneous manifestation of tuberculosis. The lesions usually contain tubercle bacilli and are characterised by painless, reddish nodules, which are smooth and shiny and which assume an "apple-jelly" colour when viewed through a glass slide pressed firmly on the lesions. Lupus vulgaris usually begins on the face or neck and the lesions heal by scar formation and cause gross disfigurement.

Scrofulodermia.—In this case the tuberculous infection begins in the lymph glands and subcutaneous tissue; usually of the neck. The skin is secondarily involved by ulceration. Treatment of lupus vulgaris and scrofulodermia is with standard antituberculous chemotherapy.

The commonest "tuberculid" is erythema induratum (Bazin's disease), which almost invariably involves the calves of young women. It is characterised by painless, red, indurated nodules that may ulcerate or disappear spontaneously.

Leprosy.—The skin is usually involved in both forms of leprosy. In tuberculoid leprosy there is a vigorous inflammatory response and the bacilli are localised; in this form the lepromin test is positive. In lepromatous leprosy the disease is generalised because there is a poor inflammatory response and the lepromin test is negative. The simplest skin lesions of leprosy are depigmented dry areas which are anaesthetic. Later the area may become indurated and the skin feels thickened as well as dry. In the lepromatous type the skin is even thicker and becomes nodular. Frequently the eyes and nose are involved.

Mycosis fungoides.—Is a form of reticulosis which only involves the skin. It occurs as reddish plaques or nodules, later generalised exfoliation may occur.

Reiter's[161] disease.—The cutaneous manifestation of this disease is keratodermia blennorrhagica; it is nearly always accompanied by iritis, arthritis and urethritis. The rash resembles psoriasis and most commonly involves the palms and soles although any site may be involved.

Porphyria.—The characteristic skin lesions are blisters, which are exacerbated by exposure to sunlight.

Raynaud's[162] phenomenon.—Raynaud's phenomenon characteristic-

161. HANS REITER (1881–1970). Berlin bacteriologist.
162. MAURICE RAYNAUD (1834–1881). Paris physician.

ally consists of episodic attacks of pallor, cyanosis and hyperaemia of the fingers and toes, usually accompanied by pain. Nevertheless many cases of otherwise classical Raynaud's phenomenon do not begin with initial pallor of the affected digitis. Occasionally the arterial spasm which causes the initial pallor may be so severe or sustained that local gangrene results. Causes of Raynaud's phenomenon include arteriosclerosis, cervical rib, scleroderma, systemic lupus erythematosus, cryoglobulinaemia, haemolysis due to cold agglutinins, heavy-metal poisoning, disuse atrophy of a limb and excessive vibration (such as in pneumatic drilling).

It should be noted that cervical "ribs" are not always seen on x-rays, as the vestigial rib may consist only of a band of fibrous tissue. If the subclavian artery is narrowed by a cervical rib there may be post-stenotic dilatation, and within the dilated portion of the artery turbulent as opposed to laminar flow occurs, predisposing to thrombus formation; a murmur is often audible over the subclavian artery. Intermittent emboli occluding the digital arteries may simulate Raynaud's phenomenon.

Gangrene of the fingers in the absence of occlusion of the larger arteries to the arm may occur in rheumatoid arthritis, ergotism and visceral malignancy.

Raynaud's disease.—Raynaud's disease is Raynaud's phenomenon occurring in women between puberty and the menopause. Attacks occur on exposure to cold, and emotional stress. They are often worse at the menses and are usually symmetrical in distribution.

Raynaud's disease should be distinguished from acrocyanosis in which there is a chronic dilatation of the capillaries. The condition has no age or sex predilection and is painless. Erythromelalgia is a painful, intermittent vasodilatation associated with excessive warmth of the affected part.

Infections.—Many systemic infections may have cutaneous manifestations such as typhoid fever (rose spots), meningococcal septicaemia, subacute bacterial endocarditis and the exanthemata.

Palmar erythema.—This occurs with cirrhosis of the liver ("liver palms"). Other skin manifestations of liver disease are spider naevi (also seen in pregnancy, weather-beaten faces and oestrogen therapy), gynaecomastia and leuconychia (white spots on the nails).

Acanthosis nigricans.—Consists of dark brown pigmentation with thickening of the skin which eventually has a velvety appearance. The lesions are bilateral and commoner in flexures, especially the axillae. In older patients the disease is always associated with visceral malignancy (usually stomach). Other cutaneous manifestations of visceral malignancy include pigmentation, dermatomyositis, thrombophlebitis migrans, pemphigoid, gynaecomastia and tylosis palmaris (thickening of the skin of the palms seen in carcinoma of the oesophagus); urticarial, eczematous and psoriasiform lesions are very occasionally associated with visceral malignancy.

Drug eruptions.—Drug sensitivity may result in almost any type of rash; the commonest are morbilliform (like measles), urticarial and vesicular. The skin may be involved if the drug causes jaundice, thrombocytopenia (purpura) or agranulocytosis (infections).

PIGMENTATION

The commonest causes of pigmentation are physiological (race, pregnancy and exposure to sunlight). Pathological pigmentation is due to deposition in the skin of bilirubin, melanin, haemosiderin or foreign substances.

Causes of deposition of haemosiderin include erythema ab igne, chronic stasis (the cause of pigmentation in varicose ulcers), excessive scratching and haemochromatosis (in which there is also excessive deposition of melanin, the cause of which is unknown).

Conditions which may be associated with excessive melanin deposition in the skin include x-ray therapy, chronic irritation, Addison's disease, cachexia (malignancy, starvation and malabsorption), Cushing's syndrome, acromegaly, thyrotoxicosis, diabetes, pellagra, reticulosis, von Recklinghausen's disease and subacute bacterial endocartditis.

Substances which may be deposited in the skin, causing discolouration, include: mepacrine, heavy metals (lead, mercury, silver, gold), arsenic and break-down products of carotene. Conditions which may simulate pigmentation are ochronosis and acanthosis nigricans.

CUTANEOUS MANIFESTATIONS OF MALIGNANCY

Virtually every known skin disorder has been described as a rare manifestation of internal malignancy. The ones that a non-dermatologist should expect to see occasionally are:

1. Acanthosis nigricans.
2. Dermatomyositis.
3. Severe irritation and xeroderma sometimes progressing to prurigo.
4. Dermatitis herpetiformis.
5. Urticaria.
6. Erythema multiforme.
7. Exfoliation (erythrodermia).
8. Tylosis palmaris.

PRURITUS

Pruritus may be due either to a disease of the skin or may occur as a manifestation of a systemic disorder. Local conditions which may cause pruritus are: pediculosis, scabies, eczema, *Candida albicans*, thread-worms and senile atrophy of the skin. Systemic disorders causing pruritus include: diabetes, uraemia, jaundice, carcinomatosis, leukaemia, Hodgkin's disease and gout.

CAUSES OF ULCERATION OF THE LEGS

1. Arterial insufficiency.
2. Trophic ulcers due to loss of sensation, e.g. tabes dorsalis and peripheral neuropathies. The ulcers of diabetes are due to a combination of arterial insufficiency and reduced sensation.
3. Hypostatic ulceration associated with varicose veins and oedema. It is usually complicated by varicose eczema and pigmentation (mainly haemosiderin from stasis-induced red cell destruction) and lichenification.
4. Rheumatoid arthritis.
5. Severe ulcerative colitis.
6. Haemolytic anaemias—particularly sickle-cell anaemia.
7. Bazin's disease (erythema induratum).
8. Necrobiosis lipoidica diabeticorum (only about 50 per cent have diabetes).
9. Syphilitic gumma.
10. Yaws and leishmaniasis.

REFERENCES

BORRIE, P. F. (1967). *Third Symposium on Advanced Medicine*, Royal College of Physicians of London. Ed. Dawson, A. M. London: Pitman.
HARE, P. J. (1966). *Basic Dermatology*. London: H. K. Lewis & Co.
MACKENNA, R. M., and COHEN, E. L. (1964). *Dermatology*. London: Baillière, Tindall & Cox.
Roxburgh's Common Skin Diseases (1967). Revised by Borrie, P. London: H. K. Lewis & Co.

ENDOCRINOLOGY

THE THYROID

Iodine is absorbed mainly from fish and iodised salt by the small intestines, it is then trapped by the thyroid gland so that the concentration of iodide in the thyroid is at least twenty times that in the serum. The trapping of iodide is inhibited by perchlorate and thiocyanate, probably by competition for binding sites in the thyroid. Within the gland, iodide is oxidised to iodine which is coupled on to mono- and di-iodotyrosines forming tri-iodothyronine (T3) and thyroxine (T4). This coupling probably takes place within the colloid of the gland, in which the amino acids are attached to the protein thyroglobulin and stored as such in the colloid. When required T3 and T4 are split off the thyroglobulin by proteolytic enzymes, and then diffuse into the blood stream; the same proteolytic enzymes also split thyroglobulin into mono- and di-iodotyrosines, these are also freely diffusible. However, they do not normally appear in the blood because dehalogenase enzymes split off the iodine from them which is then conserved in the thyroid. In the absence of dehalogenase, mono- and di-iodotyrosines enter the blood stream and are excreted by the kidneys, resulting in loss of iodine from the body and severe iodine deficiency—this is known as "tinker's disease"—so-called because it was discovered in a band of Scottish tinkers.

In the serum, a small amount of thyroxine exists free, but most of it is bound to an alpha globulin—thyroxine-binding globulin or TBG, which is normally about 20 per cent saturated. The protein-bound iodine (PBI) will rise as the concentration of free thyroxine rises in the serum. However, if the amount of TBG increases (as in pregnancy) more thyroxine will be carried bound to it, although the quantity of free thyroxine in the serum remains the same. Thyroid-binding globulin is also increased in prolonged phenothiazine and clofibrate administration. It is lowered in hypoproteinaemias, nephrotic syndrome, hydantoin and anabolic steroid therapy. In pregnancy, the PBI is raised, but the metabolically active free thyroxine is normal. This also occurs in oestrogen therapy and is, therefore, of relevance, when women are taking oral contraceptives because their PBI may be higher than normal.

Thyroid-stimulating hormone (TSH) has an effect on all the aspects of thyroxine production from the uptake of iodides to the release of thyroxine from the thyroglobulin by the proteolytic enzymes. Anti-thyroid drugs such as thiouracil and Neo-Mercazole prevent the binding of iodine to the tyrosines while thiocyanate and perchlorate prevent the uptake of iodide by the gland.

Test of Thyroid Function

Radioactive iodine (I^{131}) has a half-life of eight days, it is rapidly absorbed from the stomach; about one-third is taken up by the thyroid and two-thirds are excreted by the kidneys so that after about 24 hours there is almost no radioactive iodine in the blood. After 24-48 hours, the radioactivity in the blood rises again when thyroxine containing radioactive iodine is split off thyroglobulin and released into the circulation. There are several ways in which this cycle can be measured. The rate of uptake by the gland can be measured in two ways:

1. By the volume of plasma "cleared" of radioactivity in a given time.

2. By the proportion of radioactivity in the thyroid compared with the administered dose at a given time. The output of the gland can be estimated by measuring the amount of thyroxine incorporating radio-active iodine (I^{131}) which is bound to TBG at a given time (PBI^{131}).

There are a number of factors which affect the interpretation of these tests: renal function must be normal, otherwise more radioactive iodine than normal will be taken up by the thyroid; iodine deficiency makes the thyroid more avid for iodine and will increase the rate of uptake, and similarly excess iodine will diminish the rate of uptake. Following partial thyroidectomy, thyroxine is turned over more rapidly in what little thyroid remains, resulting in a rapid uptake and a rapid discharge of the radioactive iodine.

In practice, two radioactive isotopes are used to assess thyroid function. The 2-hour uptake of I^{132} (half-life 2·3 hours) or the 4-hour uptake of I^{131} are used to confirm a diagnosis of hyperthyroidism, and the 24- or 48-hour uptake of I^{131} are used to confirm the diagnosis of myxoedema. In myxoedema, initial iodine trapping by the gland may be relatively normal, hence the necessity for measuring the activity at 24 or 48 hours.

A rapid 4-hour uptake due to iodine deficiency can be detected by giving the patient potassium iodide for two weeks and repeating the test. In thyrotoxicosis the rate of uptake will be the same, whereas in iodine deficiency, the rate of uptake will have fallen to normal. Similarly in iodine deficiency tri-iodothyronine will suppress the increased TSH production, reducing the stimulation of the thyroid and hence the 4-hour uptake, whereas in autonomous thyrotoxicosis, altering TSH will not alter the 4-hour uptake of radioactive iodine. There are three aspects of the tri-iodothyronine (T3) suppression test, which have great clinical importance:

1. Patients who have ocular signs of Graves' disease without other signs of thyrotoxicosis usually fail to suppress with T3.

2. A few patients have undoubted thyrotoxicosis but also have normal radioactive iodine uptake. However, when thyrotoxicosis is present the normal radioactive iodine uptake is not suppressed by T3.

3. Occasionally a patient who is euthyroid and has a nodular goitre has a radioactive iodine uptake which is not suppressed by T3, this is assumed to be due to a single "hot" nodule which is not under pituitary control but which is producing enough thyroxine to keep the patient euthyroid; such patients eventually develop thyrotoxicosis.

The PBI is a measure of the thyroxine bound to TBG—in the normal the rate of secretion of thyroxine from the thyroid is exactly matched by the uptake of thyroxine by the tissues; in thyrotoxicosis the output is greater than the uptake of thyroxine, hence the PBI rises. The PBI is a difficult estimation to perform and is probably not the best method of diagnosing minor degrees of thyrotoxicosis. The PBI^{131}, 24 hours after an oral dose of I^{131}, is a much more accurate guide to the rate of thyroxine output.

Thyroxine-binding globulin (TBG) has a much greater affinity for thyroxine than tri-iodothyronine; certain resins will absorb free tri-iodothyronine. The basis of the T3 uptake test is that some I^{131}-labelled tri-iodothyronine will be taken up by the patient's TBG, the remainder will be attached to the resin; the more T3 there is bound to the resin, the less has been taken up by TBG. This means that the binding sites on TBG are almost fully saturated with thyroxine, i.e. a high resin uptake of T3 indicates high thyroxine levels in the blood. Conditions which increase the PBI (e.g. pregnancy and oestrogen administration) are accompanied by a higher level of free thyroxine, hence the T3 uptake tends to be low in those conditions in which the PBI is raised. Free thyroxine index is the product of T3 uptake and PBI and is used as a means of getting over the diagnostic problem of a raised PBI being due to conditions other than thyrotoxicosis. The normal value of the free thyroxine index (PBI × T3 uptake) is 2·2–7. The index is the best method of confirming thyrotoxicosis during pregnancy when radioactive tests are not advisable.

A common clinical problem is to confirm a diagnosis of thyrotoxicosis in a patient who has taken iodides many of which take some time to be eliminated; potassium iodide takes about two weeks whereas some iodine-containing radiological contrast materials take up to a year to be eliminated. A large body-pool of iodides will interfere with iodine uptake tests, causing a diminished uptake by the gland, suggesting that hypothyroidism is present; however, a careful history may disclose the fact that iodine-containing compounds have been consumed. There are three tests which may be of value in this situation:

1. PBI and total body iodine. The PBI is a measure of the iodine contained in thyroxine, a large discrepancy between this and the total body iodine indicates an increase in inorganic iodine in the body.

2. T3 uptake test is a measure of thyroxine bound to TBG and will not be affected by excess inorganic iodine.

3. An increased urinary excretion of iodine suggests excess iodine ingestion.

The remainder of the thyroid function tests are more useful in confirming myxoedema than thyrotoxicosis. These are:

1. Level of serum cholesterol above 8 mmol/l.

2. Basal metabolic rate (BMR) is still sometimes used to confirm hypothyroidism. It is also lowered in Addison's disease, obesity and the nephrotic syndrome.

3. Delayed relaxation of tendon jerks.

4. TSH stimulation test.

5. Creatine phosphokinase (CPK) usually high in myxoedema and low in thyrotoxicosis.

Radioactive iodine uptake and secretion rates are not as suitable for diagnosing hypo- as hyperthyroidism. However, they are useful in distinguishing primary and secondary myxoedema; in myxoedema due to destruction of the thyroid, the level of endogenous TSH will be high in an effort by the pituitary to stimulate the flagging thyroid. Under these circumstances, there will be no change in the radioiodine tests following an injection of TSH, as the patient is already producing his own TSH. Failure to alter radioiodine tests following an injection of TSH indicates myxoedema due to a damaged thyroid and not secondary to hypopituitarism. It is essential to note that in myxoedema due to pituitary failure there is no TSH being secreted, and under these circumstances injected TSH will increase radioactive iodine uptake.

One fairly common clinical problem is that patients suspected of suffering from myxoedema are given thyroxine without the diagnosis having been confirmed. The TSH stimulation test will confirm whether or not the thyroid can take up radioactive iodine; if it can then myxoedema is probably not present. The alternative is to stop the thyroxine and repeat the PBI at monthly intervals for three months—a normal thyroid will be suppressed by the administered thyroxine but will slowly recover, causing a progressive rise in the PBI. In true myxoedema the PBI will remain low.

Scintillation scanning of the thyroid is useful in distinguishing toxic nodular goitre from diffuse enlargement, in detecting a "cold" nodule which may be due to carcinoma or a cyst, and in the detection of thyroid tissue some distance from the gland. This is nearly always due to malignant disease, but may occur as a congenital abnormality when ectopic thyroid tissue usually occurs in the course of the thyroglossal duct.

Other parameters of thyroid function:

1. Circulating antibodies to thyroglobulin, colloid or microsomes.
2. Thyroid gland biopsy.
3. Circulating level of long-acting thyroid stimulator (LATS) which is an immunoglobulin recovered with IgG.

It is now possible to measure by radioimmuno-assay circulating TSH levels. These are always raised in hypothyroidism except in the rare instance of hypothyroidism being due to pituitary failure. The TSH-releasing hormone (TRH) is produced in the hypothalamus, it is easily synthesised, is available commercially and is of great value in the diagnosis of thyroid disease. Thyroid hormones (T4 and T3) interfere with the TSH-releasing action of TRH in hyperthyroidism; TSH production is reduced and cannot be stimulated by injecting TRH. In hypothyroidism TSH levels are already raised and can be further increased by injecting TRH. The 20-minute TSH level is generally sufficient.

THYROTOXICOSIS (HYPERTHYROIDISM)

A simple feature of thyrotoxicosis, which is often overlooked, is that it may be due to two conditions. The first is a diffuse hyperplasia of the gland which is known as Graves' disease[163] and the second is a toxic nodule (adenoma) which may occur alone or in a gland in which there are multiple nodules. There are a number of working rules with regard to this classification which are useful for clinical purposes (but to which there are exceptions):

1. Eye signs only occur in Graves' disease, as do certain other manifestations, such as acropachy and pretibial myxoedema.
2. Patients who have Graves' disease (diffuse toxic goitre) may develop nodules in the gland as a result of repeated hyperplasia and regression.
3. In the absence of hyperthyroidism at the time, patients with some of the extrathyroid manifestations of Graves' disease eventually develop true hyperthyroidism.
4. Graves' disease when accompanied by high levels of antithyroid antibodies usually burns itself out and is best treated with antithyroid

163. ROBERT JAMES GRAVES (1786–1853). Dublin physician.

drugs rather than partial thyroidectomy, as this will be accompanied by a high incidence of post-operative myxoedema.

One of the cardinal symptoms of thyrotoxicosis is weight loss; however, it is worthwhile noting that this is not invariable—occasionally an increase in appetite is stimulated more than the increased metabolism and the patient may actually gain weight. Other features which are common to hyperthyroidism due to Graves' disease or a toxic nodule are diarrhoea, pigmentation, osteoporosis, myopathy and myasthenia. Features which are associated only with Graves' disease are an increased incidence of Addison's disease, eye signs and thyroid acropachy. The acropachy consists of clubbing and periostial new bone formation, it is almost invariably associated with pretibial myxoedema and eye signs and is much commoner in males.

The eye signs of Graves' disease may occur in the absence of hyperthyroidism although hyperthyroidism is usually present at some stage of the disease, either before or after the eye signs. The commonest eye sign is lid retraction—this may be present all the time and account for the staring appearance and wide separation of the upper and lower lids or it may be present only when the patient attempts to look upwards (lid lag). In this case, the superior rectus muscle is always weak and the levator palpebrae superioris is over-stimulated; both muscles are supplied by the oculomotor nerve and it has been postulated that an abnormal number of impulses pass down the nerve in an attempt to overcome the weakness of the superior rectus; the increased number of stimuli causes the levator palpebrae superioris to over-react.

Actual protrusion of the eyeball (exophthalmos or proptosis) is much rarer than lid lag, but when exophthalmos is present there is an increase in the amount of fat within the orbit which may cause swelling in the supra- and infra-orbital subcutaneous tissues. Ophthalmoplegia refers to weakness of the extra-ocular muscles, particularly the superior rectus, it is present to a minor degree in most cases of Graves' disease. Later, the eyes may become congested and papilloedema or optic atrophy may occur (malignant exophthalmos). Malignant exophthalmos is a rare condition and the definitive treatment is open to dispute, however, two procedures which may save the eyes are tarsorrhaphy and surgical decompression of the orbit in which as much orbital tissue as possible is removed from behind the eye. Local treatment should include Predsol eye-drops (N.B.: occasionally Predsol eye-drops increase the intra-ocular pressure), or guanethidine eye-drops (a "medical Horner's syndrome" is produced). The patient should sleep sitting upright. Other more controversial treatments are:

1. Thyroxine, on the grounds that TSH or other exophthalmos-producing substances may be inhibited.

2. Irradiation of the orbit.

3. High doses of corticosteroids as soon as the malignant exophthalmos begins to get worse.

4. Total ablation of the thyroid on the grounds that an antigen from the thyroid acting in the orbit causes an inflammatory reaction and exophthalmos.

5. Hypophysectomy.

6. Resection of Muller's muscle which is the smooth-muscle component of the levator palpebrae.

7. Decompression of the orbit into the ethmoid sinuses.

The cause of the eye signs of Graves' disease is not known for certain; the serum often contains exophthalmos-producing substance (EPS) which is probably a gamma globulin. TSH and long-acting thyroid stimulator (LATS) may also be responsible. However, eye signs do not occur in myxoedema, in which TSH output is very high.

Treatment of Hyperthyroidism

Graves' disease is usually intermittent and sometimes self-limiting; it can always be controlled with antithyroid drugs. However, these are accompanied by disadvantages which sometimes preclude their use.

The advantages of antithyroid drugs are:

1. Hypothyroidism is readily reversed.

2. Convenience and avoidance of a major operation.

3. In pregnancy, they control symptoms and are not harmful to the foetus in therapeutic doses, although in large doses they may produce goitre in the foetus.

The disadvantages of antithyroid drugs are:

1. Treatment is long-term, and close supervision is essential.

2. The gland is not reduced in size, hence pressure effects on the trachea will not be relieved and may be made worse. Antithyroid drugs should not be used if a retrosternal goitre is present.

3. Recurrent thyrotoxicosis is more resistant to drug treatment than the first attack of thyrotoxicosis.

4. The risk of side-effects from the drugs is always present.

Partial thyroidectomy is more suitable if there is a large goitre, a single nodule, tracheal distortion or relapse following drug treatment. The disadvantages are: damage to parathyroids, recurrent laryngeal nerve palsy and possible hypothyroidism, which is severe and will require life-long substitution therapy. Hypothyroidism developing many years after partial thyroidectomy is much more common than is generally appreciated. Its incidence is much the same as that following radioactive iodine treatment for hyperthyroidism.

In the immediate post-operative period after partial thyroidectomy the main problems are:

Laryngeal oedema.

Haemorrhage.

Stridor due to recurrent laryngeal nerve palsy.

Tetany due to hypocalcaemia as a result of damage to the parathyroid, although this is usually transient.

Thyrotoxic crisis. This is now very rare, but when it does occur it is treated with hydrocortisone, fluid replacement, Lugol's[164] iodine and large doses of chlorpromazine.

Radioactive iodine is selectively concentrated in the hyperplastic gland and is a convenient way of irradiating it. It is conventional to give radioactive iodine only to patients over the age of 45 or if the patient suffers from some other disease which limits life expectancy to less than 20 years, although there is no evidence of an increased incidence of carcinoma or leukaemia following radioiodine. Radioiodine is usually the treatment of choice for retrosternal goitre or for a recurrence of thyrotoxicosis following a partial thyroidectomy. The risk of myxoedema is more than with drugs or partial thyroidectomy, and about a third of patients develop transient myxoedema. The incidence of hypothyroidism increases each year following the treatment, hence patients need long-term follow up.

Radioactive iodine may be used for treating a single toxic nodule without any danger of myxoedema, because only the "hot" nodule will take up the radioiodine; the remainder of the thyroid being quiescent, it will not take up the radioiodine and will receive little or no irradiation. The disadvantage of treating "hot" nodules in this way is that it takes up to a year for the nodule to disappear.

Once it has been decided to treat thyrotoxicosis by antithyroid drugs the most suitable drug to use is carbimazole (Neo-Mercazole), which inhibits the organic binding of iodine to iodotyrosines in the formation of thyroxine. Other drugs such as thiouracil are used only if the patient develops side-effects to carbimazole. Potassium perchlorate is a drug which prevents the uptake of iodide by the gland; very occasionally a combination of perchlorate and carbimazole is used to treat a recalcitrant case. The starting dose of carbimazole is usually about 40 mg and this is continued for one month; thereafter the dose is reduced when the patient is euthyroid as judged by weight gain, normal pulse rate and improvement in thyrotoxic symptoms; 5 mg a day are given for 2–3 months. The symptoms do not usually begin to improve for two weeks after the drug has been started. It is obviously of great importance to tell the patient this.

164. JEAN GUILLAUME AUGUSTE LUGOL (1786–1851). Paris physician.

In order to reduce the incidence of myxoedema, thyroxine is some-times given with carbimazole; this has the disadvantage that much larger doses of carbimazole have to be used, with a consequent increase in side-effects which on the standard dose are minimal. The most im-portant side-effects are agranulocytosis and aplastic anaemia. When the patient has remained euthyroid on the minimum dose for two months the drug can be stopped and a PBI estimation performed after a further two months. Thereafter, the patient should return if there is a recurrence of symptoms.

Carbimazole is used to make patients euthyroid before partial thyroidectomy, and it is given four weeks before the operation is due; iodide is given two weeks before the operation to reduce the vascularity of the gland which carbimazole causes as well as for its antithyroid effect. It is important to note that if iodine is given for a longer period, the vascularity of the gland increases again.

Biochemical evidence of thyroid activity following antithyroid drugs can be obtained by estimating the PBI two months after the drugs have been stopped. Radioactive iodine uptake by the thyroid is increased after antithyroid drugs and may remain so for some time even if the patient is euthyroid. However, evidence of suppression of I^{131} uptake with tri-iodothyronine indicates that the thyroid is under the influence of TSH and that the patient is probably euthyroid.

Some Special Problems

1. *Diagnosis and treatment during pregnancy.*—The Free Thyroxine Index is the best guide to the presence of thyrotoxicosis. Treatment with antithyroid drugs in the correct dose is generally better than thyroid-ectomy. Hypothyroidism during pregnancy should be treated with tri-iodothyronine (T3) rather than thyroxine (T4) because it crosses the placenta better.

2. *Diagnosis of thyrotoxicosis in patients who have taken iodide therapy or who have had iodide contrast material in their tissues.*—The best tests are the PBI, in which the iodine is mainly that contained in thyroxine, the T3 uptake test, and the urinary excretion of iodine.

Diagnosis of thyrotoxicosis in patients on antithyroid drugs.—The PBI is usually low during antithyroid treatment because the gland produces more T3 than normal and this is not bound to TBG. The radioactive iodine uptake tests after $2\frac{1}{2}$ hours are affected by the anti-thyroid treatment; however the 20-minute radioactive uptake tests are *not* affected by treatment. Thyrotoxic patients who have gone or will go into remission will have a normal tri-iodothyronine suppression test. Non-suppressibility of the gland after six months' antithyroid treatment indicates that sustained remission is unlikely and this is an indication for ablative thyroid therapy, either partial thyroidectomy or radio-active iodine therapy (Alexander *et al.*, 1967).

4. *Thyroid function after thyroidectomy.*—Free Thyroxine Index is the most reliable guide.

HYPOTHYROIDISM

The causes of hypothyroidism are:

1. Primary failure of the thyroid (primary myxoedema).
2. Autoimmune thyroiditis (Hashimoto's disease).
3. Secondary failure of the thyroid due to pituitary failure (second-ary myxoedema).
4. Prolonged iodine deficiency.
5. Antithyroid substances in the diet or given therapeutically.
6. Inherited enzyme defects.
7. Thyroidectomy or radioactive iodine therapy.

Primary Myxoedema and Hashimoto's Disease

The histology of the gland in these two conditions is very similar and the incidence of antithyroid antibodies in Hashimoto's disease is nearly 100 per cent, while in primary myxoedema it is about 60 per cent. The antithyroid antibodies are antibodies against thyroglobulin and an antigen within the thyroid cells. In Hashimoto's disease, the patient may be euthyroid or hypothyroid; there is a high output of TSH and if the gland is not too badly damaged it can be stimulated to produce enough thyroxine to keep the patient euthyroid at the expense of developing a goitre—the alternative is a goitre with some hypo-thyroidism. However, in the end the patient always develops myxoe-dema. Occasionally, the patients with thyrotoxicosis have antithyroid antibodies and histological changes in the thyroid similar to those of Hashimoto's disease—these patients always end up eventually with myxoedema, and are usually treated with antithyroid drugs rather than partial thyroidectomy, because the drugs can be stopped as soon as the patient is euthyroid or hypothyroid. The diagnosis of Hashimoto's disease can be confirmed by the high levels of antithyroid antibodies and biopsy of the thyroid gland. The treatment of Hashimoto's disease is replacement therapy with thyroxine, which will inhibit TSH and re-duce the size of the gland. If the gland remains large after thyroxine treatment, partial thyroidectomy is performed. Corticosteroids are not normally used.

The cause of Riedel's thyroiditis is not known. The gland is usually very fibrotic and the fibrosis may involve other structures in the neck.

Myxoedema Secondary to Pituitary Failure and Iodine Deficiency

Myxoedema due to pituitary failure is usually accompanied by a deficiency of ACTH and consequent adrenal hypofunction, as well as a failure of TSH secretion. Unlike other forms of myxoedema, the serum cholesterol is usually normal. The condition can be separated from myxoedema due to thyroid damage by the TSH stimulation test. If the thyroid itself is damaged, TSH will not affect radioiodine uptake, whereas if the thyroid itself is normal, exogenous TSH will stimulate it to take up radioiodine normally. In pituitary failure there is usually absence of body hair, and the skin is of fine texture despite the myxoedema. Occasionally when pituitary failure has been present for a long time, the thyroid itself may atrophy and will sometimes not respond to TSH.

Treatment of secondary myxoedema is by replacement with thyroxine. It is of the utmost importance to treat any coincidental adrenal hypofunction first, as treatment of myxoedema in the presence of adrenal hypofunction will precipitate an Addisonian crisis.

Prolonged iodine deficiency results in compensatory thyroid enlargement in an attempt to utilise all available iodine in the blood—the thyroid is extremely avid for iodine. Following this compensated state, frank hypothyroidism may ensue. The Medical Research Council have suggested that all table salt in this country should have iodide added to it.

Antithyroid substances.—Thyroid enlargement and hypothyroidism can occur with PAS, phenylbutazone, resorcinol and antithyroid drugs. Occasionally, excess iodides can cause hypothyroidism—the cause for this is not known. Certain foods and contaminants are goitrogenic, particularly the Brassica group of vegetables (cabbage and kale), swedes and turnips.

Inherited enzyme defects.—These are uncommon causes of myxoedema and goitre, but interesting from the point of view of inborn errors of metabolism. They are all inherited as autosomal recessives—the homozygote has goitre and hypothyroidism, whereas the heterozygotes usually have a goitre with normal thyroid function.

The enzyme defects are:

(i) Iodide trapping defect.

(ii) Defect in binding iodine with tyrosine: this is associated with congenital deafness (Pendred's syndrome).

(iii) Defect of coupling iodotyrosines to form thyroxine and tri-iodothyronine.

(iv) Dehalogenase deficiency (tinker's disease) in which excess loss of iodine occurs in the urine.

(v) Abnormal thyroxine-binding globulin, which is metabolically inactive and is unable to bind thyroxine.

Clinical Features of Myxoedema

The "myxoedema" is an accumulation of mucoprotein and water; an increase in body fat is not a cardinal clinical feature of myxoedema and the apparent obesity is due to the mucoprotein accumulation. Because of the lowered metabolic rate the patients are intolerant of cold, and their temperature is often subnormal. The slight yellow colour of the skin is due to deposition of carotene; normally carotene is converted to vitamin A, but in hypothyroidism the reduced metabolism slows this conversion so that carotene tends to accumulate. In the gastro-intestinal tract, motility is slowed so that constipation occurs and absorption across the intestinal mucosa is slower than normal resulting in a flat glucose tolerance curve.

The heart is involved in several ways: atheroma and coronary artery disease are more common, a pericardial effusion may occur, the myocardium itself may be damaged resulting in a diffuse fibrosis and a cardiomyopathy, and finally, adequate thyroxine is necessary for the proper metabolism of myocardial cells. The electrocardiogram may show a generalised reduction in voltage which is sometimes, but not invariably, due to a pericardial effusion, or there may be non-specific wave inversion and bradycardia. Most of the ECG changes are rapidly reversed when thyroxine is administered.

Anaemia is common in myxoedema and is due to several factors:

1. Diminished peripheral oxygen requirements result in a physiological reduction in the red cell mass causing a normochromic normocytic anaemia.

2. Accompanying achlorhydria may contribute to an iron deficiency microcytic, hypochromic anaemia.

3. Pernicious anaemia occurs more commonly in myxoedema than in normals.

One of the most useful and constant signs of myxoedema is delayed relaxation of the tendon jerks. Occasionally the carpal tunnel syndrome is a feature due to pressure from mucoprotein on the median nerve where it passes under the flexor retinaculum in the wrist. One presentation of myxoedema of great practical importance is a non-specific psychosis—"myxoedematous madness".

Myxoedema coma is accompanied by hypothermia (defined as a rectal temperature below 90°F. or 32°C.)—the ordinary clinical thermometer does not read below 95°F. so that a special low-temperature thermometer should be used in a suspected case.

Any case of hypothermia should be suspected of suffering from myxoedema; hypothermia may also be precipitated by infection, chlorpromazine, Tofranil and other antidepressant drugs. The important physiological disturbances of hypothermia are (Cooper, 1968):

1. Intense muscular rigidity which impairs ventilation of the lungs leading to an accumulation of carbon dioxide and respiratory acidosis. The respiratory centre is driven by the anoxic stimulus, hence oxygen therapy alone may be harmful.

2. Metabolic acidosis due to accumulation of metabolites in muscles. This may be more severe during rewarming, when muscular activity may be greatest due to the onset of shivering.

3. The cardiac output is reduced but the blood pressure is often normal due to intense vasoconstriction, the viscosity of the blood is also markedly increased. The characteristic J-wave may be seen in the ECG.

4. Renal and hepatic function are impaired.

5. There is an inability to utilise glucose, despite high blood levels of both glucose and insulin.

It is important to note that the normal methods of measuring blood gases and acid-base balance may be misleading. These estimations are normally performed at 37°C. Table VII (Hockaday and Fell, 1969) shows that in hypothermia the true value is different from the apparent laboratory level.

TABLE VII

	27°	37°
pH	7·19	7·32
P_{CO_2}	80	52
P_{O_2}	85	43
O_2 saturation	95·6	92
(HCO_3)	29·5	32·5

In the treatment of hypothermia it is recommended that rewarming should take place gradually in old people—the patient is put in a warm room and covered with blankets. In the case of young patients who have suffered from immersion in cold water, it is suggested that rewarming should be faster, and the patient should be placed in a warm bath. If respiratory acidosis is present, mechanical ventilation either via a tracheostomy or endotracheal tube will be required; respiratory stimulants such as nikethamide are justified in milder cases. Hydrocortisone and glucose are given intravenously, even though the blood glucose is sometimes high; there is probably always some adrenal insufficiency in the presence of hypothermia. Adrenal failure and hypoglycaemia will certainly be present if hypothermia is due to pituitary failure. The metabolic acidosis is corrected with parenteral bicarbonate.

Hypothermia due to myxoedema is treated with a small dose of tri-iodothyronine, in addition to the other supportive measures. Arterial blood only should be used for the determination of electrolytes and blood gases, as venous blood is virtually completedly stagnant in severe cases.

Confirmation of myxoedema.—The laboratory diagnosis of myx-oedema is much less precise than that of hyperthyroidism. No one test is entirely suitable, and in practice reliance is usually placed on the clinical features, PBI, serum cholesterol and CPK. The presence of anti-thyroid antibodies is suggestive of thyroid damage, although the titre of antibodies is no guide to the severity of the thyroid lesion. Radio-iodine tests alone are of limited value; however, used in conjunction with TSH stimulation, they are probably about the best laboratory tests.

Treatment of Hypothyroidism

L-thyroxine is given in a dose of 0·1 mg daily for 2–4 weeks and then is gradually increased until the patient is euthyroid. The usual maintenance dose is 0·2–0·4 mg daily. Elderly people, and those with coronary artery disease, should be started on a lower dose and the dose increased more gradually, with frequent monitoring of the patient's symptoms and ECG: there is great danger of precipitating angina and cardiac failure if the condition is corrected too rapidly. The patient is judged to be euthyroid on clinical grounds and by the sense of well-being. PBI estimations are higher than the clinical state of the patient would suggest, due to binding of the administered thyroxine by TBG. If the PBI continues to be low, then it is fair indication that the dose of thyroxine should be increased. It is, of course, axiomatic that treatment is life-long.

Carcinoma of the Thyroid

Thyroid cancers are quite rare but they are important because they can often be cured and they are fascinating because of the logic with which they are treated. Most thyroid cancers are well-differentiated into papillary (with long columns of cells) and follicular in which almost normal thyroid follicles are seen. The minority of carcinomas are undifferentiated or anaplastic; these are commoner in the elderly and are treated with external irradiation and surgery if they are compressing the trachea or other structures in the neck.

Papillary carcinomas are unlike all other carcinomas in that they are equally common in all age groups and furthermore they are not more malignant in the younger age groups. Some thyroid carcinomas are dependent on TSH, hence the administration of thyroxine which will reduce endogenous TSH leads to regression, and this is particularly true of the papillary type. Papillary carcinomas tend to metastasize to local lymph glands and to be very slow growing—the primary may be exceedingly small. Follicular carcinomas are commoner in the older age groups and metastasize via the blood vessels, the contralateral lobe of the thyroid is involved in over half the cases. They commonly develop in a previous long-standing goitre.

Well-differentiated (papillary and follicular) carcinomas and their metastases do take up a small amount of radioiodine, but very much less than normal thyroid tissue. For this reason, any "cold" nodule, i.e. one which does not take up much radioiodine, should be assumed malignant until proved otherwise—a benign cyst will also appear as a "cold" nodule on a thyroid scan.

As a general rule, well-differentiated thyroid carcinoma is treated with total removal of the thyroid and the local lymph glands if they are involved with growth. Following thyroidectomy, radioiodine scanning and excretion tests are performed. The scan will reveal any radioiodine accumulation in carcinoma remnant or metastases and the excretion test will measure the amount of radioiodine retained in the remnants.

One of the greatest problems is that both primary and metastatic thyroid carcinomas only concentrate a small amount of radioactive iodine; however, they can be made to take up more radioactive iodine by:

1. Removing all normal thyroid tissue.
2. Stimulation with TSH.
3. Administration of carbimazole, which increases the vascularity of the tumours.

Normal thyroid tissue is removed either by thyroidectomy or a dose of radioiodine. Opinions differ as to which is the best way of promoting the tumours and their metastases to take up iodine; whichever method is employed large doses of radioiodine are given once the tumours have been made as iodine-avid as possible. Further doses of radioiodine may be necessary if excretion and uptake tests indicate that tumour deposits are still present.

THE ADRENAL CORTEX

One of the problems which has bedevilled adrenal physiology for the non-expert is the varied terminology used for the adrenal steroids. The steroids produced by the adrenal are mainly derived from cholesterol (itself a steroid) and they are classified as:

1. Glucocorticoids (hydrocortisone).
2. Mineralocorticoids (aldosterone).
3. Androgens.

The important steps in the production of the steroid hormones in men and women are:

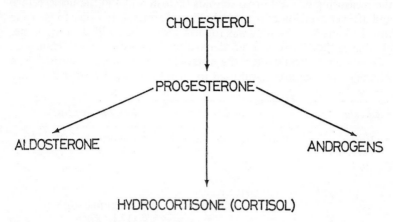

Once released from the adrenals, all the steroids are bound to plasma proteins: hydrocortisone is 95 per cent bound to an alpha globulin (transcortin) and albumin. Only the free steroid in the blood is metabolically active although the protein-bound steroid is a constant reservoir for replenishing free steroid. Aldosterone is only loosely bound to serum albumin, so that when the albumin is diminished, as in cirrhosis or the nephrotic syndrome, there is an increase in free aldosterone in the serum.

Hydrocortisone (cortisol) is not soluble in water, but in the liver it is broken down to four different substances (all steroids) which are conjugated with glucuronic acid. As such, they are water soluble, not bound to plasma proteins, and are excreted by the kidneys. Thus, in the urine there may be four breakdown products of cortisol, all conjugated with glucuronic acid. Androgens are broken down in the liver to two breakdown products which are also conjugated with glucuronides and excreted in the urine in precisely the same say way that four conjugated breakdown products of cortisol are excreted. Aldosterone is loosely bound to plasma albumin and is mainly excreted by the liver; less than one per cent is excreted unchanged by the kidneys.

The androgen metabolites in the urine are not only derived from adrenal androgens but also from ovaries or testes. The androgen metabolites are measured by a test known as the Zimmerman reaction and the substances measured are 17-oxo steroids (previously called 17-ketosteroids). The metabolites of cortisol used to be measured by converting them to 17-oxo steroids and subtracting the quantity of 17-oxo steroids derived from androgens already present in the urine;

measured by this means, the metabolites of cortisol are called 17-ketogenic or oxogenic steroids. This method of estimation necessitated the measuring of the 17-oxo steroids (ketosteroids) in the urine before and after conversion of the metabolites of cortisol. In order to get over this difficulty, a substance was found which, when added to the urine, eliminates the 17-oxo steroids derived from androgens; unfortunately, this substance slightly alters the metabolites derived from cortisol. The Zimmerman reaction is still used to measure these altered metabolites

Adrenal Steroid	Measured in Urine as	Previous nomenclature
Androgens	17-oxo steroids	17-ketosteroids (17 K.S.)
Cortisol	1. 17-hydroxy-corticosteroids (17 OHCS) 2. 17-oxogenic steroids 3. Cortisol can be measured in the blood as 17 OHCS or less commonly as 11 OHCS.	17-ketogenic steroids (17 KGS)

which are called 17-hydroxycorticosteroids or 17-hydroxycorticoids. Thus, 17-oxogenic steroids and 17-hydroxycorticoids both measure breakdown products of cortisol, but both measure slightly different substances (Mills, 1964). In practice, the results correlate well with each other, but because of the ease of estimation it is now customary to measure only the 17-hydroxycorticoids as a measure of cortisol. The 17-oxo steroids (17-ketosteroids) are still used as a measure of androgens.

The estimation of these substances in the urine is affected by glycosuria, renal impairment and meprobamate administration. Administration of paraldehyde, quinidine and colchicine affect the estimation of the blood 17 OHCS, giving false high values.

It is possible to separate the urinary steroids by chromatography but this is mainly used in research. It is also possible to measure directly the plasma levels of cortisol and aldosterone.

CUSHING'S[165] SYNDROME

Like malabsorption this is a condition in which a high clinical index of suspicion is important if mild cases are not going to be missed. The

165. HARVEY WILLIAMS CUSHING (1869–1939). Boston surgeon.

incidence of the well-known manifestations varies in different series but most of them agree that in over 75 per cent of the cases obesity, hypertension, glycosuria and hirsutism will be present. Other impressive initial features are muscular weakness, depression and osteoporosis. One point worth emphasising is that the disease often fluctuates and spontaneous improvement may occur. Suggestive simple laboratory investigations are a diminished lymphocyte and eosinophil count, elevated blood sugar and a hypokalaemic alkalosis.

The diagnosis of Cushing's syndrome falls into three parts: 1. suspicion; 2. confirmation; 3. finding the cause.

Cushing himself described the clinical features of excess cortisol excretion which he attributed to a pituitary basophil adenoma causing excess ACTH production. The exact role of the pituitary in the pathogenesis of bilateral adrenal cortical hyperplasia is not certain. Histological changes in the basophil cells of the pituitary can occur following corticosteroid therapy and small pituitary tumours can be demonstrated in up to half the patients with Cushing's syndrome (Mattingly, 1968).

Cushing's syndrome is caused by:

1. Bilateral adrenal hyperplasia usually due to excess pituitary ACTH.
2. Benign adenoma.
3. Adrenal carcinoma.
4. Carcinoma elsewhere.
5. Rarely, adrenal hyperplasia occurs in the absence of excess pituitary ACTH.

Numerically bilateral adrenal hyperplasia due to excess ACTH is responsible for about three-quarters of the cases.

Confirmation of the Clinical Diagnosis of Cushing's Syndrome

The fundamental abnormality is increased secretion of cortisol (hydrocortisone) from the adrenal cortex. Cortisol secretion rates can be estimated using radioactive labelled steroids but this is still a research tool and is not available for general use. Other measurements are used as circumstantial evidence of increased cortisol production. The most important of these are:

1. Serum level of cortisol at any one time.
2. Serum level of hydroxycorticoids (direct breakdown products of cortisol).
3 24-hour urinary excretion of 17-hydroxycorticoids (17 OHCS).
4. 24-hour urine excretion of 17-ketogenic steroids (17 KGS).

There is a diurnal variation in the rate of cortisol secretion by the adrenals; at night, during sleep, the need for adrenal steroids is low; at the beginning of the day the secretion and, therefore, the blood level is high. In Cushing's syndrome this diurnal variation is lost and output of cortisol is more or less constant throughout the day and night.

Most laboratories estimate the 24-hour urinary excretion of 17-hydroxycorticoids and 17-ketogenic steroids to confirm the diagnosis of Cushing's syndrome; however, it is worth pointing out that these estimations may miss about 20 per cent of patients who have Cushing's syndrome (Cope and Pearson, 1965). The most conclusive evidence of Cushing's syndrome is the demonstration of failure of the diurnal rhythm of cortisol secretion, which can be demonstrated simply by finding a high level of serum cortisol or hydroxycorticoids in the late evening or at midnight (Cope, 1965). Obesity can cause a real increase in the urinary ketogenic steroids which fall to normal when the patient regains a normal weight; one point of practical importance is that ketone bodies in the urine (which may occur during strict weight reduction) may interfere with the estimation of the urinary ketogenic steroids.

Patients with Cushing's syndrome from any of the causes mentioned produce excess cortisol which is not controlled by ACTH; reduction of the plasma ACTH level will not reduce the output of cortisol from the adrenals. In the normal, cortisol production is controlled by ACTH and any reduction of ACTH causes a lowered cortisol output. ACTH output from the pituitary can be diminished by administering a powerful steroid such as dexamethasone, which has the great advantage of not being broken down to hydroxycorticoids, hence urine and blood estimation of hydroxycorticoids are not altered by the dexamethasone itself. The diagnosis of Cushing's syndrome is confirmed if there is failure to suppress the level of plasma cortisol, hydroxycorticoids or 24-hour urine excretion of 17-hydroxycorticoids with dexamethasone (2 mg daily for two days).

To differentiate between bilateral adrenal hyperplasia (which is partially responsible to ACTH) and an adrenal adenoma or carcinoma which is purely autonomous, a larger dose of dexamethasone is used (8 mg daily for two days). Using this larger dose cortisol output will fall in bilateral adrenal hyperplasia but not if there is a completely autonomous adenoma or carcinoma.

Treatment of Cushing's Syndrome

Bilateral hyperplasia.—There are two orthodox approaches, one is bilateral adrenalectomy and the other is partial pituitary ablation; pituitary ablation is the treatment of choice if there is evidence of high ACTH output or if the pituitary fossa is enlarged. The disadvantage of total adrenalectomy is that the pituitary continues to pour out ACTH and may develop a chromophobe adenoma.

Adenoma or carcinoma.—These are treated by surgical removal; the opposite adrenal will be atrophic and is not removed.

Ectopic ACTH production.—The commonest primaries to produce ACTH are bronchus and thymus. The patient is usually thin, severely pigmented and has profound uncontrollable hypokalaemia. Death usually occurs from the adrenal hyperfunction; if the prognosis of the primary tumour warrants it total bilateral adrenalectomy is indicated.

ADDISON'S[166] DISEASE

The main causes of Addison's disease are:

1. Idiopathic adrenal cortical atrophy.
2. Tuberculosis.
3. Pituitary-hypothalamic disorders such as suppression of ACTH production with therapeutic corticosteroids.
4. Other replacements of the adrenals such as amyloidosis and sarcoidosis.
5. Haemorrhage of infarction of the adrenals.

It is worth emphasising at the outset that nine-tenths of both adrenals have to be destroyed before the clinical features of Addison's disease are seen; however, people with only a small amount of functioning adrenal tissue left are able to survive without stress, but in a stress situation which demands increased steroid output they will develop features of adrenal insufficiency. It is not known how many patients develop undiagnosed adrenal insufficiency following stress situations such as an emergency operation or myocardial infarction, but it is probably more common than is generally appreciated. American workers lay emphasis on the value of an eosinophil count—in a stress situation the increased output of cortisol in a normal person will lower the eosinophils below $50/mm^3$ but in a patient with adrenal insufficiency the eosinophil count is above $50/mm^3$.

Idiopathic adrenal cortical atrophy accounts for at least half the cases of Addison's disease in this country. In this group there is a high incidence of anti adrenal and antithyroid antibodies, there is also a higher than normal incidence of thyrotoxicosis, myxoedema, diabetes, hypoparathyroidism, atrophic gastritis and pernicious anaemia.

Clinical features of importance which are so common in a gastro-enterological clinic that Addison's disease may not be suspected are weight loss, vomiting, abdominal pain and diarrhoea.

Some of the metabolic effects of cortisol are not well understood; this is partly due to the fact that cortisol has some mineralocorticoid activity like aldosterone but it is not known to what extent aldosterone

166. THOMAS ADDISON (1793–1860). London physician.

is also deficient in many cases of Addison's disease. What is known is that aldosterone is not controlled by ACTH. Cortisol seems to be essential for the proper functioning of a large number of structures, e.g.:

1. *Renal tubules:* without cortisol the renal tubules are unable to dilute the urine so they cannot excrete a sudden water load. It is possible that cortisol normally acts in competition with ADH and so in cortisol deficiency ADH can act unopposed. Cortisol appears necessary for aldosterone to be able to exert its action on the renal tubules. One of the features of prolonged Addison's disease is dehydration possibly because in the absence of cortisol aldosterone is unable to retain sodium and water. Note that Addison's disease has two effects on water excretion: on the one hand there is dehydration, possibly because of end-organ unresponsiveness to aldosterone, and on the other there is inability to excrete at a normal rate an increased water load, presumably as a result of tubular dysfunction in the absence of cortisol.

2. *Blood vessels:* cortisol is necessary for the blood vessels to respond to circulating catecholamines hence the appearance of hypotension in Addison's disease and the improvement in clinical shock that may occur when hydrocortisone is given. In Addison's disease there is failure of the normal arteriolar reflexes: despite hypotension there may be peripheral vasodilatation.

3. *Gastro-intestinal tract:* in Addison's disease there may be increased excretion of faecal fats suggesting that cortisol is necessary for the functional integrity of the small intestinal mucosa. The hypoglycaemia and weight loss of Addison's disease are also due to this mechanism.

4. *Glomerular filtration:* this is generally reduced in Addison's disease and is probably the cause of the rise in blood urea which occurs.

Diagnosis

A chest x-ray, abdominal plain x-ray and Mantoux test are necessary to pick up those cases due to tuberculosis; idiopathic atrophy of the adrenals does not cause adrenal calcification. It is important to pick up those cases due to tuberculosis because replacement therapy with corticosteroids may light up the dormant tuberculosis. As with Cushing's disease the laboratory diagnosis involves first of all confirming the clinical diagnosis and then discovering the cause.

The diagnosis of Addison's disease is confirmed by administering exogenous ACTH and estimating the steroid output before and afterwards; either the serum cortisol or hydroxycorticoids or the urinary 17-hydroxycorticoids are measured. The ACTH is usually given intramuscularly as this diminishes the incidence of allergic reactions compared with giving it intravenously. Synacthen is a synthetic preparation of ACTH which does not produce allergic effects, however, its duration of action is short.

Besides primary failure of the adrenals due to atrophy or replacement there may be adrenal insufficiency for two other reasons; first the pituitary-adrenal axis may be impaired and secondly the pituitary or hypothalamus may not be able to respond normally to stress. In pituitary-adrenal axis dysfunction the normal feed-back mechanism of cortisol is impaired, so that the pituitary does not put out more ACTH in response to a lower level of cortisol. Cortisol itself is the only substance which will inhibit ACTH secretion from the pituitary. The precursors of cortisol do not inhibit ACTH but are excreted in the urine as 17-hydroxycorticoids. Metopirone (metyrapone) is a substance which blocks the synthesis of cortisol at a late stage so that the feed-back mechanism is destroyed, but the early precursors of cortisol are still produced and excreted as 17-hydroxycorticoids. Thus, if Metopirone is given to a normal person cortisol will be diminished, ACTH will be secreted stimulating the adrenal to produce more cortisol (via its precursors), but cortisol production is blocked so that the increased precursors are excreted in the urine as excess 17-hydroxycorticoids. In a patient with pituitary-adrenal axis dysfunction the fall in cortisol after Metopirone is given does not stimulate the production of more ACTH, so that the urinary level of 17-hydroxycorticoids from cortisol precursors does not rise. It is essential to note that before the Metopirone test is performed the adrenals must be shown to function normally in response to an injection of ACTH. It should also be noted that impairment of the feed-back mechanism does not mean that the adrenals cannot respond normally to stress. The response to stress involves stimulation of the pituitary or hypothalamus which then stimulate the adrenals. The hypothalamus stimulates the pituitary to produce ACTH by a corticotrophin release factor. Lysine vasopressin is a substance which acts like the corticotrophin release factor and can be used to assess the ability of the pituitary and adrenal to respond to potentially stressful situations. Insulin-induced hypoglycaemia also stimulates the secretion of corticotrophin release factor but the hypoglycaemia has to be quite profound.

Treatment of Addison's Disease

In an Addisonian crisis the patient will require cortisol, water, saline and glucose quickly. Replacement therapy is with cortisone and fludrocortisone 0·1 mg b.d.

DIABETES

Definitions in Diabetes

The British Diabetic Association definitions are:

Potential Diabetes: A normal glucose tolerance test with

(1) Both parents diabetic.

(2) Identical twin a diabetic.

(3) One parent diabetic and the other parent having a near relative a diabetic.

(4) A woman who has given birth to a baby weighing 10 lbs or more.

Latent Diabetes: (1) A normal glucose tolerance curve which is known to have been diabetic in type during pregnancy, stress or obesity.

Asymptomatic Diabetes: No symptoms of diabetes but whose glucose tolerance test is diabetic in type.

Clinical Diabetes: A diabetic glucose tolerance test with symptoms and/ or complications of diabetes.

Pre-Diabetic: Refers to the period in the life of a diabetic before the diagnosis is made.

The Pathogenesis of Diabetes

The insulin content of the blood in patients with mild maturity-onset diabetes rises after a glucose load and continues to rise when in normals it would start to fall (Yalow and Berson, 1960); no such rise occurs in severe diabetics of long-standing. There is a reduction of the β-cell mass of the islets of Langerhans as well as increased hyalinisation of the cells in young severe diabetics (Warren and Le Compte, 1952). These findings suggest that some forms of diabetes are due to diminished amounts of insulin and other forms are due to inability to utilise normal quantities of insulin. The three aspects of inability to utilise insulin which are important are:

1. End-organ unresponsiveness.
2. Alteration in insulin structure.
3. Antagonists of insulin.

End-organ unresponsiveness.—Hyperglycaemia occurs in Cushing's syndrome and phaeochromocytoma despite normal insulin production: both glucocorticoids and adrenaline slow the rate of utilisation of glucose in the tissues. The serum levels of insulin in obese patients are frequently higher than normal suggesting end-organ unresponsiveness (Yalow *et al.*, 1965).

Alteration in insulin structure.—Insulin is secreted from the islet cells into the pancreatic vein, thence via the liver to the systemic circulation. Some alteration in the structure of insulin probably takes place in the liver (Samols and Ryder, 1961). Insulin probably becomes bound to plasma proteins in the liver and only insulin which is not bound, or "free", is effective. The high level of insulin found in maturity-onset diabetes may be due to excessive insulin binding by the plasma proteins (Antoniades *et al.*, 1964).

Antagonists of insulin.—The mechanisms by which insulin itself can be antagonised are:

(*a*) Stimulation of plasma insulin antagonist.

(*b*) Rapid destruction of insulin.

(*c*) Increased ketone-body formation (ketone bodies are insulin antagonists).

A factor derived from the serum albumin (synalbumin) antagonises the effects of insulin and is found in a higher concentration in diabetics than in normals (Vallance-Owen *et al.*, 1958).

A substance which breaks down insulin in the tissues occurs; it is presumed to be an enzyme and is, therefore, called insulinase. Insulinase is probably not important in the pathogenesis of diabetes because the half-life of injected radioactive-labelled insulin is the same in diabetics as non-diabetics (Welsh *et al.*, 1956). Antibodies to insulin occur in all patients receiving therapeutic insulin and they are occasionally responsible for chronic insulin resistance, another cause of which is excessive binding of insulin by the plasma proteins. In the treatment of insulin resistance high doses of insulin are usually necessary; sometimes corticosteroids and oral hypoglycaemics are used. The sulphonylureas stimulate production of endogenous insulin and fortunately the antibodies which are present are only effective against exogenous insulins. The biguanides may increase the peripheral utilisation of insulin. Other circulating factors which antagonise insulin are free fatty acids, ketone bodies and growth hormone.

The incidence of diabetes is increasing in the developed countries, which is probably due to the prevalence of obesity and the longer average survival of the individual, because there is a deterioration in glucose tolerance with age even in non-diabetics.

A number of factors are known to be associated with the development of diabetes and there are large numbers of undiagnosed patients who either have diabetes or who are destined to develop it. It is not yet established whether the complications of diabetes can be prevented by prompt and careful treatment of the diabetes.

Patients who have a high risk of developing diabetes are said to have "pre" or latent diabetes; the three factors which are known to increase the risk are a family history, giving birth to overweight babies and an abnormal "stress" glucose tolerance curve. Corticosteroids delay the uptake of glucose by the peripheral tissues and any tendency to develop diabetes will be reflected in an abnormally high glucose blood level after corticosteroids have been given (stress glucose tolerance test). A person who has a normal glucose tolerance test but who has had an abnormal one in a period of stress (e.g. pregnancy, infection or obesity) is also a "pre-diabetic".

The oral glucose tolerance test is still the method of choice to confirm the diagnosis of diabetes. It is influenced by a number of factors other than the presence of diabetes: a previous low carbohydrate intake will produce a diabetic type curve, there is also a small increase in blood sugar attributable to being a woman and to ageing. The level of blood sugar attained will also be affected by disorders of absorption. The intravenous glucose tolerance test has not circumvented these difficulties and in practice is no more suitable than the oral test in distinguishing diabetics from non-diabetics. In this country the two biggest diabetic surveys have been in Birmingham and Bedford (Diabetic Survey, 1962; Sharp et al., 1964).

Treatment of Diabetes

There is a tendency to underplay the importance of weight reduction in overweight maturity-onset diabetes. Many of these patients are given one of the sulphonylureas (tolbutamide or chlorpropamide) while they are still overweight—this is a mistake because the drugs increase the appetite by producing mild hypoglycaemia and if the patient continues to gain weight the drugs may lose their hypoglycaemic effect. It is a good working rule to try weight reduction in obese patients before giving them drugs. The sulphonylureas exert their action by stimulating the β-cells of the pancreas to produce endogenous insulin and later they lead to hypertrophy of the β-cells. Tolbutamide has a short duration of action and has to be given twice daily, the relapse rate is high. Chlorpropamide has a longer action and need only be given once a day—to some extent the drug is cumulative and can be present ten days after it was last administered. The effects of the sulphonylureas can be potentiated by alcohol and barbiturates; alcohol may cause flushing of the face in addition. One very important side-effect of the sulphonylureas is that they may cause hypoglycaemia—it is essential to note that as chlorpropamide is a cumulative drug hypoglycaemia may continue for several days despite intermittent use of parenteral glucose. Mild hypoglycaemia may occur at night, particularly if chlorpromazine is given as a night sedative to the elderly—if hypoglycaemia and confusion occur at night it is probably better to use the shorter acting tolbutamide. The sulphonylureas may produce gastro-intestinal disturbances and jaundice—this may be of two types: cholestatic and hepatocellular. The drugs are protein bound, hence other protein-bound drugs may interfere with the binding sites causing a rise of the free drug in the serum and precipitating hypoglycaemia; such a drug is phenylbutazone. It must not be forgotten that the thiazide diuretics tend to increase the blood sugar in diabetics and non-diabetics.

Biguanides.—The most commonly used of the biguanide drugs is phenformin; they exert their action by promoting the uptake of glucose by the tissues and they tend to promote anaerobic metabolism so that lactic acid accumulates; under normal circumstances this does not matter but if there is another cause of tissue anoxia (such as cardiogenic shock) there may be an excessive accumulation of lactic acid. Another danger of the biguanides is that in a moderately severe diabetic they may produce ketosis without a rise in blood sugar being apparent (presumably because the tissues are stimulated by the drug to continue the uptake of glucose). The biguanides have never been reported to cause hypoglycaemia. They have some mild appetite-suppressing effect and are, therefore, useful in obese diabetics who are unable to stay on a rigid diet voluntarily. They are useful when hyperglycaemia persists with the sulphonylureas alone and they may be combined with insulin with a view to decreasing insulin requirements and preventing hypoglycaemic attacks. Phenformin is excreted in the urine. It should never be used in patients who have any evidence of renal impairment.

Diabetic Ketosis

If the patient is in coma the commonest practice is to give soluble insulin 50 or 100 units intravenously and 50 or 100 units intramuscularly. It should not be given subcutaneously (as diabetics normally have it) because of the delay in absorption. Some clinicians give more or less insulin according to the level of blood sugar—a simple rule is to give 1 unit of insulin per 2 mg per cent (0·1 mmol/l) of the blood sugar; however, in practice this degree of accuracy is not necessary. There is now evidence that equally good results in the treatment of diabetic coma are obtained by giving constant infusions of relatively low doses of soluble insulin 5–10 iu/hour. The insulin is sometimes given with small amounts of added human albumin which limits the adsorption of such small amounts of insulin to the plastic syringe.

A fact which is not usually appreciated with regard to fluid and electrolyte replacement is that the high blood glucose causes an osmotic diuresis and the patient is severely dehydrated—the excess loss of water in the urine causes secondary salt depletion. Thus, patients in diabetic coma are short of both salt and water but the shortage of water is the greater. It is usually safe enough to give a litre of normal (isotonic) saline; if there is evidence of severe haemoconcentration then half a litre of saline can be given with an equal volume of distilled water. One disadvantage of giving solutions which are more dilute than plasma is that they may cause haemolysis. The usual method of giving water to a dehydrated patient in an isotonic form is to give 5 per cent dextrose (glucose) and many physicians give a mixture of 5 per cent dextrose and isotonic saline in diabetic coma. The disadvantages of giving dextrose are that it increases the blood sugar and increases the osmotic load in the plasma, promoting further diuresis—in practice neither of these disadvantages is overwhelming. It has been suggested that isotonic fructose be used instead of glucose, as fructose is rapidly metabolised by the liver and does not interfere with the estimation of the blood glucose very much.

There is now general agreement that it is wise to correct the metabolic acidosis as insulin is more effective at a neutral pH. The number of milliequivalents of bicarbonate which the patient requires is calculated by considering the level of the serum bicarbonate and hence the number of milliequivalent per litre that he is depleted, remembering that the normal serum bicarbonate is 25 mEq per litre. The bicarbonate ion is both an intracellular and an extracellular ion and it has been found empirically that bicarbonate is distributed through a volume (in litres) equivalent to one-third of the body weight in kilograms, i.e. in a 60 kg man this will be 20 litres. For example if the serum bicarbonate is 15 mEq/l then each litre is (25–15) mEq short of bicarbonate; there are 20 litres to be considered so that the patient requires $20 \times (25–15) = 200$ mEq. This can either be given as isotonic sodium bicarbonate (which contains 167 mEq of sodium and bicarbonate per litre) or as 8.4 per cent bicarbonate which contains 1 mEq of bicarbonate per millilitre.

It is essential to monitor the electrolytes, acid-base status and blood sugar at frequent intervals (at least hourly for 3–4 hours). One hour after the first dose of insulin has been given the blood sugar is repeated; if the blood sugar has risen the dose of insulin is doubled, if the blood sugar remains the same the same dose of insulin is repeated and if the blood sugar is falling insulin is withheld. After 3–4 hours most patients develop hypokalaemia so that potassium has to be given—this is best administered as potassium chloride into the infusion bottle (1 g of potassium chloride contains 13·4 mEq potassium).

In cases which require very large amounts of insulin (more than 200 units per hour) there is obvious insulin resistance, and this is most commonly due to insulin antibodies which must be saturated before any free insulin is left in the serum to correct the metabolic abnormality. Insulin-resistant cases usually respond better if 100 mg of hydrocortisone are given.

The other facets of treatment of diabetic coma are:

1. Antibiotics to counteract probable precipitating infection.
2. Gastric tube to prevent gastric atony and vomiting.
3. Catheterisation of the bladder.
4. Treatment of hypotension.

Hyperosmolar coma.—Sometimes a mild diabetic has some impairment of glucose metabolism but not enough to cause the body to turn to fat as a source of energy, and in these patients there may be a rise in blood sugar but no ketosis. The rise in blood sugar promotes an osmotic diuresis and the patient becomes severely dehydrated and eventually comatose. The hall-marks of this condition are, therefore, severe haemo-concentration (with a high serum sodium and packed cell volume), hyperglycaemia and glycosuria but little or no ketosis. These patients require large amounts of fluids and only small amounts of insulin. Occasionally mild diabetes presents as hyperosmolar coma and when the patients recover they usually give a history of a sudden onset of a craving for sweet foods (and liquids) some weeks before.

Stabilisation of Diabetes

The great problem with diabetics requiring insulin is to stabilise them with a once daily dose of insulin. There are some fairly simple rules for this: the first thing to establish is the patient's renal threshold for glucose because much of the alteration in insulin dose is going to depend on subsequent urine testing. A diabetic who also has a low renal threshold for glucose has a great risk of developing hypoglycaemia if the insulin he receives depends on uncritical urine examination, because he will have glycosuria at a low level of blood sugar.

Once the patient is out of coma he is put on a "sliding scale" of insulin according to urine tests for glucose—if the urine shows 0·5 per cent or less of glucose then no insulin is given; urine testing is gradually reduced so that it is being done three or four times a day—all this time the patient is receiving soluble insulin in accordance with the urine test. The next step is the one most frequently mismanaged, partly because so many long-acting insulin preparations are available. The aim of treatment of a severe diabetic is to give one injection of insulin a day if it is possible thereby to keep the patient normoglycaemic throughout the day. The corner-stone of treatment is insulin lente which begins to act about two hours after it is injected and has its maximum action four to six hours later, but it continues to have some action 24–30 hours afterwards. If these times of action were the same in all patients and each patient could take meals at the same time there would be no problem—insulin lente would suffice for everyone.

As an example let us assume that a diabetic patient has a normal renal threshold and takes his meals in the usual amounts at the usual times (i.e. 8 a.m., 1 p.m., 4 p.m. and 7.30 p.m.). An injection of insulin lente at 8 a.m. will begin to work about 10 a.m., will have its maximum effect about 2 p.m. and wane thereafter. The time at which he will develop glycosuria is when the insulin is wearing off and he has a meal, i.e. after his supper. In order to prevent glycosuria at this time the dose of insulin has to be increased. This can be done provided he does not develop hypoglycaemia when the insulin is having its maximum effect after lunch at about 2 p.m. If he does develop hypoglycaemia at 2 p.m. either the dose of insulin must be cut, or he must eat a larger lunch and in order to stop glycosuria after his supper he must eat a smaller supper. This is the principle by which the dose of insulin and the size of meals are adjusted. Unfortunately not everyone can alter their meals so conveniently, for example, a labourer usually has a snack lunch and a big supper and, furthermore, the duration of action of various insulins is variable. The other difficulty with a big evening meal is that in the early morning, before the 8 a.m. insulin injection, and for an hour or two after the injection, the previous day's insulin lente is wearing off and severe glycosuria may occur. In order to get over the problems of the big evening meal and early morning glycosuria longer-acting preparations are used such as insulin ultralente and protamine zinc insulin (PZI), which have an action that begins some 12 hours later and continues for 24–36 hours. PZI is less suitable than insulin ultralente because it cannot be mixed with soluble insulin, as the excess protamine in PZI converts most of the soluble insulin to PZI. When the long-acting insulins are used they are nearly always combined with a shorter-acting insulin such as insulin semilente or soluble. The most severe diabetics need to have more than one injection a day but they represent a very small minority.

Once the patient who has developed diabetic coma is stabilised on a "sliding scale" of soluble insulin, he should be started on a morning dose of insulin lente containing about three-quarters of the total number of units which he was having as soluble insulin throughout the day.

Other long-acting insulins besides insulin lente can be used. These include:

1. *Protamine zinc insulin (PZI)*. Some older diabetics are still well controlled on mixtures of PZI and soluble insulin but PZI suffers from two main disadvantages—some of the soluble insulin with which it is mixed is converted to PZI by the excess protamine and secondly it has a long duration of action and is cumulative and may produce hypoglycaemia at night.

2. *Isophane insulin*. This insulin is popular in the U.S. It does not alter the properties of any added soluble insulin; its duration of action is less than PZI but even so it may still produce nocturnal hypoglycaemia.

3. *Biphasic insulin (Rapitard)*. This contains rapid-acting porcine soluble insulin and bovine soluble insulin in a slow-release form. Its duration of action varies from 12–14 hours.

Quality of Control and the Incidence of Diabetic Complications

Probably a fair generalisation of current policy is to advise manipulation of diet and insulin so as to avoid large changes in the blood sugar throughout the 24 hours. Most studies agree that those patients who seem to have been well controlled have less vascular disease than those who have been poorly controlled (Malins, 1968). However this controversy is still unresolved; experienced diabetologists can cite good evidence to support either viewpoint.

Hypoglycaemia

At a serum level of 40 mg per cent (2·1 mmol/l) of glucose there will usually be symptoms of hypoglycaemia, although it is important to note that some normal people tolerate a blood level of 30 mg per cent (1·7 mmol/l) without developing symptoms and others develop symptoms of hypoglycaemia at a higher level if there has been a rapid fall from a previously high level.

The important causes of hypoglycaemia are:

1. Functional hypoglycaemia: this occurs two hours after a meal and is due to excessive outpouring of insulin in response to the meal. It tends to occur in the psychiatrically ill.

2. Excessive insulin or sulphonylureas.

3. Liver disease.

4. Post-gastrectomy and malabsorption states.

5. Early diabetes—in the early stages there may be attacks of spontaneous hypoglycaemia after meals. In early diabetes there seems to be a delayed response to a meal but when the response does occur excess insulin is produced causing hypoglycaemia.

6. Sensitivity to alcohol.

7. Addison's disease and pituitary failure.

8. Insulinoma.

9. Non-pancreatic neoplasms such as mediastinal or retroperitoneal sarcoma, hepatic carcinoma and adrenal tumours.

10. Inborn errors of metabolism.

Diagnosis.—As in many endocrine conditions it is necessary to confirm the clinical diagnosis biochemically and then investigate for the cause. Spontaneous hypoglycaemia is confirmed by measuring the blood sugar after a fast. The most useful tests for finding the cause of hypoglycaemia are:

1. *Tolbutamide tolerance test*—a positive test is a level of blood sugar of 40 mg per cent (2·1 mmol/l) 3 hours after intravenous injection of 1 g of tolbutamide. The test is not usually positive in reactive hypoglycamia although it is in insulinomas and liver disease.

2. *Glucagon test.* In insulinomas there is rebound hypoglycaemia but not in reactive hypoglycaemia and not usually in liver disease.

3. *Plasma insulin levels.* Single normal values do not exclude an insulinoma.

The plasma insulin level following tolbutamide is of greater diagnostic value. Other tests which are sometimes helpful in hypoglycaemia are insulin and leucine tolerance tests (Marks and Rose, 1965).

Treatment of insulinomas is total pancreatectomy unless metastases are present. Diazoxide is a thiazide drug which has no diuretic action but a strong diabetic effect; it may be very useful in preventing attacks of hypoglycaemia in malignant insulinoma or if symptoms persist after subtotal pancreatectomy.

PITUITARY AND HYPOTHALAMUS

The clinical manifestations of pituitary hormone deficiency are variable and depend on whether:
Some or all the anterior pituitary hormones are affected.
The hypothalamus is involved.
The posterior pituitary is also involved.
The cause of the pituitary failure is producing the effects of space occupation or compression.

Clinical Manifestations of Pituitary Failure

ACTH deficiency.—Features of Addison's disease without the pigmentation because of associated deficiency of MSH. Water and electrolytes may be normal since aldosterone output remains normal.

TSH deficiency.—Features of myxoedema except that there may be loss of body hair; the patient is usually not obese and the skin not greasy or thickened as in myxoedema. In women amenorrhoea is usual with hypopituitarism but in myxoedema menorrhagia is more common.

Growth hormone deficiency.—Excess sensitivity to insulin.

FSH, ICSH and LH deficiency.—Loss of libido, loss of secondary sex characteristics and fine wrinkled skin. Amenorrhoea is usual in women.

Vasopressin (ADH) deficiency.—Polyuria and thirst.

Hypothalamic deficiency.—The most usual manifestation is lack of TSH and ACTH due to deficiency of hypothalamic releasing factors. Disturbances of temperature, sleep and body weight are *not* common.

ACROMEGALY

Management

Acromegaly which is obviously progressing or is associated with evidence of compression of the optic chiasma is generally treated with surgical decompression or deep x-ray therapy. So-called "burnt out" cases are generally not treated because it is felt that the "cure" (by causing the necessity for replacement therapy) is worse than the disease, and the general impression is that acromegaly is a relatively benign disease. However, the average age of death of patients with acromegaly is around 60 and the mortality is twice that of subjects of the same age (Wright *et al.*, 1970). By treating acromegaly these authors have reduced the mortality as compared with untreated acromegalics. The increased mortality in acromegaly is due to hypertension, cardiac failure and diabetes.

A reasonable general rule would be to advise pituitary ablation (by the best local means) in otherwise well acromegalics who show evidence that growth hormone is still being produced in excess.

Methods of assessing growth hormone or "activity" of acromegaly.—
1. Serum level of GH.
2. Raised urine calcium.
3. Raised serum phosphate.
4. Augmented *insulin* tolerance test. Patients with excess GH are relatively resistant to insulin.
5. Glucose tolerance test and augmented GTT.
6. GH levels during glucose tolerance test. In normal subjects a high blood glucose suppresses growth hormone; in patients with acromegaly GH is not suppressed.

HIRSUTISM

Most androgens, which are excreted in the urine as 17-ketosteroids, are derived from the ovaries and adrenals. Testosterone is the most important androgen responsible for hair growth but it is *not* excreted in the urine in women as part of the 17-ketosteroids. Women with idiopathic hirsutism generally have a raised plasma and urinary testosterone and a ketosteroid excretion which is at the upper limit of normal.

The important causes of hirsutism and the tests used to confirm the diagnosis are:

Ovarian tumour
1. Gynaecological examination.
2. Raised urinary 17-ketosteroids.

Adrenal tumour.
1. Raised 17-ketosteroids.
2. Often raised cortisol excretion particularly with adenomas.
3. Sometimes raised dehydro-andro-episterone with adrenal carcinomas.

Congenital adrenal hyperplasia
1. Raised 17-ketosteroids.
2. Raised urinary pregnanetriol (which occurs when there is a deficiency of 21-hydroxylase enzyme, which is the commonest form of congenital adrenal hyperplasia presenting in adult life).

Cushing's syndrome   1. Clinical features.

                                         2. Raised cortisol and hydroxycorticoids.

Stein-Leventhal   1. Clinical features (infertility, amenorrhoea,
syndrome   late menarche, obesity, irregular ovulation).

                                         2. Gynaecological examination (enlarged ovaries).

                                         3. Marginally elevated 17-ketosteroids.

These are important conditions to be excluded before "idiopathic" hirsutism is diagnosed. Nevertheless idiopathic hirsutism is by far the commonest cause of hirsutism seen in general medical out-patients. In many cases of "idiopathic" hirsutism it is possible to find out evidence of mild ovarian or adrenal dysfunction or both (Nabarro, 1966). From a practical point of view no further investigation is indicated *after* the known organic disorders causing hirsutism have been excluded. Treatment of idiopathic hirsutism should be by cosmetic means in the first instance; if this fails cycles of small doses of oestrogens should be tried on the grounds that if there is an ovarian abnormality excessive stimulation of the ovaries may be suppressed with oestrogens, and that the oestrogens may have a direct affect on the hair follicles. If oestrogens are going to help they do so within 3 months. If oestrogens are ineffective it is sometimes worth trying small doses of prednisone to try and suppress possible adrenal over-stimulation. The beneficial effects of adrenal suppression may take up to a year to become apparent (Nabarro, 1966).

GYNAECOMASTIA

Causes of Gynaecomastia

Physiological   At birth and puberty

Pathological   Testicular tumours
                          Other tumours
                          Bronchial carcinoma
                          Hypernephroma
                          Hodgkin's disease

Drugs   Digitalis
                          Spironolactone
                          Phenothiazines
                          Isoniazid
                          Amphetamines
                          Corticosteroids
                          Androgens
                          Oestrogens

Endocrine	Thyrotoxicosis
disorders	Diabetes
	Acromegaly
	Addison's disease

Other	Hepatocellular failure
disorders	Starvation and wasting disorders
	Paraplegia
	Ulcerative colitis
	Rheumatoid arthritis
	Chronic renal failure
	Congestive cardiac failure.

REFERENCES

THYROID

ALEXANDER, W. D., HARDEN, R. M., SKIMMINS, J., McLARTY, D., and McGILL, P. (1967). *Lancet*, 2, 681.

COOPER, K. E. (1968). *Recent Advances in Medicine*, 15th edit. Eds. Baron, D. N., Compston, N., and Dawson, A. M. London: J. & A. Churchill.

HOCKADAY, T. D., and FELL, R. H. (1969). *Brit. J. hosp. Med.*, 2, 1083.

TROTTER, W. R. (1962). *Diseases of the Thyroid.* Oxford: Blackwell Scientific.

ADRENALS

COPE, C. L. (1965). *Second Symposium on Advanced Medicine* at the Royal College of Physicians. Ed. Trounce, J. R. London: Pitman Med. Pub. Co.

COPE, C. L., and PEARSON, J. (1965). *J. clin. Path.*, 18, 82.

MATTINGLY, D. (1968). *Recent Advances in Medicine*, 15th edit. Eds. Baron, D. N., Compston, N., and Dawson, A. M. London: J. & A. Churchill.

MILLS, I. (1964). *Clinical Aspects of Adrenal Function.* Oxford: Blackwell Scientific.

DIABETES

ANTONIADES, H. N., BOUGAS, J. A., CAMERINI-DAVALOS, R., and PYLE, H. M. (1964). *Diabetes*, 12, 230.

Diabetic Survey (1962). *Brit. med. J.*, 1, 1497.

MALINS, J. (1968). *Clinical Diabetes Mellitus.* London: Eyre & Spottiswoode.

MARKS, V., and ROSE, F. C. (1965). *Hypoglycaemia.* Oxford: Blackwell Scientific.

SAMOLS, E., and RYDER, J. A. (1961). *J. clin. Invest.*, 40, 2092.

SHARP, C. L., BUTTERWORTH, W. J., and KEEN, H. (1964). *Proc. roy. Soc. Med.*, 57, 193.

VALLANCE-OWEN, J., DENNES, E., and CAMPBELL, P. N. (1958). *Lancet*, 2, 336.

WARREN, S., and LE COMPTE, P. M. (1952). *The Pathology of Diabetes Mellitus.* London: H. Kimpton.

WELSH, G. W., HENLEY, E. D., WILLIAMS, R. H., and COX, R. W. (1956). *Amer. J. Med.*, **21**, 324.

YALOW, R. S., and BERSON, S. A. (1960). *J. clin. Invest.*, **39**, 1157.

YALOW, R. S., GLICK, S. M., ROTH, J., and BERSON, S. A. (1965). *Ann. N.Y. Acad. Sci.*, **131**, 357.

PITUITARY

WRIGHT, A. D., HILL, D. M., LOWY, C., and FRASER, T. R. (1970). *Quart. J. Med.*, **39**, 1.

HIRSUTISM

NABARRO, J. D. (1966). *Second Symposium on Advanced Medicine*, Royal College of Physicians of London. London: Pitman.

RENAL DISEASES

Clinical Features

Pain from the kidney is referred to the skin in the distribution of the 10th, 11th and 12th thoracic nerves. The pain of ureteric colic is felt in the same distribution but often extends to the cutaneous distribution of L.1 and to the testicle or labia. Tenderness from renal disease may be elicited by firm palpation posteriorly in the angle between the 12th rib and erector spinae ("renal angle").

The right kidney is 1½ cm below the left and the lower pole of the right kidney is generally higher than anticipated; it is level with a point 2½ cm above the umbilicus.

There is considerable movement of the kidneys during respiration, but for practical purposes, the hilum is considered to be at the level of L.2. Clinical examination of the kidneys should include auscultation to exclude a bruit from stenosis of the renal artery. The best sites for auscultation are in the lumbar region opposite L.2 and on the anterior wall of the abdomen, 1 in. lateral to the umbilicus; at this site, the stethoscope can be pressed firmly into the abdomen.

The course of the ureters is variable but usually lies over the tips of the transverse processes of the lumbar vertebrae and across the front of the sacro-iliac joints. The ureters are narrowed in three places: at their origin from the renal pelvis, where they pass over the pelvic brim, and at their entrance to the bladder. These sites are the most common for impaction of a renal stone.

Examination of the Urine

Proteinuria is usually due to disease of the glomeruli despite the fact that glomerular filtrate normally contains 10–20 mg/dl of protein which is reabsorbed by the tubules. "Tubular proteinuria" occurs in conditions affecting tubular function, such as the Fanconi syndrome, and heavy-metal poisoning. Urinary protein may also be present as a result of disease in the lower urinary tract; however, heavy proteinuria (5 g/l) will usually be due to a functional disorder of the glomeruli. Smaller amounts of urinary protein arise from inflammation of the lower urinary tract or blood loss. The rate of protein loss by the kidney in renal disease is fairly constant throughout the day, it is therefore important to know the specific gravity of a specimen of urine in which protein is found. A trace of protein in a dilute urine will be more serious than a trace of protein in a more concentrated urine. The presence or absence of urinary casts is helpful in deciding the site of the protein loss. Hyaline casts are complexes of albumin and other proteins secreted by the tubules and cast in the shape of the renal tubules, and if present in excess in a fresh specimen of urine, they indicate that the proteinuria is of renal origin. Epithelial casts consist of freshly shed epithelial cells from the renal tubule, and they indicate that the disease process is affecting the tubules. Granular casts are probably degenerate epithelial casts. Electrophoresis of the urinary protein may give some indication as to the site of origin: disease of the glomeruli causes loss of albumin, while disease of the tubules causes mainly loss of alpha and beta globulins.

Normal urine contains red cells, white cells and hyaline casts. Addis (1949) defined the normal excretion of them in 24 hours. Subsequently, alternative methods of expressing the rate of excretion have been devised. The average normal excretion is 0–200,000 red and white cells per hour.

RADIOLOGY OF THE KIDNEYS

A straight x-ray of the abdomen may show the shape, size and position of the kidneys, as well as renal stones or calcification within the kidneys. A lateral x-ray will help to locate the site of a radio-opaque stone; most renal stones are radio-opaque, whereas the majority of gall-stones are radiotranslucent.

Intravenous Pyelogram (Excretion Nephrogram)

Some compounds containing iodine are radio-opaque and are both filtered through the glomeruli and actively excreted by the proximal tubules. To diminish the urine flow and increase the concentration in the urine, the patient is dehydrated. Excretion from the kidneys and emptying of the ureters are delayed if external pressure is applied to the lower abdomen, which compresses the lower part of the ureters.

In the presence of renal failure and raised blood urea, a nephrogram can be performed by infusing the contrast medium intravenously over a long period and taking the x-rays at a longer time interval than usual. The conventional IVP will usually not give meaningful results if performed when the blood urea is above 150 mmol/l.

There is some variation of size of normal kidneys between the two sides and at different times. General anaesthesia and hypotension may cause a diminution in size of the kidneys. As a practical rule, the length of the long axes of the kidneys is 12–14 cm; there should not be more than 1·5 cm difference between the two kidneys. An imaginary line should always be drawn joining the tips of all the renal pyramids, and the distance between this line and the renal outline should be constant. This is known as the "renal substance". Any localised depression or bulging of the renal outline should be noted; depression of the renal outline is due to scarring and fibrosis due to infarction or infection. Occasionally in normals the outline may have a lobulated appearance, particularly at the upper poles. The renal substance may be diminished in old age, renal artery stenosis, fibrosis and back pressure on the kidney. The renal substance and length of the kidney may be increased in hypertrophy due to disease of the opposite kidney (Hodson, 1967). Hypertrophy of one kidney is suggestive of severe damage to the opposite kidney even if the radiological appearances are normal or near-normal.

The calyces drain into the renal pelvis; projecting into each calyx is a pyramid of renal tissue into which the collecting ducts drain. Any increased pressure or infection in the calyces will tend to destroy the delicate renal pyramid leading to the appearance of a rounded, enlarged end to the calyces—"clubbing of the calyces". In ureteric obstruction the rate of urine formation is diminished, the ureter and pelvis may be dilated, the calyces are clubbed and the renal substances is diminished. In its extreme form, this is the appearance of hydronephrosis. Space-occupying lesions within the kidney, such as tumours, cysts or abscesses, may cause bulging of the renal outline and displacement or distortion of the calyces. Renal arteriography should always be performed in the presence of a space-occupying lesion; carcinomas usually have an abnormal vascular pattern, whereas cysts are usually avascular. However, it is important to note that cysts may undergo malignant change, and that a carcinoma may be avascular if it is necrotic or if its nutrient artery is thrombosed (Hodson, 1967). Renal cysts do not cause hypertension, although hypernephromas may do so (Peart, 1967).

Pyelonephritis causes localised narrowing of the renal substance, due to focal scarring, and clubbing of the calyces which is at first restricted to one or two calyces. If all the calyces are involved it suggests that there is obstruction in the ureters or lower urinary tract. The pyelonephritic kidney is usually smaller than normal.

Scarring of the surface of the kidney may be due to infection or ischaemia; in general, scars due to infection will be associated with abnormal calyces whereas the calyceal pattern is usually normal in ischaemia. Rarely, scarring may be due to tuberculosis, in which case the scar is likely to be calcified and possibly associated with evidence of a tuberculous infection elsewhere in the urinary system—such as a contracted bladder.

The course of the ureters should be noted; peristalsis in the ureters may cause great variation in their apparent size. Particular attention should be paid to anatomical sites where narrowing normally occurs. In the standard IVP external abdominal compression is applied to compress the lower ureters, in order to delay the contrast leaving the renal pelvis. The abdominal pressure may distort the position of the ureters; in addition, the pressure may not affect both ureters equally so that excretion of the dye may appear to be delayed on one side, giving an appearance suggestive of renal artery stenosis. For this reason it is important not to base the diagnosis of renal artery stenosis on an IVP taken with abdominal compression. The site of narrowing of the ureters are the most likely ones for impaction of a small calculus which may be very difficult to see. In the IVP a small calculus will be seen as a filling defect. At the pelvi-ureteric junction there may be a small filling defect, due to an aberrant renal artery, such as may occur in unilateral renal artery stenosis. Rarely, such an artery may be the cause of ureteric obstruction. Reduplication of the ureters is a common cause of continuing urinary infection; the diagnosis is usually easy if the ureter drains functioning kidney, which will excrete the dye normally: however, sometimes the second ureter drains non-functioning kidney and will not fill with contrast. A second ureter draining non-functioning kidney should be suspected if there are fewer calyces on one side, if part of the kidney does not appear to have calyces or if the long axis of the kidney is altered by displacement of the kidney by an inflammatory swelling.

Retroperitoneal fibrosis causes narrowing of the ureters over a distance of several centimetres. The ureters gradually widen out again to attain the normal size. As well as being narrowed, the ureters are pulled towards the midline. The condition is almost invariably bilateral, but both sides are not always affected equally.

At the end of the IVP contrast material should be seen in the bladder, and the amount remaining in the bladder after micturition should be noted. Normally there should not be more than a small amount remaining. Incomplete bladder emptying suggests infection or obstruction at the bladder neck or in the urethra. Prostatic enlargement will cause increased trabeculation of the bladder wall and a filling defect at the lower end of the bladder. Hypertrophy of the bladder wall with lower urinary obstruction may result in diverticulae of the bladder; if large, they may give rise to the symptom of "double micturition"—a desire to pass urine twice within a short space of time. This symptom may also occur if there is reflux of urine up dilated ureters during micturition (vesico-ureteric reflux). Such reflux will be seen in the majority of patients suffering from chronic pyelonephritis if a micturating cystogram is performed. The investigation is somewhat tedious, and is usually only performed if the IVP shows a definite abnormality in the kidney.

THE MECHANISM OF CONCENTRATION AND DILUTION OF THE URINE

In the proximal convoluted tubule, the concentration of the fluid remains exactly the same; nevertheless, large amounts of water and solutes are reabsorbed but in the same proportions. With water, some sodium and chloride, and all the glucose are reabsorbed. Chlorothiazide acts on the proximal tubules, preventing reabsorption of sodium and chloride, and hence water. Fluid isotonic with plasma is delivered to the descending limb of the loop of Henle[167]; the wall of the descending limb is permeable to water but not to sodium; the distal limb of the loop of Henle actively pumps out sodium into the interstitial fluid. The resulting increased concentration of sodium in the interstitial fluid draws out water from the proximal (descending) limb of the loop. This process continues down the proximal limb—water being removed by concentrated interstitial fluid—so that urine flowing down the proximal limb becomes more and more concentrated, as does the interstitial fluid; the concentration reaches a maximum at the tip of the loop of Henle. As fluid ascends the distal limb, sodium is pumped out, causing it to become more dilute again. Near the tip of the loop the urine leaving the proximal limb is highly concentrated so that a great deal of sodium is available for pumping out into the interstitial fluid near the tip of the loop. This is the principle of the counter-current multiplier system. The points that are usually not made clear are that the system has two purposes:

1. To produce a high concentration of solutes near the tip of the loop of Henle.

2. To *dilute* the urine ascending the distal limb. It is important to note that the primary purpose of the system is to concentrate the interstitial fluid near the tip of the loop of Henle.

The microscopic anatomy of the kidney is such that the tips of the loop of Henle of all the nephrons lie close to the collecting ducts into which the distal tubules drain. Dilute urine from the distal limb of the loop of Henle enters the distal convoluted tubule and collecting ducts. This dilute urine in the collecting duct comes into contact with the areas of high concentration of solutes in the interstitial tissue. Water is withdrawn from the collecting ducts and the urine becomes more concentrated. The amount of water which crosses the collecting tubules is controlled by altering the permeability of their walls. This is done with antidiuretic hormone (ADH)—when the hormone is secreted the wall becomes highly permeable to water which is withdrawn into the inter-

167. FRIEDRICH GUSTAV JACOB HENLE (1809-1885). Göttingen anatomist.

stitial fluid leading to a concentrated urine (antidiuresis). The confusion about the counter-current system arises because the loop of Henle *taken with* the collecting duct is a mechanism for concentrating the urine, *but* the urine leaving the loop of Henle is dilute.

Functions of the Tubules

The ability to concentrate and dilute the urine is the single most important function of the tubules and the one most useful in assessing tubular function. The tubules also actively excrete potassium, hydrogen ion and ammonium salts, independently of glomerular filtration. Phosphate excretion depends on glomerular filtration, it is not actively excreted by the tubules, hence renal (glomerular) failure is accompanied by a rise in serum phosphate. Conditions which cause phosphaturia (i.e. excess loss of phosphate) are due to a defect in the tubules preventing reabsorption of phosphates from the glomerular filtrate. Similar defects are responsible for inability to reabsorb amino acids; thus, there are two ways in which tubular defects may be manifest:

1. Inability to excrete actively.
2. Inability to reabsorb.

Inability to excrete actively.—Loss of excretory function of the tubules causes an elevation of the serum potassium and an inability to excrete hydrogen ion and ammonium salts. Inability to excrete hydrogen ion may also be due to an inherited tubular defect (renal tubular acidosis). Retention of hydrogen ion leads to acidosis and a fall in plasma bicarbonate; the fall in bicarbonate is accompanied by an increase in chloride (hyperchloraemic acidosis) in order to keep the anion content of the blood constant. Often the blood urea is not much raised, and the clue to the condition is the very low plasma bicarbonate with only slight elevation of the blood urea.

Inability to reabsorb.—Sodium is largely reabsorbed in the proximal tubules; chronic renal failure may be associated with excessive loss of sodium and patients will need a high salt intake.

Sodium deficiency is a cause of renal failure and is one of the causes of uraemia in Addison's disease. Other conditions associated with loss of sodium can also cause renal failure, e.g. diabetic coma, vomiting, diarrhoea, although these are associated with dehydration as well. Normally the tubules reabsorb glucose, phosphate and essential amino acids; congenital or acquired loss of ability to reabsorb all of these is the Fanconi[168] syndrome. In addition to the collective disorder which constitutes Fanconi's syndrome, isolated tubular defects of reabsorption may occur. The most important of these are:

168. GUIDO FANCONI (b. 1892). Zürich paediatrician.

1. Renal glycosuria (inability to reabsorb glucose).
2. Renal diabetes insipidus (inability to reabsorb water due to un-responsiveness of collecting tubule to ADH).
3. Vitamin D-resistant rickets (inability to reabsorb phosphate).
4. Cystinuria (inability to reabsorb cystine).

(Cystinuria should not be confused with cystinosis which is part of the Fanconi syndrome. As well as an inherited defect of tubular re-absorption in cystinosis, there is an inherited defect of protein and amino acid metabolism, leading to accumulation of cystine in the tissues.)

Acquired disorders which may cause isolated tubular defects of reabsorption without causing more severe renal damage are:

Potassium deficiency.
Sickle-cell anaemia.
Chronic pyelonephritis.
Heavy-metal poisoning (gold, lead and copper).
Myelomatosis.

Tests of the Ability of the Tubules to Reabsorb and Excrete

Ability to reabsorb.—The ability to reabsorb water to produce a concentrated urine is the simplest test of tubular reabsorptive capacity. The test can be performed by inducing fluid deprivation or injecting ADH. The ability to reabsorb sodium can be tested by sodium depriva-tion or giving a salt-retaining hormone.

Glucose is normally completely reabsorbed in the proximal tubule. If glucose appears in the urine it is either because the blood (and hence glomerular filtrate) level is abnormally high, or because there is a con-genital defect in the ability of the tubule to reabsorb glucose (renal glycosuria). There is a point at which glucose will appear in the urine if the blood level is gradually raised, i.e. despite reabsorption from the tubule, some glucose is getting through to the urine. This is the point at which the tubule is reabsorbing maximally.

The maximum amount of glucose reabsorbed (maximum tubular reabsorption of glucose, or TM_g) will be the amount presented to the tubules less the amount in the urine in one minute, or

(glomerular filtration rate $\times$ plasma glucose) −

(urine glucose $\times$ urine volume)

The normal value is 320 mg/min (52 mmol).

Ability to excrete.—A substance actively excreted by the tubules which is easy to measure in blood and urine is para-amino hippuric acid (PAH). The maximum amount actively excreted (Tm_{PAH}) is PAH excreted in the urine less the amount filtered by the glomeruli, or

(urine PAH $\times$ urine volume) −

(glomerular filtration rate $\times$ plasma PAH)

The normal Tm_{PAH} is 70 mg/min (11 mmol).

The other tests of tubular function of importance are:

1. Ability to produce an acid urine (tested by loading with ammonium chloride).

2. Ability to conserve sodium on a low-sodium diet or with salt-retaining hormone (fludrocortisone).

3. Ability to excrete potassium (level of serum potassium).

4. Ability to conserve amino acids (chromatogram of urine for abnormal urinary amino acids).

Renal Tubular Disorders

The tubules have homeostatic functions which involve either absorption or excretion. Congenital disturbances of tubular function are usually due to an enzyme deficiency leading to increased excretion of precursors or accumulation of precursors which are toxic. As a rule toxic damage to the tubules causes failure of all tubular functions. This means that there is:

Proteinuria.
Glycosuria.
Phosphaturia.
Aminoaciduria.
Disturbed acid-base balance.

Toxic damage to the tubules can either be *congenital* as in the case of Wilson's disease, galactosaemia or cystinosis, or *acquired*, e.g. heavy-metal poisoning, multiple myeloma, drugs (expired tetracycline, streptomycin, salicylates) or hypokalaemia. Many other tubular disorders are due to a deficiency in one enzyme and hence all the tubular functions are not affected. The most important disorders of *single* tubular functions are:

1. Renal glycosuria.
2. Specific aminoaciduria
     e.g. cystinuria (cystine stones).
3. Vitamin D-resistant rickets
     (inability to reabsorb phosphates).
4. Renal tubular acidosis
     (defective reabsorption of bicarbonate).
5. Resistance to antidiuretic hormone
     (nephrogenic diabetes insipidus).

Glomerular Function

The glomeruli act as simple filters. The properties of filters which are of importance are the amount of fluid they let through, whether they stop substances which should be allowed through, or allow through substances which should be retained. Glomerular filters can fail in the same way, i.e.:

1. By a reduction in the amount of fluid which passes them—reduced glomerular filtration rate.
2. By retaining substances which should be filtered, e.g. urea and creatinine.
3. By allowing substances through which should be retained, e.g. plasma proteins.

Glomerular filtration rate.—A substance which is not absorbed or excreted by the renal tubules will appear in the urine at the same rate that it is filtered through the glomeruli. Such a substance is inulin. The fluid in the proximal tubule is isotonic with plasma, hence the concentration of a substance in the glomerular filtrate is the same as in the plasma. The glomerular filtration volume in one minute is:

$$\frac{\text{Conc. inulin in urine} \times \text{volume of urine}}{\text{Conc. inulin in plasma}}$$

In practice, creatinine clearance is used to estimate glomerular filtration rate. Creatinine is an endogenously produced substance, whose plasma concentration remains uniform throughout the day, and which is not absorbed or excreted by the renal tubules to an extent which interferes with its usefulness. Because the level of creatinine in the serum remains constant only one blood estimation is necessary. The urine is collected for 24 hours, thus minimising errors due to incomplete bladder emptying and inaccuracies of timing.

"Clearance" is an entirely theoretical concept. It may be defined as the volume of plasma which contains the amount of the substance which appears in the urine in one minute, assuming the plasma to be completely "cleared" of the substance.

If u = urinary concentration of the substance
v = urine flow per minute
p = plasma concentration of the substance

$$\text{Clearance} = \frac{uv}{p}$$

i.e. $\dfrac{\text{amount in urine (per minute)}}{\text{amount in plasma (mg. per cent)}}$

The normal creatinine clearance is 100–120 ml/minute (in effect this is the volume of the glomerular filtrate. The value normally falls with age, so that at 80 the normal creatinine clearance is 65 ml/minute. The retention of substances in the blood which should be filtered does not occur until there in a marked fall in glomerular filtration rate. The blood urea and blood creatinine on a normal diet do not start to rise until the creatinine clearance is below 50 ml/min. (i.e. 50 per cent of normal). The glomeruli allow through protein if they are damaged; however in very severe renal failure protein may disappear from the urine because of widespread loss of functioning glomeruli (i.e. the filter is completely "clogged up").

The individual components of renal function and their tests are:

Glomerular function:

Glomerular filtration rate (creatinine clearance)
Blood urea and creatinine
Proteinuria
Serum phosphate.

Tubular excretory function:

Serum potassium
Acidosis (low bicarbonate, raised chloride).

Tubular reabsorptive function:

Concentration and dilution of urine
Serum sodium (and urine sodium)
Glycosuria
Urinary amino acids.

GLOMERULONEPHRITIS

Problems of Classification[169]

Much of the confusion about nephritis has arisen as a result of failure to appreciate that there are a limited number of end results to a large number of diseases. The end results of most renal diseases are:

1. The nephrotic syndrome.
2. Renal failure (uraemia) which may be acute or chronic.
3. Hypertension.

Three aspects of glomerulonephritis are accepted as uncontroversial:

1. There is an acute form of nephritis associated with haematuria and previous streptococcal infection.

2. About 5 per cent of cases of acute nephritis develop a chronic, long-standing and eventually fatal disease.

3. There is a chronic form of nephritis associated with albuminuria and eventual renal failure in which there is no history of preceding acute nephritis.

169. SIR ARTHUR WILLIAM MICKLE ELLIS (b. 1883). Formerly Professor of Medicine at the London Hospital.

Complete recovery occurs in 90 per cent of cases of acute nephritis, a small proportion die in the acute attack from severe hypertension and anuria, the remainder develop proteinuria and hypertension which becomes chronic and they eventually die of malignant hypertension or uraemia (renal failure). Chronic nephritis usually causes symptomless proteinuria which is followed by the nephrotic syndrome. A *late* result of the nephrotic syndrome is renal failure and hypertension.

Principal Histological Features of Glomerulonephritis

The problems of clinical classification do not extend to the histological features of acute and chronic nephritis. There is general agreement as to the histological features of acute nephritis, rapidly progressive acute nephritis, and chronic nephritis, whether it be due to slowly progressive acute nephritis or chronic nephritis of insidious onset.

The main controversial points are that severe hypertensive changes are thought to indicate the slowly progressive form of acute nephritis rather than chronic nephritis of insidious onset, and that persistence of relatively normal numbers of glomeruli may indicate chronic nephritis of insidious onset, whereas in the slowly progressive form of acute nephritis the glomeruli are fewer in number because they have been destroyed by the previous acute nephritis.

The changes of acute nephritis are swelling and multiplication of the endothelial cells of the glomerular capillaries and their basement membranes, infiltration of glomeruli and interstitial tissue with polymorphs and the appearance of red cells in Bowman's[170] capsule. In the *rapidly* progressive form, the changes are more severe and are accompanied by increase in size and number of the epithelial cells of Bowman's capsule—epithelial crescent formation. Accompanying hypertension will cause necrosis of glomerular arterioles and capillaries which leads to areas of focal necrosis in the kidneys and secondary tubular damage.

Chronic nephritis, being much more long-standing, will be accompanied by more degenerative changes (replacement of renal substance by hyaline tissue and fat) which causes the characteristic pale, enlarged, featureless kidney of chronic nephritis. The glomeruli show endothelial proliferation of the blood vessels and thickening of the basement membranes. Some glomeruli are surrounded by fibrous tissue and others undergo hyaline change.

Acute nephritis.—The histological features usually resolve as the patient improves clinically. A small number (5 per cent) of patients do not improve and develop chronic glomerulonephritis. The histology of the glomeruli in these patients shows mainly "proliferative" changes;

170. SIR WILLIAM BOWMAN (1816–1892). London ophthalmic surgeon.

hence the condition is often called "proliferative glomerulonephritis". The histology of all early cases of acute nephritis shows similar although less severe changes. If the changes persist the patient has developed chronic glomerulonephritis.

Proliferative glomerulonephritis.—This is marked proliferation and reduplication of the endothelial cells of the capillaries in the capillary tufts, as well as proliferation of the epithelial cells of Bowman's capsule. There is marked polymorph infiltration and deposition of immuno-globulin in relation to the capillary and epithelial basement membrane which is often reduplicated. Occasionally these changes only affect parts of each glomerulus.

Membranous glomerulonephritis.—In this condition mainly the basement membrane is affected, hence its name. Proliferation of cells and infiltration with polymorphs is not seen.

Minimal change glomerulonephritis.—Studies by light microscopy show little or no change in the glomeruli although the electron micro-scope shows abnormalities in the foot processes of the epithelial cells.

Acute Nephritis

Acute nephritis almost invariably follows previous infection with a "nephritogenic" strain of beta haemolytic streptococcus. The most usual site of infection is the throat, although, rarely, infection in other sites may be responsible, for example streptococcal endocarditis or infected burns. The interval between infection and the onset of nephritis is usually 2–3 weeks but the limits are probably 48 hours to 4 weeks.

The disease usually starts suddenly with oliguria, oedema, haema-turia, proteinuria and hypertension. The oedema is caused by hypo-proteinaemia, due to diminished production, and by water retention due to excessive tubular reabsorption of salt. The reasons for the diminished protein production and excessive salt absorption are not known. The hypertension may cause hypertensive encephalopathy and left ventricular failure, which will be exaggerated by the fluid retention. The urine contains albumin, red blood cells, granular and cellular casts.

Treatment.—Prophylactic penicillin is given to the contacts of a patient who has developed acute nephritis. Penicillin is also given in established cases, usually for the duration of the haematuria. The main disorder of function is fluid retention and oliguria which is accompanied by a rise in blood urea. The aim of treatment is to promote a diuresis and limit the harmful effects of oliguria, hence salt, water and protein intake should be limited if oliguria and uraemia are present. Bed rest alone usually promotes a diuresis. Protein and casts may continue in the urine for several years after the acute attack. The patient should be allowed out of bed when the red cell excretion in the urine becomes constant (de Wardener, 1967). Conditions which may simulate acute nephritis are Henoch-Schönlein purpura, subacute bacterial endocarditis and acute polyarteritis nodosa.

PYELONEPHRITIS

Chronic pyelonephritis is the commonest cause of chronic renal failure. The essential feature which is often overlooked is that the infection is not only in the urine but also in the interstitial tissue of the kidneys and walls of the renal pelvis and ureters. All cases of pyelonephritis have minute abscesses within the renal substance. These abscesses heal by fibrosis and are most frequently found in the medulla near the collecting tubes which drain into the renal pelvis. The tubules are much more susceptible to damage than the remainder of the kidney. There are two other aspects of the pathology of pyelonephritis which are usually under-emphasised, the first is that there is usually marked fibrosis surrounding the glomeruli in concentric layers (periglomerular fibrosis) and the second is the frequency of vascular involvement by the inflammation, leading to secondary ischaemic changes. Involvement of the kidneys is usually bilateral except when infection arises as a result of unilateral obstruction; the involvement is also patchy so that a normal renal biopsy does not exclude the diagnosis. Progressive fibrosis leads to shrinking of the kidneys, inflammation leads to scarring and depression of the surface and involvement of the arteries leads to wedge-shaped areas of infarction which also cause depression of the renal surfaces. Infection may destroy the renal pyramids within the calyces, leading to "clubbed" calyces.

Hypertension may cause narrowing of the renal arterioles, exaggerating the areas of infarction which may occur as a result of inflammation. Pyelonephritis is common in hypertension and in other causes of renal damage, e.g. glomerulonephritis and diabetes. The main point of distinction between the IVP appearances of renal damage due to ischaemia alone and due to infection is that the calyceal pattern will be normal in ischaemia but abnormal if the renal scarring is due to long-standing pyelonephritis. In renal damage due to chronic back-pressure the calyces are dilated uniformly throughout both kidneys, whereas pyelonephritis causes patchy involvement. In essence, therefore, the structural changes in the kidneys in chronic pyelonephritis which are reflected in the IVP are:

1. Decrease in size of the affected kidney.
2. Focal scarring and decrease in "renal substance".
3. Abnormal calyces.

With regard to these changes, two other factors should be considered. It is now believed that clubbing of the calyces and focal scarring almost always occur as a result of renal infection during childhood (Hodson and Wilson, 1965). The renal changes due to pyelonephritis acquired in adulthood are diffuse interstitial fibrosis which leads to contraction of the kidneys. Coarse scars may be present if there is associated infarction due to hypertensive changes. The structural changes in the kidneys and the histological appearances of the interstitial tissue are not specific for pyelonephritis—a large number of other conditions can cause an identical histological picture. Any pre-existing renal damage predisposes to infection; the clinical significance of this is that the x-ray appearances of a small kidney with a biopsy appearance of interstitial fibrosis and evidence of infection in the urine does not mean that the structural changes in the kidneys are due to the infection. Among conditions which may cause interstitial fibrosis of the kidneys are:

1. Potassium depletion.
2. Sulphonamide excess.
3. Phenacetin excess.
4. Hypertension.
5. Radiation.
6. Ureteric obstruction.
7. Ageing.

Mechanisms of Renal Infection

There are three routes by which organisms may reach the kidneys: via the ureters from the bladder, via lymphatics from the gut or bladder, and by haematogenous routes. Of these, the most important is ascending infection from the bladder. Vesico-ureteric reflux of infected urine from the bladder will make renal infection almost inevitable; however, in some cases vesico-ureteric reflux cannot be demonstrated radiologically. There is good experimental evidence that bacteria will survive in a surface film of urine after a vessel has been emptied, also flow mechanics have shown that when fluid flows down a tube there is an upward movement of a thin layer of fluid adjacent to the wall of the tube. In the ureters this would explain infection of the kidneys in the absence of ureteric reflux.

The renal medulla is peculiarly susceptible to infection, and the main reasons for this are (Beeson, 1967):

1. High concentration of ammonia in the medulla which interferes with the antimicrobial action of complement.
2. Hypertonicity of the interstitial fluid interferes with the action of phagocytes and allows the survival of protoplasts. Protoplasts are organisms which have lost their pathogenicity because of loss of a

vital component of the cell membrane. They can only survive in hypertonic solutions, and they may become pathogenic again under suitable circumstances.

3. The blood supply of the medulla is meagre compared with the cortex. This leads to a reduced supply of phagocytes; the blood supply to the medulla can be increased by promoting a diuresis and this has been shown to prevent and eliminate infection.

4. The medulla is susceptible to damage from other causes which may predispose to stasis.

Factors Predisposing to Infection

1. Catheterisation of the bladder.
2. Urinary obstruction.
3. Disorder of micturition due to neurological reasons.
4. Diabetes mellitus.
5. Coitus and pregnancy.
6. Gout.
7. Potassium deficiency.
8. Nephrocalcinosis and nephrolithiasis.
9. Hypertension and other causes of renal damage (e.g. collagen disorders).
10. Phenacetin ingestion.
11. Sickle-cell trait.

Evidence of Infection

Infection may be present without symptoms or signs; there may be non-specific evidence (fever, leucocytosis and increased sedimentation rate). Although in pyelonephritis the essential infection is in the interstitial tissue of the kidney, the urine will provide a sample of the fluid within the interstitial tissue. Examination of the urine may demonstrate the infecting organism or evidence of renal damage. It is now well-established that careful collection of a normally voided specimen of urine will usually give evidence of infection when present. Catheterisation is not necessary for the collection of samples. One of the problems is that even with very careful cleaning, there is always some contamination. However, this problem has been overcome by the demonstration that the bacterial counts in the urine below 10,000/ml do not indicate infection, whereas counts above 100,000/ml indicate infection in 85 per cent of cases (Kass, 1957). Bacterial counts between 10,000 and 100,000/ml are equivocal and a further specimen should be examined. Further evidence of infection is the growth of a single organism; the presence of several organisms suggests contamination. Evidence of inflammation may be given by an abnormally high excretion of leucocytes and casts. It is essential to appreciate that pyelonephritis may be present in the absence of white cells or pus cells in the urine. The presence of white cells in the urine indicates inflammation but this is not necessarily due to infection. White cells in a sterile urine may indicate pyelonephritis, renal tuberculosis, typhoid fever, acute glomerular nephritis, nephrolithiasis or phenacetin nephropathy.

Normal urine contains some white cells, and the number of these in normal urine has been defined and is up to 200,000/hour (Little, 1962). There is an overlap between normals and patients with pyelonephritis; however, the excretion of white cells in a patient with pyelonephritis can be increased by an intravenous injection of 40 mg of prednisone phosphate (Little, 1965). Further evidence of structural renal damage is the presence of proteinuria and an inability to concentrate and dilute the urine, due to involvement of the distal tubule which is more susceptible to damage than the glomeruli; the patient may develop nocturia and an inability to concentrate the urine before there is any rise in blood urea or impairment of creatinine clearance. Rarely, a salt-losing syndrome due to tubular damage in the presence of a normal blood urea is the presenting feature.

The orthodox indications for an IVP examination in the presence of clinical evidence of a urinary infection are:

1. A severe attack of pyelitis in a woman.
2. A second attack of "mild" pyelitis in a woman.
3. A first attack of pyelitis in a man or boy.

Treatment

Preventative
Avoid catheterisation where possible.

Prophylactic
1. Detection of any structural or obstructive abnormality in the urinary system.
2. Instil antibiotics into the bladder following catheterisation.
3. Detection of asymptomatic bacteriuria.

Urine is an almost ideal culture medium for the most common organism responsible for urinary infection—*E. coli*. Its pH, glucose content, osmolality and lack of humoral and cellular antibacterial substances make it a good reservoir for bacteria (Asscher *et al.*, 1966). This is analogous to the situation in chronic bronchitis in which the sputum is an ever-present home for potentially pathogenic bacteria. *Symptomatic* renal and lower urinary tract infections are undoubtedly associated with infection and micro-abscess formation within the tissues of the urinary tract. It follows from the above that successful treatment of symptomatic urinary infections or infections in which there is other evidence of tissue infection demands a high tissue level of antibiotic to which the organism is sensitive *and* steps to render the urine a less comfortable home for the offending organisms. However, another issue follows—if the urine is such a suitable place for the organisms to grow perhaps they grow there doing *no* harm; it is certainly true that bacteriuria is very common in the absence of any symptoms or other evidence of infection.

Evidence of *tissue* infection would be leucocytosis, raised sedimentation rate, pus cells, increased urinary enzymes (lactic dehydrogenase and glutamic oxaloacetic transaminase) and an increased titre of circulating antibodies to organisms grown from the urine. It has already been indicated that there are nearly always some pathogenic organisms in all urine—less than 10,000 per ml is regarded as normal, more than 100,000 organisms per ml indicates urinary infection in 85 per cent of cases —this is regarded as "significant" bacteriuria. It is accepted that *transient* "significant" bacteriuria is common in normal women and girls; an "abnormality" is only likely in an asymptomatic patient with no renal damage when "significant" bacteriuria is *persistent*, i.e. has occurred in *three* successive specimens of urine. In the presence of urinary symptoms or other evidence of urinary infection, of course, one urine specimen containing 100,000 organisms is highly significant and should be treated (v.i.). Pyuria (i.e. 5+ white cells per high power field) when present usually indicates *tissue* infection; however, *tissue infection can be present in the absence of pyuria.*

In the absence of symptoms bacteriuria should not be considered significant unless there are more than 100,000/ml in at least *three* specimens; furthermore, pus cells may be absent from the urine even though infection is significant. Because:

1. Pyuria is often intermittent.
2. The concentration of pus cells is very dependent on rate of urine flow.
3. Pus cells may be lysed in the urine.
4. Pus cells are often absent from the urine even in clinically obvious pyelitis.

If there is doubt about the significance of pus cells a prednisolone provocation test may be indicated. *Absence* of pus cells from the urine in the presence of bacteriuria should *not* lead to complacency.

In order to try and resolve some of the difficulty about the significance of persisting bacteriuria attempts have been made to establish whether infection is involving renal parenchyma. The ways of doing this are (Reeves and Brumfitt, 1968):

1. Serum antibodies to the O antigen of *E. coli* found in the urine only occur when infection is involving the renal parenchyma.

2. Urine concentration. Ascending renal infection affects the efficiency of the collecting ducts and distal tubule leading to impairment of concentrating ability.

3. Excretion of enzymes in the urine known to result from inflammation of renal medulla, e.g. SGOT and LDH.

4. The presence of "glitter" cells.

5. Ureteric catherisation.

6. Renal biopsy culture.

7. Urine obtained by Fairley techniques (Fairley *et al.*, 1967). This is a method of obtaining urine direct from the kidneys. The bladder is catheterised and sterilised with neomycin and well irrigated with sterile water. Samples are taken via the catheter every 10 minutes after inducing a diuresis.

The clinical importance of these techniques is to help assess whether recurrent asymptomatic bacteriuria is really due to infection within the kidneys or whether the organisms are harmless parasites or are contaminants.

The preliminary investigation of urinary infection should include an IVP and a micturating cystogram if there is a relapse or reinfection. It is usually not possible to eradicate organisms from the urine if there is anatomical abnormality in the urinary system.

One of the great enigmas about repeated urinary infections is the frequency with which they are followed by progressive renal damage and chronic pyelonephritis; and another whether persistent significant bacteriuria in the absence of other evidence of infection is to be regarded as a true urinary *tract* infection. Most authorities agree that *repeated* urinary *tract* infections during childhood often lead to chronic pyelonephritis. In adults opinion is divided; some authorities regard *asymptomatic bacteriuria* in the absence of other evidence of infection as a benign condition (Petersdorf, 1966; Kimmelstiel, 1966). Other authorities have evidence that persistent significant bacteriuria does lead to chronic renal damage (Beard and Roberts, 1968; Kunin, 1968).

Undiagnosed, asymptomatic pyelitis is widely regarded as a "missing link" between the frequent finding of chronic pyelonephritis at autopsy and the absence of any symptoms during life. However, the incidence of chronic pyelonephritis is equal in the two sexes, while bacteriuria and urinary infections are much commoner in women; many other diseases other than repeated urinary infections can lead to histological appearances identical to pyelonephritis.

The incidence of chronic pyelonephritis is less common than was formerly believed and is of the order of 3 per cent, which corresponds with the incidence of undiagnosed structural disorders of the urinary tract which no one denies do lead to damaging infection and chronic pyelonephritis. Nevertheless despite the conflicting evidence ten working rules can be laid down for the clinician dealing with urinary tract infection:

1. Asymptomatic bacteriuria *alone* may indicate chronic pyelonephritis.

2. Repeated urinary infections *can* lead to progressive renal damage in the adult.

3. Repeated urinary infections *do* lead to progressive renal damage in children.

4. Patients who have *recurrent* urinary infections frequently have a structural abnormality of the urinary tract.

5. Suppression of recurrent asymptomatic bacteriuria *can* prevent progressive renal damage if given early, although successful supression does not *always* prevent progressive damage.

6. Asymptomatic bacteriuria and urinary tract infections of pregnancy are associated with foetal prematurity and subsequent attacks of acute pyelonephritis in a quarter of women affected (Whalley, 1967).

7. Persistent significant bacteriuria does not *always* mean infection in the kidney; infection may be localised to the bladder.

8. Asymptomatic bacteriuria with *any* evidence of tissue infection should be treated vigorously.

9. Hypertension complicates an unknown but probably small number of chronic renal infections.

10. Pyuria is *not* always present in urinary tract infections.

Following antibiotic treatment the incidence of a further infection either with the same or different organism is very high. The rate of reinfection is not related to the length of the course of antibiotics; the rate of reinfection is 70–80 per cent regardless of whether the acute infection is treated for 14 days or 18 months (Little and de Wardener, 1966). It is worth emphasising that the symptoms of pyelitis usually subside spontaneously even though bacteriuria and pyuria continue unchanged.

Numerous series have shown that recurrence rate following an acute urinary infection is around 80 per cent either with the original infecting organism or a different organism. For this reason it is *absolutely mandatory* that any patient with a urinary infection should be followed up for a minimum of 2 years with urine cultures every month for 6 months, then every 3 months for 18 months. *The available evidence does not in any way support the common practice of discharge of an asymptomatic patient after one or two token out-patient visits.*

Over 70 per cent of urinary infections are due to *E. coli* and 15 per cent to *Proteus vulgaris*. Sulphonamides are the drugs of choice for a first infection. In this country the evidence suggests that for the first symptomatic urinary infection short sharp courses of chemotherapy are as good (or bad!) as continuous treatment. In America Kass believes that urinary infections in pregnancy should be treated with chemotherapy continuously until delivery; in this country there is a tendency not to use continuous chemotherapy *provided* there is *no* persistent bacteriuria. There is general agreement that pyelitis and continuing bacteriuria during pregnancy predispose to toxaemia and prematurity. It is also agreed that a high proportion (probably 20–30 per cent) of women who have symptomatic or asymptomatic bacteriuria of pregnancy will develop acute pyelonephritis and will have an abnormal IVP after pregnancy—it is not yet known what proportion of these women had bacteriuria (or urinary infection) before the pregnancy started.

The exact risk of developing renal damage with persistent bacteriuria is not known; however, it is known that *some* patients with persistent bacteriuria develop renal impairment and chronic pyelonephritis; furthermore this can happen when the bacteriuria is being actively treated. It should follow that an attempt should be made to eliminate persistent bacteriuria; however, there is genuine dispute as to whether the proportion (how small or large is not known) of patients who do develop progressive renal damage justifies routine treatment of asymptomatic bacteriuria in the remainder. It is suggested that those who develop renal damage will do so whether the bacteriuria is treated or not (Petersdorf, 1966; Kimmelstiel, 1966). There are several pieces of evidence that are difficult to interpret.

1. Bacteriuria occurs commonly in young girls without leading to renal damage.

2. Bacteriuria occurs very commonly (20–30 per cent) in elderly hospital patients.

3. Urinary infections are much commoner in women but the incidence of pyelonephritis at postmortem is equal in men and women.

4. The histological features of "pyelonephritis" can be caused by agents other than bacterial infection.

Recurrence of symptoms, significant bacteriuria or other evidence of infection is an indication for further *short* courses of chemotherapy.

In some centres facilities are available for measuring the circulating antibody titres to *E. coli* organisms which are grown from the urine. The antibody titre falls to zero within 6 weeks when the infection has been eliminated. Persistence of a raised titre indicates persisting infection or relapse of the original infection. Recurrence of infection due to a different organism is strong presumptive evidence of a structural abnormality of the urinary tract which should be fully investigated. One of the commonest causes of frequent relapses (due to the original infecting organism) or recurrence of an infection (i.e. due to a different organism) is reflux of urine from the bladder up the ureters—this may be demonstrated by a micturating cystogram. Evidence of dilatation of the calyces of the *upper* poles of the kidneys is particularly common with ureteric reflux.

Repeated recurrence of infection due to a different organism is an indication for long-term, continuous chemotherapy. This is best given continuously in the early stages; later it may be possible to give intermittent chemotherapy (e.g. for one week in three). The same antibiotics should be used continuously or for the intermittent courses. It is *not* recommended that alternating courses of different antibiotics be given as this is a sure way of producing antibiotic-resistant organisms. Nalidixic acid given with an acidifying agent such as mandelic acid is often suitable as a urinary antiseptic when recurrences are frequent. High concentrations are reached in the urine but not in the tissues; however, this may not matter if ascending infection on the urine is the route by which the organisms reach the kidneys.

Treatment of acute urinary infection.—Sulphonamides are the initial drug of choice for most urinary infections; a loading dose of 3·0 g is followed by 1·0 g 6-hourly for 10 days. A long-acting sulphonamide such as sulphamethoxine 0·5 g can be given once daily instead. One disadvantage of a long-acting sulphonamide is that should the patient develop a hypersensitivity reaction, such as the Stevens-Johnson syndrome, the adverse reaction is usually more severe than with the shorter-acting drugs. All sulphonamides are bound to the plasma proteins but to a variable extent; the more free drug there is in the serum the higher is the effective tissue concentration of the drug. Sulphonamides are excreted by the kidneys after they have been acetylated; however, the acetyl derivative has no antibacterial properties. The drugs of choice in urinary infection are: sulphadimidine, sulphamethizole (Urolucosil) and sulphafurazole (Gantrisin). Sulphamethizole and sulphafurazole are less bound to plasma proteins and are only about half acetylated, the remainder of the drug being excreted unchanged and hence in an active form in the urine.

Sulphonamides should be used with care if there is renal impairment. If one kidney is more damaged than the other, most of the drug will be excreted by the best kidney; hence almost no effective drug concentration will occur in the urine of the most damaged kidney.

Sulphadiazine is hardly bound at all to the plasma proteins and hence reaches a high tissue concentration; the concentration in the CSF may be 80 per cent of that in the blood, making it the drug of choice in the treatment of meningococcal meningitis. Unfortunately the solubility of the acetyl derivative is low, which makes the risk of crystalluria very high particularly if there is oliguria. It should not be used in urinary infections.

The sulphonamides are most effective and the risk of crystalluria minimal if the urine is kept *alkaline* for *E coli* infections. For *Str. faecalis* infections they work better in an acid urine.

If the sulphonamides fail to control infection or if there is symptomatic or bacterial evidence of a relapse they should be followed by 10-day courses of the following chemotherapeutic agents provided the organisms cultured have been shown to be sensitive to them:

1. Septrin or Bactrim—a synergistic mixture of trimethoprim and a sulphonamide (urine pH should be alkaline).
2. Ampicillin 500 mg *q.d.s.* (unaffected by urinary pH).
3. Nitrofurantoin (unaffected by urinary pH).

The relapse rate following successful treatment of acute urinary infection is high; 60 per cent of patients relapse within 6 months and 80 per cent within 18 months. It therefore follows that all patients who have an acute urinary infection should be followed at *monthly intervals* for 6 months and 3-*monthly intervals* for a *further* 18 *months*.

Other antibiotics are sometimes necessary for the treatment of severe and persistent acute infections. The pH of the urine may be important because the effectiveness of the antibiotics is often pH-dependent. In all urinary infections the patient should be persuaded to have a high fluid intake—this creates the least hospitable environment for the organisms; the dilution of the antibiotics in a dilute urine is less important than the production of other factors hostile to the infecting organisms.

Urinary pH for optimum antibacterial effect

Alkaline	*Acid*	*Unaffected by pH*
Sulphonamides (and trimethoprim)	Tetracycline	Nitrofurantoin
Penicillin	Novobiocin	Ampicillin
Streptomycin	Cycloserine	
Erythromycin		
Kanamycin		
Gentamycin		
Colistin (Colomycin)		

RENAL FAILURE

Renal failure implies failure of normal function of both glomeruli and tubules. By convention, isolated congenital or acquired tubular defects are not included. Chronic renal failure is not synonymous with irreversible renal failure, because chronic renal failure can sometimes be reversed by removing the cause, e.g. obstruction of the urinary tract or eradication of infection.

Functional Disturbances

One feature of renal failure which should be emphasised is that the glomeruli and tubules usually fail together. Any reduction in glomerular filtration due to disease affecting the glomeruli generally results in a diminution of blood supply to the tubules, resulting in a combination of glomerular and tubular failure ("total nephron failure").

Water excretion.—A reduction in glomerular filtration rate of solutes results in a rise in the serum concentration of urea, uric acid, urochromogen, phosphates and sulphates. These substances greatly increase the osmotic load and induce an osmotic diuresis, which results in polyuria and dehydration if water intake is not increased. Secondary tubular impairment (due to total nephron failure) results in inability to concentrate the urine, although the urine can often still be diluted if the kidney is presented with a water load. Inability to concentrate the urine results in nocturia,. as the normal kidney concentrates urine at night. Later the kidney loses its ability to dilute, so that the urine has a fixed specific gravity—isosthenuria. Despite the ability to dilute the urine, the kidney is unable to excrete a water load as quickly as in a normal person because the total number of functioning nephrons is reduced. Patients with chronic renal failure are, therefore, vulnerable from the point of view of both overtransfusion and dehydration from vomiting and diarrhoea.

Acidosis.—Hydrogen ion is excreted in three forms:

1. Combined with ammonia (NH_3) to form ammonium (NH_4) salts.
2. Combined with bicarbonate ($NaHCO_3$) to form carbonic acid (H_2CO_3).
3. Combined with disodium hydrogen phosphate (Na_2HPO_4) to form sodium dihydrogen phosphate (NaH_2PO_4).

The lowered glomerular filtration rate results in retention of phosphates which are then not available in the tubules for the formation of NaH_2PO_4. Tubular failure results in inability to produce ammonia and causes a leakage of bicarbonate, which is therefore not available for the formation of carbonic acid.

The increased hydrogen ion concentration in the blood is probably partly buffered by calcium buffers derived from the bones as well as the normal bicarbonate/carbonic acid buffers. Retention of hydrogen ion tends to cause a reduction in serum bicarbonate and hence a compensatory reduction in carbonic acid; CO_2 is blown off by hyperventilation (Kussmaul or acidotic breathing).

Sodium excretion.—Tubular impairment results in inability to re-absorb as much filtered sodium as normal. In the later stages of renal failure, overt sodium depletion may be present, which can be treated by increasing the dietary intake of sodium. However, this should be done carefully, because by this stage the kidney will have lost its ability to excrete increased amounts of solutes.

Potassium excretion.—Potassium is excreted by active tubular excretion as well as by glomerular filtration. Total nephron failure results in diminished filtration as well as impairment of active tubular excretion. Rarely, diseases which affect the renal tubules more than glomeruli (Fanconi syndrome and pyelonephritis) result in tubular damage and failure to reabsorb any filtered potassium, resulting in "potassium-losing nephritis". Hypokalaemia itself may cause tubular defects and increase the susceptibility to nephritis.

Calcium metabolism.—(See p. 443).

Anaemia.—There are many factors responsible for the anaemia of renal failure. The most important are:

1. Increased haemolysis.
2. Bone marrow depression due to reduced production or inhibition of erythropoietin.
3. Failure to incorporate iron bound to transferrin into red cells.
4. Bleeding due to ulceration of the gastro-intestinal tract and purpura due to a platelet deficiency or increased capillary fragility.

The treatment of the anaemia of uraemia is unsatisfactory, as repeated blood transfusions have only a transient beneficial effect and sometimes they are positively harmful. When the haemoglobin level is raised by transfusion (and the PCV rises), the proportion of plasma in the blood falls; in chronic renal disease, the renal blood flow is usually fixed, so that less plasma will be flowing through the kidneys, and so the blood urea may rise.

Non-metabolic disturbances which may occur in uraemia are: pericarditis, "uraemic lung", peripheral neuropathy, coma, epilepsy, and hypertensive encephalopathy if there is associated hypertension.

Nephrotic Syndrome

The syndrome consists of proteinuria, hypoproteinaemia and oedema. There is often, but not invariably, a rise in serum lipids (cholesterol) and a fall in serum calcium which may lead to tetany. The calcium is normally carried bound to the plasma albumin, but if the amount of circulating albumin is reduced, less calcium can be transported. The hypoproteinaemia and fluid retention cause oedema which results in secondary hyperaldosteronism which occasionally causes hypokalaemia. The nephrotic syndrome does *not* include a rise in blood urea or hypertension.

Causes of Nephrotic Syndrome

1. Glomerulonephritis.
2. Pyelonephritis.
3. Diabetes.
4. Amyloid disease.
5. Systemic lupus erythematosus and polyarteritis nodosa.
6. Renal vein thrombosis.
7. Drugs, such as Tridione, gold and mercury.
8. Rare causes such as: malaria, renal carcinoma and hypersensitivity states.

The nephrotic syndrome is treated with a high protein intake (to compensate for renal loss of protein) and no added salt diet (to diminish fluid retention due to hypoalbuminaemia and salt retention). Thiazide diuretics, frusemide and Aldactone are used to reduce fluid retention. Potassium supplements may not be necessary if potassium retention accompanies the glomerular failure. Gross oedema may result in hypovolaemia; occasionally a diuresis can be induced with a plasma expander such as dextran—the benefit is usually short-lived.

The use of steroids and immunosuppressives in the nephrotic syndrome.
The indication and effectiveness of these drugs in the nephrotic syndrome have not been clearly defined. They may be valuable in some cases of chronic glomerulonephritis. They are almost certainly of less value when the nephrotic syndrome is secondary to pyelonephritis, diabetes, amyloidosis and renal vein thrombosis. There are two main ways of judging the prognosis and assessing the functional abnormality in chronic glomerulonephritis, viz:

1. The severity of changes in the renal biopsy.
2. Whether the loss of protein is selective or unselective.

With regard to assessing the effect of treatment there are three main considerations:

1. Immediate improvement in renal function.
2. Effect of the treatment on the structural damage.
3. Whether the duration or rate of progress of the disease is affected.

Selectivity of proteinuria.—The renal clearance of normal proteins with different molecular weights is compared with the clearance of one protein (transferrin). If smaller amounts of high-molecular-weight proteins than low-molecular-weight proteins appear in the urine the proteinuria is said to be "selective". If large amounts of high- and low-molecular-weight proteins appear in the urine the proteinuria is said to be "unselective".

The quantity of protein in the urine does not correlate with selectivity of proteinuria, nor does the quantity of proteinuria give any indication as to the outcome of the attack; alteration in the daily output of protein either spontaneously or as a result of treatment does not alter the selectivity of proteinuria. There is a correlation between severity of biopsy appearances with selectivity of proteinuria—the less damage to the glomeruli the more selective the proteinuria; however, there are many exceptions; occasional cases of severe proliferative glomerulonephritis have a highly selective proteinuria. If the biopsy shows epithelial crescent formation this is always associated with unselective proteinuria. There is a good correlation between a response to steroids and a selective proteinuria (Cameron, 1966).

The M.R.C. trial of corticosteroids in the nephrotic syndrome indicated that only patients with "minimal change" glomerular lesions are *likely* to respond to steroids; also, steroids can be harmful in other forms of glomerulonephritis (Rose and Black, 1967; Cameron, 1968). However, individual patients with more severe glomerular changes can be improved. Patients with membranous changes and unselective proteinuria given steroids may have improved renal function and develop remission in the nephrotic syndrome although without improving the histological appearances of the glomeruli. The steroids may have to be given for as long as six months before deciding that they are not going to help (Rastogi *et al.*, 1969).

Use of immunosuppressive drugs.—For proliferative glomerulonephritis it is worth trying either azathioprine or cyclophosphamide; these patients hardly ever respond to steroids alone although steroids given with immunosuppressives may permit a higher dose of the latter to be given without producing serious side-effects (White *et al.*, 1966).

For patients with minimal change or membranous glomerulonephritis who fail to respond or become resistant to steroids a trial of azathioprine or cyclophosphamide should be considered. There is general agreement that nephrotic syndrome secondary to other conditions such as diabetes, renal vein thrombosis, pyelonephritis and amyloidosis is unlikely to respond to either steroids or immunosuppressives. These cases almost invariably have an unselective proteinuria; in the rare instance of proteinuria being selective these drugs should probably be considered.

Acute Renal Failure

The main causes are:

1. Acute or chronic renal failure.
2. Cardiogenic or septicaemic shock.
3. Ureteric obstruction.
4. Electrolyte imbalance (as in severe vomiting).
5. Poisons.
6. Mismatched blood transfusion.

One practical problem when confronted with a patient who is oliguric and uraemic is to decide whether dehydration and hypovolaemia are the cause, or whether there is damage to the kidney itself. This is an extremely important distinction, for in the one fluids will be required, and in the other they will be contra-indicated.

The clinical features may be vital in establishing the cause of the oliguria. It is essential to note:

1. Any cause for dehydration (vomiting, diarrhoea, intestinal fistulae, excessive diuretics or diabetes).

2. Duration of oliguria.

3. Previous history of renal disease (pyelonephritis, nephritis and polycystic kidneys) or urinary symptoms particularly of prostatism or cystitis.

4. Presence of any cause of acute renal failure, for example shock, blood transfusion reaction, renal infarction or urinary infection.

If definite answers can be given to the above then it is usually easy to decide whether oliguria is due to dehydration or acute renal failure superimposed on normal or previously diseased kidneys. However, often reliable answers are not available and one has to rely on circumstantial evidence for obtaining the necessary information. The following information is necessary on all patients who are being treated for oliguria:

1. A definite decision as to whether dehydration is present or not. (It should be remembered that persistent vomiting is a cause of dehydration and acute uraemia is a cause of vomiting. The presence of dehydration does not necessarily mean that the dehydration is due to the vomiting.)

2. Previous information with regard to renal function is available, for example a routine blood urea taken at an earlier admission.

3. A careful record of the exact volume of urine passed.

4. Examination of the urine will help decide whether oliguria is due to dehydration or damage to the kidneys, for example the presence of casts on microscopic examination.

    (a) *Concentration*—If the specific gravity is above 1015 severe renal damage can usually be ruled out. The colour of the urine is *no* indication as to its concentration. Urochrome pigments are excreted even in renal failure and may make the urine very dark in colour even though it is dilute.

    (b) *Urine urea.*—Over 2 g per cent suggests normal kidneys, less than 1 g per cent suggests renal damage.

    (c) *Urine sodium.*—On a normal diet the normal urinary sodium is roughly 100 mmol/l. In oliguria due to dehydration or circulatory failure the urinary sodium is usually very *low* (less than 20 mmol/l); this is because aldosterone secretion is stimulated and is causing sodium retention; the fact that the kidneys are able to respond to aldosterone and conserve sodium means that renal damage is not severe. In the presence of *oliguria* a urine sodium of more than 80 mmol/l suggest renal damage because the kidneys are not responding to aldosterone.

(d) *Urine osmolality and specific gravity.*—The specific gravity of plasma without the plasma proteins is approximately 1010. In acute renal failure any urine passed has approximately this specific gravity. In prerenal oliguria the urine passed is much more concentrated due to the affect of ADH secretion. The specific gravity depends on the weight of dissolved substances regardless of their osmotic potential: osmolality measures the osmotic potential. Glucose, urea and other substances increase the specific gravity much more than the osmotic potential. It is more accurate to measure osmolality than specific gravity. The osmolality of plasma is 330 mOsm/l in prerenal ureamia; with maximal ADH secretion the osmolality of the urine should reach at least 1200 mOsm/l. In acute renal failure the osmolality of any urine passed is around 300 mOsm/l.

(e) *Urinary casts.*—A large number of casts suggests renal damage.

(f) *Culture of the urine.*—A heavy growth of a single organism suggests renal infection.

(g) *Urinary protein with electrophoresis.*—Large amounts of albumin (low molecular weight) suggest glomerular damage. Large amounts of globulin (high MW) suggest inflammation in the lower urinary tract.

5. Serum electrolytes and urea. It should be noted that an increase in all the electrolytes may indicate haemoconcentration and, therefore, dehydration.

6. Haemoglobulin and packed cell volume (PCV). Chronic renal damage often causes anaemia. Changes in the PCV are one of the ways of assessing the extracellular fluid state.

7. Plain x-ray of the abdomen to demonstrate kidney size and the presence or absence of a calculus which may be causing ureteric obstruction. The presence of one small kidney will indicate long-standing renal disease. If oliguria is due to unilateral ureteric obstruction the affected kidney may be slightly larger than normal.

8. Daily or twice daily ECG.

9. Routine weighing of the patient if possible. An increase of weight is an indication of fluid retention.

Management of Acute Renal Failure

The management of acute renal failure is based on the premise that provided the cause is removed acute renal failure is potentially reversible. However, the accumulation of metabolites and waste products may cause death before the kidneys have a chance to recover. The most important substances which accumulate are:

Water.
Urea.
Electrolytes, particularly potassium.
Acidic metabolites such as sulphates.

Under normal circumstances, approximately 1,000 ml water is lost in the sweat and faeces. However, many of the metabolic processes of the body produce water as a waste product—"water of metabolism"; usually this is about 500 ml but it may be considerably more in hypercatabolic renal failure (v.i.). This means that up to about 500 ml water can be given even if the patient has complete anuria.

The basal calorie requirement of the body at rest is about 1,000—this is essential for voluntary and involuntary muscular movements etc. If the patient is starved, body protein will be broken down to provide these basal calorie requirements, hence adequate carbohydrates must be given in order to prevent the harmful breakdown of body protein. There is evidence that by giving an excess of calories as carbohydrate or fat almost no body protein need be metabolised. The importance of sparing body protein is that patients who lose weight rapidly due to protein loss are prone to develop systemic infection and complicated electrolyte disturbances, and acidosis. Another important reason for preventing protein breakdown is that more urea and electrolytes are produced. The aim of treatment is, therefore, to conserve as much of the body's own protein as possible.

If a condition is present which is likely to cause acute renal failure (for example, shock, surgical operation, burns) there is now good evidence that administration of mannitol given prophylactically will prevent acute renal failure. It increases extracellular fluid volume and renal blood flow; its osmotic action is probably not important.

Mannitol can also be used to determine whether renal failure is due to dehydration. Infusion of 100 ml 20 per cent mannitol over 15 minutes should result in a diuresis of 100 ml in the next 2 hours in the presence of dehydration but not if there is renal impairment.

Fluids.—500 ml plus the previous 24-hour urine volume.

Electrolyte requirements.—If the patient is passing no urine at all no electrolytes are needed. The sodium and urea content of all urine passed should be measured if possible. Electrolytes should be replaced according to the amount lost in the urine.

Diet.—The diet should contain the basal quantity of calories plus an excess in order to spare endogenous protein breakdown. In addition certain essential amino acids can be given which do not cause a rise in blood urea when they are synthesised to body proteins. The Giordano-Giovanetti diet contains all the essential amino acids except that methiomine and tyrosine have to be added.

The Giordano-Giovanetti diet has been modified to suit British palates; such a diet contains 2,000 calories, 500 ml water, 12 mmol of sodium, 16 mmol of potassium. If it is not possible to give a patient the proper Giordano-Giovanetti diet his protein intake should be restricted to 20 g protein diet per day, unless he is being dialysed, when the protein intake can be increased. If the patient is unable to take solid food by mouth a concentrated form of glucose can be given which contains 400 calories per 100 ml (Hycal).

Parenteral fluids and nutrition.—If the patient is too ill to take any fluids by mouth he will have to be fed entirely intravenously and the great problem is to give sufficient calories without an excess of fluid.

20 per cent glucose or 20 per cent fructose will produce 800 cals/litre. Although both solutions are hypertonic and acidic, fructose is preferable because it possibly causes less thrombophlebitis, it is rapidly metabolised in the absence of insulin and does not escape into the urine.

Fats have a higher calorific value per gramme than carbohydrates (9 cals/g as against 4 cals/g for carbohydrates and protein). Solutions of emulsified fat are available for intravenous use *BUT* at least $\frac{2}{3}$ of the calories administered have to be given as carbohydrate (1 litre of 20 per cent Intralipid will provide 1,800 cals).

Examples of suitable parenteral regimes:

(a) Complete anuria.
     500 ml 40 per cent fructose (800 cals).
(b) Oliguria (500 ml urine in previous 24 hours).
     1,000 ml 20 per cent 40 per cent or fructose (800 or 1,600 cals).
(c) Oliguria (1,000 ml urine in previous 24 hours) entering the diuretic phase.
     1,500 ml 20 per cent or 40 per cent fructose (1,200 or 2,400 cals).

Because the parenteral solutions used are hypertonic they must be given into a large vein. In addition heparin 1,000 units per litre of fluid is usually given.

Anabolic steroids.—Protein breakdown can be reduced by giving anabolic steroids and it is customary to give norethandrolone 10 mg for the duration of the acute renal failure.

Hyperkalaemia.—This is the most dangerous complication of acute renal failure because it causes cardiac arrhythmias. The changes in the ECG which occur in hyperkalaemia are:

Tall T waves.
Widening of the QRS complex.
Prolongation of the PR interval.
Disappearance of the P waves.

In an emergency the effects of potassium on the heart can be counter-acted by intravenous calcium gluconate (20 ml of 10 per cent solution). The serum potassium can be temporarily lowered by giving insulin which promotes potassium transfer into the cells. 20 units of soluble insulin are given with 100 ml of 50 per cent glucose. Potassium can also be removed from the body by sodium ion exchange resin (Resonium-A). 40 g daily is given either by mouth or as a retention enema.

Other requirements.—(a) Vitamins should be given.

(b) Dry mouth can be prevented by sucking ice cubes, chewing gum or small pieces of lemon.

(c) *Severe* anaemia should be corrected with blood transfusion but it must be noted that stored blood contains a large amount of potassium and protein.

Should these methods fail to control the metabolites before the patient begins to pass urine, then dialysis (either haemo or peritoneal) is con-sidered. The main indications for dialysis are:

1. Hypercatabolic renal failure (rise in urea of more than 6·5 mmol/l per day).
2. Blood urea 45 mmol/l.
3. Serum potassium above 6·5 mmol/l.
4. Serum bicarbonate below 15 mmol/l (indicating acidosis).
5. Clinical deterioration and bleeding.

Peritoneal dialysis is usually the treatment of choice in the manage-ment of acute renal failure. It can be performed even if the patient has had a recent abdominal operation. It is particularly suitable for patients in whom it would be hazardous to perform haemodialysis, for example in those with a bleeding diathesis, poor cardiac output (e.g., after cardiac infarction), and in those patients who have an uncommon blood group for whom sufficient blood is not available for haemodialysis. Peritoneal dialysis is relatively simple to manage and requires the minimum of equipment and staff. Only two solutions are necessary, each contains the necessary concentration of electrolytes except potassium which has to be added. The solutions only differ in the amount of dextrose which they contain: one contains an excess of dextrose so that if the patient is overhydrated water will be absorbed into the fluid; the other solution which is used routinely is iso-osmolar with normal plasma (although, of course, not with plasma containing a high concentration of urea). The fluid is run into the peritoneum in hourly cycles, and is left in for 45 minutes before being siphoned out.

Potassium is added to the dialysis fluid if the patient is becoming hypokalaemic. The peritoneum exudes a certain amount of protein into the fluid and this can be replaced by allowing the patient to have some first-class protein in the diet, or by giving plasma or Aminosol. Each day, a sample of the dialysate is cultured after dialysis and if infection is present it is treated with the appropriate antibiotic. The incidence of infection is low and seems to be even less if the dialyses are kept down to 6–8 per day.

The main dangers of management to be avoided are:

1. Delay in starting dialysis until the patient has clinically deteriorated.

2. Inadequate care with catheterisation: technique should be irreproachable, and daily bladder washouts with antibiotic (neomycin usually) should be performed.

3. Over-enthusiasm once peritoneal dialysis is started: it is better to aim to dialyse for short periods and control the urea, potassium and hydration, than to aim for complete normality.

After all, the aim of this treatment is only to tide the patient over; the number of dialyses should be kept to a minimum.

4. Stopping too soon. Once the diuretic phase has started, it is important to keep the dialysis tube in place until the blood urea and potassium are falling and the sodium and urea concentrations in the urine are rising.

Treatment of Chronic Renal Failure

It is worth emphasising two important functional differences between chronic and acute renal failure: in chronic renal failure the patient usually excretes too much water and too much sodium—the complete opposite to acute renal failure. *But* in the nephrotic syndrome, before chronic renal failure develops, there is hypoproteinaemia which leads to fluid retention and sodium retention—this is why it is essential to grasp the difference between the nephrotic syndrome and chronic renal failure, and to appreciate that the nephrotic syndrome may terminate as chronic renal failure, necessitating alteration of treatment.

In other respects, acute and chronic renal failure cause similar functional disturbances, viz. rise in blood urea, rise in serum potassium acidosis and anaemia. Hypertension may complicate chronic renal failure.

The important aspects of the management of chronic renal failure are:

1. Ensure adequate water intake—give the patient some idea by saying that he must fill a 2-litre container with urine each day.

2. Ensure adequate sodium intake.

3. Control acidosis by prescribing oral sodium bicarbonate each day.

4. Prevent uraemic symptoms and protein breakdown by giving a modified Giovanetti diet which contains a known amount of first-class protein, and essential amino acids. Restrict the intake of other proteins.

5. Control gently the blood pressure, urinary infections and anaemia if possible.

Before the stage of chronic renal failure in the nephrotic syndrome, the patient will usually require increased protein in the diet to compensate for excessive loss in the urine, but sodium intake should be restricted because the patient will have fluid retention due to hypoproteinaemia. If the blood urea begins to rise in the nephrotic syndrome or chronic renal failure develops, then protein intake will need to be restricted.

Fluid and Electrolyte Balance

It is possible to cope with any practical problem of fluid, electrolyte and acid-base imbalance if certain simple concepts and rules are applied (see p. 104 for discussion of Acid-Base Balance). The first of these is to remember the approximate volumes of the fluid compartments which are, in a 70 kg person:

Extracellular volume = 15 litres = 20 per cent of the body weight
Plasma volume   = 3 litres = 4 per cent of the body weight
Intracellular volume = 30 litres = 40 per cent of the body weight
Total body water   = 48 litres = 60 per cent of the body weight

Water is freely diffusible between extra- and intracellular compartments. Sodium is restricted to the extracellular compartment and potassium to the intracellular compartment; bicarbonate occurs in both.

Milliequivalents (Millimoles) and Available Solutions

One atom of hydrogen reacts with one atom of chloride which reacts with one atom of sodium. The weight of one atom of hydrogen is the unit, the weight of sodium is then 23 and of chloride is 35. Hence, 1 gram of hydrogen will react with 35 g of chloride, which reacts with 23 g of sodium. The weight of a substance which reacts with 1 g of hydrogen is known as the "gram equivalent weight". 23 g of sodium will combine with 35 g of chloride, but only one atom of chloride reacts with one atom of sodium, therefore, 35 g of chloride and 23 g of sodium each contain the same number of atoms (or "particles"). It is the number of "particles" present that determines the osmotic potential and the pH of solutions, and not the relative weight of the particles.

In chemical solutions which contain known weights of ions, we need to know, for physiological purposes, the number of "particles", in order to keep the pH and osmotic potential constant.

1 gram of hydrogen is equivalent to 35 g of chloride which is equivalent to 23 g of sodium.

1 gram equivalent (of hydrogen) is equivalent to 58 grams (23 + 35) of sodium chloride.

1 milligram equivalent of hydrogen is equivalent to ·058 g or 58 milligrams of sodium chloride.

1 milligram equivalent is called a milliequivalent (mEq) or a milli-mole (mmol).

∴   1 mEq or millimole = 58 milligrams of NaCl.
∴   1,000 mEq or millimoles = 58 g of NaCl.
∴   1 gram NaCl contains 1,000/58 mEq or millimoles = 17 mEq or millimoles (mmol).

We can, therefore, say that a gram of sodium chloride contains 17 milliequivalents of sodium and chloride. We need to know the number of milliequivalents in 1 gram of other salts, the most important of these are:

potassium chloride	13
sodium bicarbonate	12
calcium chloride	9

To summarise:

We need to bother with milliequivalents or millimoles for these reasons:

(i) All simple salts contain equal numbers of milliequivalents or millimoles of their constituent ions (but different weights of each ion).

(ii) To be at a neutral pH solutions must contain equal numbers of milliequivalents or millimoles of anions and cations, and not equal weights of each.

(iii) Solutions containing the same number of milliequivalents of different ions will be iso-osmotic with each other.

If we had to remember the number of milligrams of sodium which reacted with the number of milligrams of chloride or bicarbonate etc., it would be a monumental task to work out the amount of each ion that had to be given to combine with the other, and it would need separate calculations to work out the osmotic strength of the solution and whether its pH has changed.

Expressed simply, the pH and osmotic potential depend on the number of ionised "particles" present, and not on the weight of the "particles". Furthermore, simple salts consist of one "particle" of one ion joined to one "particle" of another ion, the relative weights of each "particle" do not matter.

In normal plasma mmol/l of anions = mmol/l of cations = 150.

All parenteral solutions aim to be the same concentration (isotonic) as plasma. To achieve this, slightly different *concentrations* of each salt are necessary, for example, sodium chloride has to be a 0·9 per cent solution, and sodium bicarbonate a 1·4 per cent solution to be isotonic with plasma (i.e. 0·9 grams per 100 ml of NaCl and 1·4 grams per 100 ml of $NaHCO_3$).

It is convenient to consider all solutions in litres rather than in units of 100 ml, therefore a 0·9 per cent solution of sodium chloride will contain 9 grams per litre, and a 1·4 per cent solution of sodium bicarbonate, 14 grams per litre.

We already know that 1 gram of sodium chloride contains 17 mEq or mmol of sodium and chloride, therefore 9 grams will contain 153 mEq or mmol, i.e. a litre of isotonic (0·9 per cent) solution of NaCl will contain 153 mEq or mmol of sodium and chloride. Similarly, a litre of 1·4 per cent $NaHCO_3$ will contain 167 mEq or mmol of sodium and bicarbonate.

It is not recommended that complicated prepared intravenous solutions such as Ringer's, Hartmann's or Darrow's solutions be used, as the exact electrolyte content of each is not usually widely known.

Fluid Compartments of the Body

In a 70 kg person these are roughly:

Extracellular volume = 15 litres. = 20 per cent of the body weight.
Plasma volume   = 3 litres = 4 per cent of the body weight.
Intracellular volume = 30 litres = 40 per cent of the body weight.
Total body water   = 48 litres = 60 per cent of the body weight.

CORRECTION OF DISTURBED ELECTROLYTE BALANCE

Sodium and Water

1. Depleted serum sodium.—This can be due either to (a) excessive water, or (b) a reduction in the amount of sodium (almost invariably accompanied by loss of water as well). Excess water is present if there is reduced excretion of water, for example acute renal failure, severe oedema or an excess of intake over excretion (for example, over-transfusion).

An excess of intake over excretion of pure water may result in *water-intoxication*. The excess water is evenly distributed throughout both compartments. A small excess in circulating volume and extracellular fluid is not important but a small excess of intracellular water gives rise to water intoxication; it is the brain cells which are most sensitive to this increase in water, hence most of the symptoms are cerebral and the patient becomes stuporous and eventually comatose with convulsions.

Reduction of the serum sodium due to excessive loss of sodium is almost invariably accompanied by loss of water; when water is lost from the body (dehydration) it is first lost from the extracellular fluid in an attempt to conserve both the intracellular water and the circulating blood volume; if the loss continues water is removed from the intra-cellular compartment and finally from the circulating volume. The physical signs of dehyration reflect this sequence of salt and water loss.

Loss from extracellular compartment:
    dry tongue;
    dry skin and loss of skin elasticity;
    reduced intra-ocular pressure.
Loss of intracellular fluid: drowsiness;
    pyrexia.
Loss of circulating fluid: tachycardia;
    reduced blood pressure;
    constricted veins.
Other signs of dehydration: reduced flow of concentrated urine;
    high packed cell volume (increased
      haematocrit);
    increased blood urea.

Summary.—A low serum sodium with
  (a) signs of dehydration means loss of salt and water;
  (b) absence of signs of dehydration with disturbance of cerebral function means water intoxication.

2. Increased serum sodium.—In practice this means (a) excess loss of water over sodium or (b) over-transfusion with saline. Excess loss of water occurs in fistulae or excessive sweating and will be accompanied by the signs of dehydration. Over-transfusion with salt and water will result in an increase in volume of the extracellular and vascular com-partments (not the intracellular, because sodium only occurs in the extracellular compartment). Excess fluid in the extracellular compart-ment affects mainly the lung, resulting in pulmonary oedema; later, oedema of the sacrum and finally the ankles may occur. Excess fluid in the vascular compartment results in elevation of the jugular venous pulse.

Summary.—An increased serum sodium
   (a) with signs of dehydration means excessive water loss;
   (b) without signs of dehydration but with elevation of the jugular venous pulse or pulmonary oedema means over-transfusion.

Treatment

A low serum sodium.—(a) With signs of dehydration (indicating loss of excessive salt and some water), give:
   i hypertonic saline (NaCl 5 per cent) which contains 855 mEq (mmol/l) of sodium and chloride;
   ii sodium bicarbonate (1·4 per cent) which contains 167 mEq (mmol)/l of Na and 167 mEq (mmol)/l of HCO_3.
   (b) Without signs of dehydration but with disturbance of cerebral function (water intoxication). The aims of treatment are to reduce the cerebral oedema and promote the loss of water. This is best achieved by 20 per cent mannitol.

A high serum sodium.—(a) With signs of dehydration (indicating excess loss of water over sodium), give:
   i normal saline (0·9 per cent) NaCl which contains 154 mEq (mmol)/l of NaCl, that is, isotonic with plasma;
   ii dextrose/saline—NaCl (0·18 per cent) and 4·3 dextrose (called "fifth normal saline"—note that 0·18 is $\frac{1}{5}$ of 0·9); this contains 31 mEq (mmol)/l of sodium and chloride;
   iii rarely, if water loss is truly excessive, dextrose 5 per cent. The sugar is metabolised leaving behind pure water.
   (b) Without signs of dehydration usually means over-transfusion. The infusion should be stopped and a diuretic given (frusemide 40 mg intramuscularly).

How much of these solutions should be given?—The cardinal points to remember are the size of the compartments, the normal electrolyte content of plasma, and the fact that water is freely diffusible through both compartments but that sodium is found only in the extracellular compartment.

If the serum sodium is high it means that water has been drawn out from the cells to attempt to dilute the concentrated extracellular fluid; hence, sufficient water has to be given to dilute the serum so that the serum sodium returns to normal, and enough has to be given to replace that which has been drawn out from the cells. Hence, enough water has to be given to dilute the *total body water*—which is approximately 60 per cent of the body weight. Thus, if the observed serum sodium is

160 mmol/l it means that every litre of body water is concentrated to the same extent (although in the cells sodium will not be the ion which accounts for the concentration). Every litre, therefore, contains 20 mEq too much sodium.

∴ if the normal serum sodium is 140 mEq (mmol) every litre contains 20/140 more sodium than normal;

∴ to bring the serum sodium back to normal concentration each litre must be increased by 20/140 (that is, 1/7).

However, it has already been stated that every litre of body water has to be considered,

∴ the total amount of water required will be in litres
1/7 × 60 per cent of the body weight (kg);

that is, in hypernatraemia due to water and salt loss the amount of water required will be:

$$\frac{[Na] - 140}{140} \times \tfrac{3}{5} \text{ body weight in litres.}$$

If the serum sodium is low in the presence of loss of sodium and water it means that water has been drawn into the cells so that the total body water is available for diluting any administered sodium.

Assuming the serum sodium is 120 mEq (mmol)/l, each litre will be 20 mEq (mmol) of sodium short. Hence, to increase the sodium content of the extracellular fluid to normal it must be assumed that the excess water in the cells is also available for diluting the administered sodium, that is, every litre of body water is 20 mEq (mmol) of sodium short, hence the amount of sodium which needs to be given is

20 × 60 per cent body water in mEq (mmol).

In practice in combined salt and water loss:
(a) if the serum sodium is 120–160 mEq (mmol)/l normal saline is given;
(b) if the serum sodium is less than 120 mEq (mmol)/l, 1 litre hypertonic saline is given;
(c) if the serum sodium is more than 160 mEq (mmol)/l, 3 litres 5 per cent dextrose is given.

Potassium

The serum level of potassium is a poor guide to potassium balance since potassium is found mainly inside the cells and the level in the serum will depend partly on the amount of water in the extracellular and vascular compartments. In addition potassium may leak out of cells in conditions causing an acidosis (for example, uraemia and diabetes) producing a high level in the serum due to depletion of normal intracellular potassium. Potassium depletion is best confirmed with an ECG (hypokalaemia causes lowering and inversion of T waves, prominent U waves and prolongation of the QT interval). Potassium depletion may cause:

(a) cardiac arrhythmias;
(b) excessive sensitivity to digitalis;
(c) muscle weakness;
(d) renal damage.

Significant hypokalaemia is always accompanied by an alkalosis (hydrogen ion is lost by the kidney in an attempt to conserve potassium; hydrogen ion also passes into the cells to compensate for leakage of potassium leading to an intracellular acidosis). Accompanying water depletion may cause apparently normal serum levels of potassium due to haemoconcentration.

Hypokalaemia may only become obvious when the dehydration is treated. Similarly a metabolic acidosis may mask the accompanying alkalosis due to potassium depletion.

Potassium depletion occurs:

1. During loss of large volumes of intestinal contents (vomiting, diarrhoea, fistula).

2. During starvation (an adequate intake of glucose is essential for the functional integrity of cell membranes).

3. During hypercatabolic states when potassium is lost in the urine together with large amounts of endogenous protein.

4. During diuretic therapy.

5. In potassium-losing nephritis.

6. In hyperaldosteronism (primary and secondary).

7. In severe salt and water depletion in which large amounts of aldosterone are produced causing sodium retention at the expense of potassium.

8. In renal tubular disorders and certain rare potassium-losing tumours of the large intestine.

9. In Cushing's syndrome.

10. Familial periodic paralysis.

Correction of hypokalaemia.—If potassium deficiency is suspected, potassium should be administered in 5 per cent dextrose or 4·3 per cent dextrose/fifth normal saline. 1 g potassium chloride contains 13 mEq of potassium. It is seldom necessary to give more than 1–2 g per hour.

(For a discussion of acid-base disturbance, see p. 104.)

Parenteral nutrition.—For patients who are unable to take any food by mouth, prolonged intravenous feeding may be necessary. The greatest problem is to ensure that the patient has enough calories without receiving too much fluid. Most patients require at least 3,000 calories daily; if this is not provided in the form of carbohydrate, body protein is broken down to supply calories, leading to weight loss, decreased muscle size and wasting. If wasting becomes severe, the patient is more prone to develop infections and electrolyte disturbances. It is, therefore, advisable to supply the patient with his full daily need of calories and amino acids and so prevent breakdown of his own proteins. He should also receive nitrogen in a form that can be easily metabolised, in order to compensate for "wear and tear" and prevent further breakdown of body proteins. Carbohydrate given in the form of 5 per cent dextrose produces 200 calories per litre so that 15 litres would need to be given in order to fulfil the calorie needs of the body. Glucose can be given as a 20 per cent solution, but this is very irritant to the veins, so instead, 20 per cent solution of fructose is used (which provides 800 calories/litre). Fructose also has the advantage that it is less irritant to veins and is not excreted in the urine, and so does not produce an osmotic diuresis as does glucose. Both fructose and glucose solutions suffer from the disadvantages that relatively large amounts of fluid have to be administered, and that the solutions are very acid (pH about 4). Intralipid consists of an emulsion of fats obtained from soya beans. One litre of a 20 per cent solution of Intralipid provides 1,800 calories; the pH of the solution is normal and the solution is isotonic with plasma.

Nitrogen products can be administered in the form of a solution of amino acids (Aminosol). This does not provide any calories, but one litre of 10 per cent Aminosol contains 160 mEq (mmol) of sodium. An electrolyte-free form of amino acid solution is available (Trophysan). It is worth emphasising that at least 60 per cent of calories should be given as carbohydrate, less carbohydrate than this will still result in protein breakdown, also the carbohydrate should be given before the amino acid solution and Intralipid. None of these solutions contains potassium, so that potassium chloride should be added (2 g per litre). In addition, of course, vitamins will be required. Parenteral nutrition is only needed in serious illness, such as severe ulcerative colitis, septicaemia, burns, and post-operative states.

Hypercatabolic renal failure.—Following any severe trauma, such as burns, road accidents, major surgery and sepsis, there is a vast increase in metabolism of the whole body resulting in rapid breakdown of protein and carbohydrates; coupled with this, there is diminished excretion of sodium and water. Sudden and rapid loss of weight such as occurs after trauma, surgery, burns or exacerbations of ulcerativecolitis leads to:

1. Reduced wound healing.
2. Electrolyte disturbances, particularly hyponatraemia.

3. Disturbed acid-base balance.
4. Marrow depression.
5. Reduced resistance to infections.

Hypercatabolic renal failure is a condition which has not received sufficient emphasis in the past, and the likelihood of infections and electrolyte disturbances in patients who lose weight rapidly after major trauma tends to be overlooked and the easily-preventable cause remains untreated.

Design of intravenous diet.—The problem is to get 2000–3000 calories per 24 hours into a patient in as small amount of fluid as possible together with as much nitrogen (in the form of amino acids) as is being metabolised. A rough guide to the rate of metabolism of nitrogen is given by the number of grams of urea excreted in 24 hours—this is an essential measurement when planning intravenous nutrition. It is important to remember the following:

2 g urea is equivalent to 1 g nitrogen which is equivalent to 10 g amino acids. In hypercatabolic states the 24-hour urine urea is usually about 20 grams, hence approximately 100 grams of amino acids are needed.

An example of a suitable parenteral diet for a moderately severe hypercatabolic stage is shown below:

Infusion Period	*Solutions*
8 hours	$\frac{1}{2}$ litre Aminosol 3·3%, fructose 15%, ethanol 2·5%, plus 26 mEq KCl (2 g) $\frac{1}{2}$ litre 20% Intralipid plus 5000 units heparin
8 hours	$\frac{1}{2}$ litre Aminosol 3·3%, fructose 15%, ethanol 2·5%, plus 26 mEq KCl $\frac{1}{2}$ litre 10% Aminosol
8 hours	$\frac{1}{2}$ litre Aminosol 3·3%, fructose 15%, ethanol 2·5%, plus 26 mEq KCl $\frac{1}{2}$ litre 20% Intralipid plus 5000 units heparin

(from Peaston, 1968)

The contents of this diet are:

Nutrition Solution	*Total Volume (ml)*	*Water (ml)*	*Calories*	*Carbo-hydrate (g)*	*Alcohol (g)*	*Amino acids*	*Fat (g)*	*Nitro-gen (g)*	*Electro-lytes (mEq)*
Aminosol 10%	200	475	165	—	—	50	—	6·375	Na 160
Aminosol fructose ethanol	1500	1275	1750	225	37·5	50	—	6·375	Cl 120
Intralipid 20%	1000	750	2000	—	—	—	200	—	K 0·4
Total	2700	2500	3915	225	37·5	100	200	12·75	

Note that electrolyte requirements must be assessed separately; with this parenteral diet about one-third of the necessary sodium and chloride and less than half a gram of potassium are being supplied.

Forced Diuresis

Many drugs are bound to the plasma proteins or rapidly bound in the tissues. However, with many of these, some free drug is present in the serum in equilibrium with the bound drug, so that if the free drug can be excreted the bound drug will follow. Any drug which is partly excreted by the kidney either by glomerular filtration or tubular excretion can be excreted more rapidly if urine flow is increased. Unfortunately, many drugs are detoxicated only by the liver, and their excretion will not be influenced by forced diuresis.

Altering the pH increases the ionisation, and hence excretion, of some drugs, e.g. the long-acting barbiturates (phenobarbitone) are more rapidly excreted in an alkaline urine, and amphetamines are more rapidly excreted in an acid urine. The short- and intermediate-acting barbiturates are excreted mainly by the liver, and excretion is not greatly increased by alkaline diuresis. The excretion of salicylates is increased very markedly in an alkaline urine.

Salicylates have a very complicated effect on the acid-base balance:

1. Most salicylates are acidic and ingestion of large quantities may produce a metabolic acidosis.

2. They are respiratory stimulants and so increase the rate of breathing, causing a respiratory alkalosis.

3. Later, when the patient becomes comatose, respiratory depression occurs, causing a respiratory acidosis.

4. Prolonged unconsciousness and lack of food may lead to ketosis and metabolic acidosis.

Thus following salicylate poisoning there may be almost any alteration of the acid-base balance depending at which stage the patient is seen.

Many schemes have been proposed for forced alkaline diuresis. It is probably better not to promote an osmotic diuresis until after the first hour, as dehydration may be present which may be aggravated by an osmotic diuresis. It is reasonable to promote a water, as opposed to an osmotic, diuresis first as this will automatically correct any dehydration.

A simple scheme for forced alkaline diuresis is:

1. Blood for the levels of salicylates and barbiturates, electrolytes and blood urea, pH, Po_2, Pco_2, bicarbonate and blood sugar. It is important to take a blood sugar in case the patient is a diabetic and is either in diabetic or hypoglycaemic coma.

2. First two hours: 2 litres of isotonic saline.

3. At the end of 2 hours, 20 mg frusemide, 200 ml of 8·4 per cent of bicarbonate and 2 g of potassium chloride.

4. Give in each subsequent hour an amount of fluid equal to the volume of urine passed in the previous hour, add 2 g of potassium chloride to every litre of fluid. After the first two hours, give alternate bottles of 4·3 per cent dextrose/1/5N saline, and isotonic saline.

5. Repeat 8·4 per cent bicarbonate every 2 hours until the urine pH is 8.

(Notice all the "2"s.)

In general, gastric lavage is not recommended in comatose patients unless the tablets have been taken within two hours of admission. Respiratory depression will be indicated by a raised Pco_2 and a low Po_2; as an emergency, 100 per cent oxygen is given but the patient will need artificial ventilation. Antibiotics are not usually administered routinely but only if pneumonia develops; some antibiotics may be preferentially metabolised by the same enzymes which metabolise the drug and so may impair drug excretion by the liver.

In the presence of severe shock, rapid fluid replacement, preferably with blood or plasma, may be necessary. In salicylate overdose, vitamin K should be given routinely, because aspirin causes hypoprothrombinaemia, gastric erosions and a thrombocytopenia. Prolonged unconsciousness may cause hypothermia, which should be treated along the lines suggested on p. 343.

Retroperitoneal Fibrosis (Saxton *et al.*, 1969)

The most common presenting feature is hypertension, although weight loss, loin pain, urinary symptoms and low backbache are also common symptoms. The condition is not confined to the retroperitoneal area: involvement of the pancreas may lead to diabetes, of the heart to heart block and conduction defects, of the liver to portal hypertension, of the mediastinum to vena cava and oesophageal obstruction, and of the lungs to pulmonary fibrosis. The sedimentation rate is usually elevated; the IVP shows narrowing of the mid-point of the ureters which are generally deviated medially. It is important that the whole of both ureters be seen on the IVP. Drugs which are reported to cause the condition are methysergide, dexamphetamine, ergotamine and hydrallazine. Other sclerosing conditions such as sclerosing cholangitis, Riedel's thyroiditis and fibrotic contractures of the fingers are reported to have been associated. Retroperitoneal lymphomas can cause widespread fibrosis. Injection of sclerosing substances for haemorrhoids and varicose veins have been suggested as possible causes.

REFERENCES

ADDIS, T. (1949). *Glomerular Nephritis*. New York: Macmillan Co.

ASSCHER, A. W., SUSSMAN, M., WATERS, W. E., DAVIS, R. H., and CHICK, S. (1966). *Lancet*, **2**, 1037.

BEARD, R. W., and ROBERTS, A. P. (1968). *Brit. med. Bull.*, **24**, 44.

BEESON, P. B. (1967). In *Renal Disease*. Ed. Black, D. A. Oxford: Blackwell Scientific.

CAMERON, J. S. (1966). *Proc. roy. Soc. Med.*, **59**, 512.

CAMERON, J. S. (1968). *Brit. med. J.*, **4**, 352.

FAIRLEY, K. F., BOND, A. G., BROWN, R. B., and HABERSBERGER, P. (1967). *Lancet*, **2**, 427.

HODSON, C. J. (1967). In *Renal Disease*. Ed. Black, D. A. Oxford: Blackwell Scientific.

HODSON, C. J., and WILSON, S. (1965). *Brit. med. J.*, **2**, 191.

KASS, E. H. (1957). *Arch. intern. Med.*, **100**, 709.

KIMMELSTIEL, P. (1966). *Controversy in Internal Medicine*, p. 313. Eds. Ingelfinger, F. J., Relman, A. S., and Finland, M. Philadelphia: W. B. Saunders Co.

KUNIN, P. W. (1968). *Urinary Tract Infection*, p. 235. Eds. O'Grady, F., and Brumfitt, W. London: Oxford Univ. Press.

LITTLE, P. J. (1962). *Lancet*, **1**, 1149.

LITTLE, P. J. (1965). *J. clin. Path.*, **18**, 556.

LITTLE, P. J., and de WARDENER, H. (1966). *Lancet*, **2**, 1277.

PEART, W. S. (1967). In *Renal Disease*. Ed. Black, D. A. Oxford: Blackwell Scientific.

PEASTON, M. J. (1968). *Brit. J. hosp. Med.*, **1**, 708.

PETERSDORF, R. G. (1966). *Controversy in Internal Medicine,* p. 302. Eds. Ingelfinger, F. J., Relman, A. S., and Finland, M. Philadelphia: W. B. Saunders Co.

RASTOGI, S. P., HART-MERCER, J., and KERR, D. N. S. (1969). *Quart. J. Med.*, **38**, 335.

REEVES, D. S., and BRUMFITT, W. (1968). In *Urinary Tract Infection*. Eds. O'Grady, F., and Brumfitt, W. London: Oxford Univ. Press.

ROSE, G. A., and BLACK, D. A. K. (1967). *Quart. J. Med.*, **36**, 607.

SAXTON, H. M., KILPATRICK, F. R., KINDER, C. H., LESSOF, M. A., McHARDY-YOUNG, S., and WARDLE, D. F. (1969). *Quart. J. Med.*, **38**, 159.

DE WARDENER, H. E. (1967). *The Kidney*. London: J. & A. Churchill.

WHALLEY, P. (1967). *Amer. J. Obstet. Gynec.*, **97**, 723.

WHITE, R. H., CAMERON, J. S., and TROUNCE, J. R. (1966). *Brit. med. J.*, **4**, 853.

10

SHOCK

Shock results from complicated circulatory disorder affecting:

1. The pumping function of the heart.
2. Blood distribution (arterioles).
3. Microcirculation (capillaries).
4. Capacitance vessels (veins).
5. Physical properties of the blood.
6. The pulmonary circulation and lungs.

One of the simplest and most inclusive definitions of shock is a *clinical state in which the cardiac output is insufficient for tissue requirements*; the main tissue requirements are an adequate supply of oxygen and nutrients *and* adequate removal of the waste products of metabolism. Shock may be accompanied by or caused by acute heart failure; but all cases of heart failure are not necessarily shocked, because the dominant feature may be congestion behind the pump rather than forward failure of the pump and inadequate vascular compensation (Friedberg, 1966).

Causes

A. **Reduced venous return**

1. Haemorrhage.
2. Dehydration:
    Vomiting and diarrhoea
    Diabetic ketosis
    Addison's disease
    Heat stroke.
3. Endotoxin shock.
4. Anaphylaxis.
5. Neurogenic shock (abdominal and testicular trauma, paracentesis).
6. Psychogenic shock.
7. Acute peritonitis, pancreatitis and perforation.
8. Burns.

B. **Reduced cardiac output (cardiogenic shock)**

1. Myocardial infarction.
2. Pulmonary embolism.

3. Myocarditis.

4. Dysrhythmia.

5. Cardiac tamponade.

6. Ruptured valve cusp, papillary muscle, interventricular septum or chordae tendineae.

7. Tight aortic or mitral stenosis.

Haemorrhage and loss of circulating fluid.—Following a sudden loss of blood or fluid from the intravascular compartment the cardiac output is maintained by an increase in the heart rate. Vasoconstriction of the arterioles occurs in such a way that perfusion of privileged tissues (brain and heart) is maintained while blood is diverted from less essential tissues. In the later stages of shock due to fluid loss there is a decrease in venous return, a fall in central venous pressure, a diminution in stroke volume and eventually a fall in blood pressure. The oxygen available to the tissues is very little reduced by a fall in haemoglobin of 30 per cent. The emphasis is swinging away from the rule "blood for blood lost". The most important factor is restoration of circulating volume. If dehydration has not reached the stage of causing a reduction in circulating volume electrolyte solutions can be used for rehydration. These will pass immediately into the dry extracellular space. If dehydration has progressed to the stage of diminished intravascular fluid volume as well as diminished extracellular fluid volume early replacement is best made with solutions with a high oncotic pressure, i.e. the osmotic pressure is due to colloids (whole blood, plasma, albumin or dextrans). Later electrolyte solutions can be used to rehydrate the extracellular compartment.

If electrolyte solutions are given to patients in whom dehydration has diminished the extracellular and vascular compartments most of the administered fluid passes straight into the extracellular compartment.

Endotoxin or Gram-negative shock.—The endotoxin responsible for the peripheral circulatory failure in septicaemia due to Gram-negative organisms is a lipopolysaccharide within the cell wall of the organisms. The endotoxin has an intense sympathomimetic effect resulting in vasoconstriction of arterioles of the bowel, kidneys and lungs. The sympathomimetic effect is also partly due to release of endogenous catecholamines and the combination of the endotoxin with some substance in the blood producing an unknown sympathomimetic agent. The most usual organisms responsible are *E. coli*, *Str. faecalis* and *Pseudomonas aeruginosa* (*pyocyanea*). It is important to be aware that Gram-positive septicaemia can result in similar haemodynamic disturbances, although less commonly. The incidence of Gram-negative septicaemia is increasing due to increased use of intravenous infusions, corticosteroids, immunosuppressive drugs, surgery in neonates and the elderly, increasing awareness of the complication and the fact that many Gram-negative organisms are becoming resistant to antibiotics. Pulmonary oedema occurs more readily in septicaemia than other forms of shock even in the absence of left ventricular failure (Riordan and Walters, 1968); pulmonary hypertension also occurs more frequently.

Anaphylaxis.—Anaphylactic shock results from an antibody-antigen reaction which occurs on the surface of the mast cells releasing vaso-active substances such as histamine, 5-hydroxytryptamine, bradykinin and other kinins. These cause contraction of bronchial smooth muscle and airways narrowing, dilatation of the microcirculation and pooling of blood; increased capillary permeability and loss of intravascular fluid. Sympathomimetic drugs are beneficial in the early stages of anaphylactic shock.

Neurogenic shock.—Sudden trauma to sensitive autonomic ganglia (e.g. a blow to the abdomen or testicles) can result in temporary dysfunction of the autonomic control of blood vessels. There is good evidence that some of the effects of shock due to pulmonary embolism and myo-cardial infarction is due to stimulation of local afferent nerve fibres and inappropriate response by peripheral blood vessels (Sleight, 1964).

Psychogenic shock (vasovagal syncope).—Sudden emotional "shock" can cause widespread peripheral arteriolar dilatation and pooling of blood with a low cardiac output. Usually this is quickly reversible but occasionally it persists. Signs of disordered autonomic function including disturbed vascular reflexes are sometimes part of disordered emotional behaviour after sudden or sustained psychogenic shock (e.g. "battle-fatigue"). During the Second World War the use of immediate sedation after a harrowing experience reduced the incidence of subsequent hysterical behaviour. The situation is complicated if a patient has been physically injured *and* is suffering from psychogenic shock. This is seen in civilian practice when an injured driver sees his passenger mutilated in a road traffic accident. Severe pain and fear also gives rise to disordered vascular function through neurogenic or psychogenic mechanisms. For these reasons sedation and analgesia should be given to conscious casualties as soon as possible after injury. Morphia is given for its analgesic and sedative properties—if a casualty in an accident is not in pain morphia is still indicated for its sedative properties. It should generally be given intravenously because of irregular absorption from intramuscular sites in states of shock.

Intra-abdominal emergencies and burns.—The causes of shock in these situations are due to several factors; fluid, protein and electrolyte loss, sudden pain, neurogenic factors and Gram-negative septicaemia.

Cardiogenic shock.—This is characterised by a sudden fall in cardiac output which brings into operation protective mechanisms similar to those in all other situations in which effective cardiac output is reduced.

The response of the peripheral circulation to an inadequate cardiac output is the same whether it is due to Gram-negative septicaemia, anaphylaxis, haemorrhage and fluid loss, myocardial infarction, pulmonary embolism or dysrhythmia. In the case of cardiogenic shock two other adverse factors are in operation: one is the fact that the pump itself is damaged, and the other is the variable part played by neurogenic mechanism in impairing peripheral circulatory function. It is thought that impulses from the injured myocardium or coronary arteries travel in afferent sympathetic pathways—probably via the vagus nerve—and disturb peripheral vascular responses (Agress, 1962; Aviado and Schmidt, 1955; Sleight, 1964). In acute cardiac failure there is often a simultaneous reduction in venous return so that pulmonary congestion does not always occur (Mathes, 1962).

Pathophysiology of Shock

All blood vessels contain both types of adrenergic receptors—α and β. In general, stimulation of the α receptors results in constriction of arterioles, capillaries and veins, while stimulation of the β receptors results in vasodilation. The relative numbers of α and β receptors varies in different blood vessels, hence the exact response to adrenergic receptor stimulation differs in different parts of the body. Stimulation of β receptors of the heart results in an increase in myocardial contractility (inotropic action); β receptors predominate in the heart.

The capillaries are freely permeable to water and electrolytes. Flow through capillaries is controlled by sphincter mechanisms at both ends—the pre- and post-capillary sphincters. The pre-capillary sphincter tend to open in response to accumulation of local metabolites. The post-capillary sphincters respond to catecholamines both directly and via the sympathetic nervous system. A rise in catecholamines results in constriction of post-capillary sphincters. Control of capillaries is such that only one third of all the capillaries is open at any one time. If all the capillaries in the body opened at the same time the capillary circulation could contain two to three times the circulating blood volume.

All types of shock are associated with a high level of circulating catecholamines. In the early stages this is beneficial and is responsible for maintaining the central blood pressure and allowing perfusion of privileged tissues, particularly the brain and heart. This is possible because the arterioles of muscle, skin and splanchnic beds are richly innervated with α receptors—the vessels of the brain and heart are poorly innervated with α receptors. As a result of sustained catecholamines production the peripheral resistance increases. The pressure of fluid in a closed system is equal to the flow times the resistance ($P = F \times R$). If the blood pressure is kept constant and the peripheral resistance is increased by catecholamines or sympathomimetic drugs then it follows that flow must decrease. Decreased flow of blood in the microcirculation is responsible for the invariably fatal outcome of severe shock. Modern forms of therapy aim at preventing prolonged reduction of flow to the microcirculation particularly in the splanchnic organs. It is convenient to consider the pathophysiology of shock in two stages. Stage I is the stage in which increased catecholamines production is a temporary necessity which is beneficial if it is not prolonged. Stage II is the stage in which catecholamine production is prolonged and harmful resulting in irreversible damage within the microcirculation.

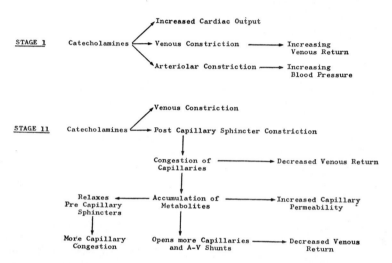

Stage I: Catecholamines result in an increase in cardiac output due to direct stimulation of the heart. This is offset later because the increased work of the heart must be carried on by anaerobic metabolism leading to local acidosis which reduces contractility (Bloch *et al.*, 1966; Aviado, 1965). Catecholamines cause constriction of the capacitance vessels (veins) which contain 80 per cent of the circulating blood volume and so they temporarily increase venous return. Catecholamines also cause differential arteriolar constriction causing preferential perfusion of privileged tissues.

Stage II: Sustained catecholamine production causes further vein constriction which now acts as an *obstruction* to further venous return. They also constrict the post-capillary sphincters leading to capillary congestion and a further fall in venous return. Capillary congestion allows the local metabolites of anaerobic metabolism to accumulate leading to:

1. Precapillary sphincter *relaxation* and more capillary congestion.
2. Opening of some of the two-thirds of capillaries which are norm-

ally closed at any one time causing further pooling of blood and direct shunting from the arterial to venous side and by-passing of the micro-circulation. These changes further decrease venous return and tissue perfusion.

3. Increased capillary permeability and loss of intravascular fluid into the extracellular compartment.

4. Further cell damage causes release of vasoactive substances (hist-amine, 5-hydroxytryptamine and other kinins) causing further pooling in the microcirculation.

In the later stages of shock, intravascular clotting probably occurs (Hardaway, 1968).

Physiological and Metabolic Disturbances of Shock

Catecholamines.—The concentration of endogenous catecholamines in the plasma increases proportionately with the degree of hypotension, leading to vasoconstriction, particularly in the splanchnic, renal and cutaneous vessels.

Blood volume.—The blood volume has been monitored during the bleeding of animals. At the stage of maximum blood loss, the volume of blood remaining in the circulation is greater than the amount calculated from the original blood volume and the amount in the reservoir. This is due to fluid passing from extracellular compartments into the circulation. Towards the end of the critical stage of four and a half hours and the beginning of the stage of irreversible shock, the blood volume falls sharply as fluid is removed from the effective circulation by pooling in the splanchnic bed. Normally only one-third of the capillary bed is open, in man. Acidosis or anoxia cause the remaining two-thirds to open, leading to a 10 to 15 per cent loss of effective circulating blood (Rush-mer, 1955). As stagnant anoxia within the microcirculation continues, ulceration causes intravascular fluid to be lost into the gut.

Plasma haemoglobin.—The stagnant anoxia causes haemolysis of the red cells and some of the liberated haemoglobin is released into the circulation, causing a rise in free plasma haemoglobin.

Blood flow.—Measurements of the blood flow in the superior mes-enteric artery indicate that during hypotension the flow is reduced to 10 per cent of normal. If the superior mesenteric artery is perfused with blood at a normal pressure in a hypotensive dog the state of irreversible shock does not occur, nor do the other metabolic and physiological disturbances. It is suggested that the hypotension of irreversible shock is due to endotoxins from Gram-negative organisms in the blood as a result of loss of gut wall resistance (Aub, 1944). However, the hypo-tension still occurs when the gut is sterilised with antibiotics and the animals are kept in a germ-free atmosphere.

On the basis that the stagnant anoxia may be exaggerated by coagulation of the blood in the microcirculation, heparin has been given. However, there is no decrease in mortality (Hardaway, 1968).

Protein metabolism.—In the early stages of hypotension, the blood urea rises, due to catabolism of muscle proteins. Later, in the stage of irreversible shock, the urea falls, due to diminished formation by the anoxic liver. Because of the liver anoxia there is loss of the ability to deaminate the amino acids, which accumulate in the plasma. The blood ammonia also rises but never to toxic levels in clinical shock.

Carbohydrate metabolism.—The blood sugar is generally elevated in clinical shock, probably because of the increase in catecholamines. In the stage of irreversible shock, hypoglycaemia occurs, partly due to reduced gluconeogenesis in the anoxic liver, and partly to increased tissue uptake of glucose.

Renal function.—Following an episode of hypotension oliguria may occur when the renal blood flow is again normal. Although total renal blood flow may be normal, the blood is shunted through the juxtamedullary glomeruli and the renal cortex becomes ischaemic (Trueta *et al.*, 1947). The volume of glomerular filtrate may be normal but there is often widespread necrosis and destruction of the renal tubules. This allows fluid to leak into the interstitial tissue of the kidneys (Oliver *et al.* 1951). There is usually metabolic acidosis in shock but occasionally in endotoxin shock there is respiratory alkalosis, probably the result of stimulation of the respiratory centre by endotoxins (Simmons *et al.*, 1960).

Viscosity and coagulation of blood.—The flow properties of blood are such that at slow rates the viscosity is 10 times that at normal flow rates. This is due to the formation of aggregates between red cells and the plasma proteins, particularly fibrogen and globulins which may be increased in shock (Merrill *et al.*, 1963; Lewis *et al.*, 1950). This increase in viscosity in the slow-moving blood will tend to increase the stagnation in the congested capillaries.

In the initial stages of shock the blood is hypercoagulable and there is increased fibrinolysis. There may be intravascular clotting within the microcirculation. However, later there is a hypocoagulation state, possibly because the clotting factors have been consumed in the capillary clotting.

Management

The treatment of shock must aim at increasing effective blood flow through the microcirculation. To this end the fundamental considerations are the ability of the heart to pump, of the arterioles to distribute to the microcirculation and of the microcirculation to distribute to the cells. Other important considerations are the flow properties of the blood, the function of the lungs and the kidneys, acid-base balance, and correction of the *cause* of the shock.

Physical Examination and Observations

1. *Assessment of pump function:*

    i Ability to pump blood forward (state of the peripheral circulation).
    ii Ability to prevent blood draining back behind the pump (central venous pressure and evidence of pulmonary oedema).
    iii Evidence of impaired function from examination of the pump itself:
        (a) Gallop rhythm.
        (b) Reversed splitting of the second sound due to left ventricular dysfunction.
        (c) Papillary muscle or valvular dysfunction.
        (d) Pericardial friction rub or tamponade.

2. *Assessment of peripheral circulation:*

    i Pulse volume and blood pressure. (It is important to note that as the arterioles are the main resistance vessels the pulse may appear of good volume in the proximal arteries without necessarily indicating adequate forward flow and tissue perfusion.)
    ii Skin colour and temperature.
    iii Speed of filling of superficial veins on the dorsum of the hands and feet. As a rule filling of veins within 5 seconds of emptying them indicates adequate tissue perfusion *of the part examined.*
    iv Skin capillary circulation. Blanching the skin should be followed by return of colour 3 seconds later if tissue perfusion is adequate.

3. *Central venous pressure.*—This is a most useful method of monitoring the venous return. It is *not* a substitute for careful clinical observation of the jugular venous pulse. Its value lies in the fact that it can be measured by the nurses at frequent intervals, and that it can be measured when the patient is flat or on a respirator. It cannot be emphasised strongly enough that the central venous pressure measures not one parameter but three, viz:

    i The ability of the pump to prevent fluid damming back.
    ii The blood volume.
    iii The tone of the veins and "size" of the microcirculation.

These three have to be assessed independently and by other means before the significance of changes in the central venous pressure is known. In general two of these factors do not change at the same time *but they may*.

4. *Urine output:*
   i Volume. An output of 50 ml/hour usually indicates adequate renal function.
   ii Colour. Dark coloured urine is not always a concentrated urine. Urochrome pigments may be excreted in severe oliguria.
   iii Concentration. Specific gravity above 1015 *usually* indicates an ability to concentrate the urine, and if associated with a low urine output indicates prerenal uraemia; however, again there are exceptions. Occasional cases of cortical necrosis and acute glomerular nephritis are associated with a urine concentration above 1015.
   iv Urine urea. A urine urea concentration above $1 \cdot 0$ g/l indicates that renal function is adequate.
   v Urine sodium. This can be misleading: complete inability to concentrate the urine is associated with a near-absence of sodium from the urine whereas severe cortical necrosis causes leakage of plasma through the kidneys and hence a urine sodium of 140 mEq (mmol)/l. As a rule a urine sodium concentration between 30–80 mEq (mmol)/l indicates adequate renal function.
   vi Urine and plasma osmolality. Urine osmolality twice that of the plasma, or over 500 osmoles per litre, indicates adequate renal function.

5. *Blood cultures* are mandatory in *all* forms of shock.

6. *Blood gases and acid-base balance.*—Most cases of shock are accompanied by a metabolic acidosis. Some cases of septicaemic shock have a respiratory alkalosis presumed to be due to stimulation of the respiratory centre by endotoxin.

7. *ECG monitoring.*

8. *Daily chest x-rays.*—It is important to note that the appearances of pulmonary oedema on the chest x-ray can be misleading. It is occasionally seen in the absence of a raised and diastolic left ventricular pressure (i.e. left ventricular failure) (Nixon and Taylor, 1968). It may take 24 hours to disappear after left ventricular failure has been reversed and it may take 24 hours to appear after left ventricular failure. Nevertheless frequent chest x-rays are essential because in some instances they are the only sign of left ventricular or left atrial failure. Portable chest x-rays may be misleading with regard to pleural fluid— large effusions can be missed if the portable is taken with the patient lying flat or nearly flat. Dilated upper lobe veins even in a portable film may be valuable pointers to pulmonary venous hypertension. Blurring

of the outline of hilar vessels may be the only sign of pulmonary oedema.

9. *Blood volume and cardiac output measurements* are not widely available. If they are they may give information which is helpful but not usually essential to the proper management of shock. It is important to note that the necessary blood volume may be 50 per cent more than the calculated normal value in patients with shock because of the widespread pooling in the microcirculation.

There are two aspects of the management of shock about which there is no disagreement, namely transfusion for haemorrhage and fluid loss, and antibiotics for septicaemia.

Intravenous fluids

Blood is the best fluid for shock due to haemorrhage. Saline or plasma are better if the haematocrit is over 55 per cent and if fluid has been lost from extensive burns or dehydration. As a rule saline is indicated if there is depletion of salt and water from extracellular fluid; solutions with a high oncotic pressure are indicated for expansion of the vascular compartment. It is important to note that in dehydration the vascular compartment is affected after the extracellular *but* when saline is given most of it passes into the extracellular compartment before the vascular compartment is expanded.

Dextrans.—Low-molecular-weight dextrans (Rheomacrodex, average molecular weight 40,000) are of special value in cardiogenic shock and in situations where the flow properties of the flood are impaired, e.g. severe dehydration, polycythaemia and slow flow rate. Rheomacrodex improves the flow properties of blood by:

1. Preventing aggregation of red cells.
2. Expanding the circulating plasma volume.
3. Reducing intravascular clotting.

For these reasons dextrans have a place in the managment of acute arterial insufficiency and Rheomacrodex is of proven value in the prophylaxis of deep vein thrombosis and pulmonary embolism (Lambie *et al.*, 1970). Because the average molecular weight of Rheomacrodex is 40,000 and the renal threshold for dextrans is around 50,000 Rheomacrodex is excreted into the urine—most of it within 6 hours; it therefore has some value as an osmotic diuretic.

Mannitol (25 per cent) should be given as early as possible in cardiogenic and septicaemic shock because of its known beneficial effect in delaying acute renal failure to which patients with septicaemia are particularly prone. Not more than 200 ml should be given if the patient does not appear dehydrated and does not pass 50 ml urine in the first hour after the infusion.

Antibiotics in Shock

Gram-negative septicaemia (endotoxin) shock should be suspected if there is a history of recent operation or urological instrumentation. Other suspicious findings are leucocytosis fever, petechiae, jaundice and cyanosis. Endotoxin shock should always be considered if there is no other obvious cause for the shock. Urine and blood cultures should be taken before treatment is started.

The most suitable antibiotics for Gram-negative septicaemia are shown in Table VII.

TABLE VII

ANTIBIOTICS IN GRAM-NEGATIVE SEPTICAEMIA

Antibiotics	Dose	Adverse Reactions
Colistin (Polymyxin E)	5 M.U. daily (400 mg)	Neuromuscular blockade Hypokalaemia Renal impairment
Gentamycin	80 mg 8-hourly I.M.	Vestibular damage Cochlear damage Neuromuscular blockade Renal damage
Kanamycin	250 mg 6-hourly	Cochlear damage Vestibular damage Neuromuscular blockade Renal damage
Carbenicillin	1 g 4-hourly	Hypersensitivity Nephrotoxicity Haemolytic anaemia } in high doses Epilepsy
Chloramphenicol	2 g daily	Marrow aplasia Optic neuritis
Tetracycline	2 g daily	Liver damage—probably only in pregnancy Renal damage if out-of-date

Attention to the Pump

In cardiogenic shock or shock accompanied by cardiac failure it is important to consider all the drugs which have an inotropic action (i.e.

improved heart muscle contractility). The important drugs are:

1. *Digoxin.*—All patients with moderately severe shock should be given digoxin but the drug should not be repeated if the blood urea is over 100 mg per cent.

2. *Isoprenaline.*—The heart contains a rich supply of β receptors which when stimulated improve myocardial contractility. Isoprenaline is an almost pure β stimulator and so as well as having an inotropic action on the heart has some vasodilator properties. It is given in a dose of 2–4 mg/ml (1–2 mg isoprenaline in 500 ml 5 per cent dextrose).

3. *Hydrocortisone* in a pharmacological dose (50–100 mg/kg body weight).

4. *Glucagon.*—As well as raising the blood sugar, glucagon stimulates the adenylcyclase enzyme system responsible for β receptor activity (Brogan *et al.*, 1969).

Attention to the Peripheral Circulation

The therapeutic spectrum in shock extends from α stimulation through β stimulation to α blockade. Stimulation of the α receptors and arteriolar, capillary and venular constriction in shock is associated with an almost 100 per cent mortality. The place of sympathomimetic drugs in the treatment of shock is now seriously questioned (*Lancet*, 1967). α Stimulation does nothing to improve the flow through the microcirculation. β Stimulation (with isoprenaline) has a mildly beneficial effect which varies in different individuals. The beneficial effects of β stimulation on the peripheral circulation are weak because most blood vessels contain more α than β receptors and also because the level of circulating catecholamines is high.

The harmful effects of an excess catecholamine drive cannot be over-emphasised.

Effects of Noradrenaline (α Stimulation) in Shock

Noradrenaline has a strong vasoconstrictor action on the blood vessels (arterioles and venules) of the kidneys, splanchnic organs and skin. There is also some vasoconstriction of the coronary, cerebral, skeletal muscle and pulmonary vessels. There is an increase in blood returning to the heart as the veins contract initially; however, as they remain contracted, venous return, and therefore cardiac output, falls.

The blood pressure is increased but the pulse pressure narrows, due to raised pressure in the arterioles; blood flow is therefore reduced. Blood pools in the capillaries, leading to local ischaemia and acidosis. More capillaries open, more fluid passes through their walls to the extravascular spaces. The viscosity of the blood increases. Under these conditions the arterioles dilate but the venules remain closed; this leads to further rise in hydrostatic pressure in the capillaries and more loss of fluid to the extravascular compartment. Some blood shunts across the capillary bed, especially in the splanchnic area, so allowing no exchange of gases or metabolites. Irreversible changes occur in the now severely ischaemic viscera (Nickerson, 1964).

A direct stimulation effect of noradrenaline on the heart is offset by the fact that there is no increase in coronary blood flow. The increased work by the heart must be carried out by anaerobic metabolism leading to local acidosis which produces contractility.

It can be seen, therefore, that when noradrenaline (or its analogues) are given in established shock, no physiological improvement occurs. Because of the largely unsuccessful result that this treatment gives, attention is now directed to drugs which block the effect of adrenaline on alpha receptors. The group includes phentolamine, tolazoline and phenoxybenzamine. Although phentolamine is used its action is short. Phenoxybenzamine is the α blocking drug of choice for use in the treatment of shock.

Phenoxybenzamine (Dibenyline)

The recommended dose in the treatment of shock is 1 mg/kg body weight, diluted in 250 to 500 ml of five per cent glucose or normal saline. It should be given over about one hour (Goodman and Gilman, 1965). The maximal effect is not reached until one hour later because metabolic activity is necessary to produce the active constituent. The alpha receptor blockage is long-lasting. The overall effect is one of vasodilatation, the coronary, pulmonary and systemic vessels being dilated. This effect is not influenced by acidosis. The vasodilatation leads to a fall in blood pressure and for this reason *these drugs must only be used when there has been adequate replacement of lost circulating blood volume*. Both the known loss of fluid and the fluid lost into the extravascular space and extracapilliary bed must be estimated. The vascular capacitance may be increased by 25 per cent of the calculated normal value for the given patient. Most workers have used measurements of the central venous pressure (CVP) to control the rate of volume of fluid replacement. *Transfusion is continued until the CVP rises to 12 cm of water.*

Though there is a fall in blood pressure with phenoxybenzamine it appears that if the total blood volume is adequate and there is dilatation of the microcirculation, a mean blood pressure of 70 mm mercury is adequate to maintain circulation of the blood and tissue perfusion.

The alpha adrenergic blockade leads to arteriolar and venular relaxation so that hydrostatic pressure in the capillaries falls and less fluid is lost to the extravascular space.

Phenoxybenzamine has other actions which are beneficial but which are generally weak, viz.:

1. Fluid tends to move from the interstitial to the vascular compartment.
2. Suppresses dysrhythmias.
3. "Anti-endotoxin effect."

In therapeutic doses it produces a slight tachycardia and sometimes pupillary constriction.

Isoprenaline

This drug is an almost pure β stimulator. The main reason for using it in clinical shock are for its beneficial inotropic stimulating effect on the myocardium. However, its β blocking properties will be beneficial on those blood vessels which are supplied with β receptors. In general it produces a slight rise in systolic pressure. It is given in doses of 2–4 μg/ml (1–2 mg/500 ml dextrose). The combination of isoprenaline and phenoxybenzamine was found to be the most effective form of treatment in dogs with experimental endotoxin shock (Vick *et al.*, 1965). This combination is also recommended for use in man (Lillehei *et al.*, 1964). Isoprenaline should always be considered in septic shock particularly if there is evidence of myocardial failure (Wosornu and Easmon, 1970).

Corticosteroids

There is general reluctance to use corticosteroids in septicaemic and cardiogenic shock on the grounds that the circulating level of endogenous glucocorticoids and mineralocorticoids is usually high in these types of shock. The increased physiological amounts of corticosteroids have three important functions:

1. They have a direct inotropic action on the myocardium, probably by facilitating the transfer of ions across cell membranes.
2. They enable the mineralocorticoids to exert their effect on the distal renal tubules and are therefore important in regulating fluid losses.
3. In physiological doses they potentiate and revive the effects of circulating catecholamines on the blood vessels. In the early stages of shock this has an important beneficial action.

In pharmacological doses of the order of 50 mg per kg of hydrocortisone corticosteroids have different, definite, but often poorly explained effects (Sambhi *et al.*, 1964). In pharmacological doses they:

1. Cause a fall in peripheral resistance (mild α blocking effect).
2. Influence the tone of veins.
3. Increase splanchnic blood flow.
4. "Protect" against the effects of bacterial endotoxin.
5. "Protect" against the effects of excess catecholamines.

Oxygen and Positive Pressure Ventilation

Positive pressure ventilation is so important in the management of shock that it is suprising that the reluctance to use it is so widespread. Hypoxia is virtually always present in clinical shock. Positive pressure respiration is the most suitable means of increasing blood Po_2 if hypoxia persists after the patient breathes 100 per cent oxygen through a properly fitted Ventimask. Pulmonary oedema is so common in all types of shock that so ready a means of diagnosing and treating as a positive pressure ventilator should be welcomed wholeheartedly by physicians. Pulmonary oedema increases the stiffness of the lungs; most positive pressure respirators deliver gas at a predetermined pressure. The volume of gas (the tidal volume) delivered at this pressure is usually 500–600 ml per cycle. If the machine creates a constant pressure any increase in stiffness of the lungs will mean that a smaller volume of gas is delivered. A check on the tidal volume should be made and recorded every 30 minutes: at a fixed pressure a fall in the tidal volume means increased resistance to flow of air into the lungs of which the commonest causes is pulmonary oedema. The fall in tidal volume is often the earliest evidence of pulmonary oedema.

Positive pressure ventilation can play an important part in treating pulmonary oedema once it has developed by:

1. Increasing intra-alveolar pressure preventing interstitial fluid entering the alveoli.

2. Reducing venous return (by increasing the amount of air in the chest and so diminishing the amount of blood which can enter).

3. Allowing fluid to be sucked out of the airways through the endotracheal tube or tracheostomy.

Hyperbaric oxygen.—Oxygen at a high pressure causes an increased solution of molecular oxygen in a physically dissolved form in the blood so that relatively more oxygen is delivered to the tissues. Hyperbaric oxgen has been used in the treatment of dogs with experimental shock. In one series, improvement only occurred if it was given early, in the less severe stage of shock (Blair *et al.*, 1965). Other workers (Young and Clark, 1965) showed a reduction in mortality in dogs with shock exposed to oxygen at two atmospheres pressure. However, only 50 per cent of the extra oxygen was utilised.

Depression of cardiac output has been shown to occur at increased tensions of inspired oxygen; vasoconstriction is also seen. These effects offset the improvement in oxygenation of the tissues and hyperbaric oxygen probably is not indicated in the treatment of shock in man.

Correction of Acidosis

The administration of 8·4 per cent sodium bicarbonate which contains

1 mEq (mmol)/ml is a convenient way of combating excess metabolic acidosis in shock. Correction of acidosis is usually not possible until shock has been reversed by other methods. It is important to remember that acidosis is occasionally a cause of shock.

Heparin in Shock

There is considerable evidence that the later stages of shock are accompanied by a hypocoagulable state thought to be due to consumption of the clotting factors in widespread intravascular clotting within the microcirculation (Hardaway, 1966). Heparin may prevent this harmful intravasular clotting; it is probably also indicated as a prophylaxis against deep venous thrombosis.

The haemolytic uraemic syndrome, characterised by renal failure and micro-angiopathic haemolytic anaemia, is due to widespread intravascular clotting causing ischaemia and necrosis. Bleeding occurs and is due to consumption of coagulation factors. The renal failure is due to thrombosis of renal arterioles. The intravascular coagulation is initiated by Gram-negative endotoxin. Heparin is the only treatment which can prevent the intravascular clotting. The syndrome occurs more commonly in severe Gram-negative shock than is usually appreciated. It used to be regarded as a disease of children but examples are quite often seen in adults with severe shock.

REFERENCES

AGRESS, C. M. (1962). *Heart Bull.*, **11**, 25.
AUB, J. C. (1944). *New Engl. J. Med.*, **231**, 71.
AVIADO, D. M. (1965). *Ann. intern. Med.*, **62**, 1050.
AVIADO, D. M., and SCHMIDT, C. F. (1955). *Physiol. Rev.*, **35**, 247.
BLAIR, E., OLLODART, R., ATTAR, S., and COWLEY, R. A. (1965). *Amer. J. Surg.*, **110**, 348.
BLOCH, J. H., DIETZMAN, R. H., PIERCE, C. H., and LILLEHEI, R. C. (1966). *Brit. J. Anaesth.*, **38**, 234.
BROGAN, E., KOZONIS, M., and OVERY, D. C. (1969). *Lancet*, **1**, 482.
FRIEDBERG, C. K., (1966). *Diseases of the Heart*, 3rd edit., p. 443. Philadelphia: W. B. Saunders.
GOODMAN, L. S., and GILMAN, A. (1965). *The Pharmacological Basis of Therapeutics*, 3rd edit., p. 618. New York: Macmillan Co.
HARDAWAY, R. M. (1966). *The Syndromes of Disseminated Intravascular Coagulation*. Springfield, Ill.: Chas. C. Thomas.
HARDAWAY, R. M. (1968). *Clinical Management of Shock*. Springfield, Ill.: Chas. C. Thomas.
LAMBIE, J. M., BARBER, D. C., HALL, D. P., and MATHESON, M. A. (1970). *Brit. med. J.*, **3**, 144.
Lancet (1967). **1**, 830.

SHOCK 427

LEWIS, L. A., PAGE, I. H., and GLASSER, O. (1950). *Amer. J. Physiol.*, **161**, 101.
LILLEHEI, R. C., LONGERBEAM, J. K., BLOCH, J. H., and MANNAX, W. G. (1964). *Ann. Surg.*, **160**, 682.
MATHES, K. (1962). In *Shock: Pathogenesis and Therapy*, p. 253. Ed. Bock, K. D. Berlin: Springer-Verlag.
MERRILL, E. W., GILLILAND, E. R., COKELET, G., SHIN, H., BRITTEN, A., and WELLS, R. E. (1963). *J. appl. Physiol.*, **18**, 255.
NICKERSON, N. (1964). *Circulat. Res.*, **15**, Suppl. 2, 130.
NIXON, P. G., and TAYLOR, D. J. (1968). *Lancet*, **1**, 1230.
OLIVER, J. MacDOWELL, M., and TRACEY, A. (1951). *J. clin. Invest.*, **30**, 1307.
RIORDAN, J. F., and WALTERS, G. (1968). *Lancet*, **1**, 719.
RUSHMER, R. F. (1955). *Cardiac Diagnosis. A Physiologic Approach*, p. 59. Philadelphia: W. B. Saunders.
SAMBHI, M. P., WEIL, M. H., UDHOJI, V. N., and SHUBIN, H. (1964). In *Shock*, Ed. Hershey, S. G. Boston, Mass.: Little, Brown.
SIMMONS, D. H., NICOLOFF, J., and GUZE, L. B. (1960). *J. Amer. med. Ass.*, **174**, 2196.
SLEIGHT, P. (1964). *J. Physiol. (Lond.)*, **173**, 321.
TRUETA, J. R., BARCLAY, A. E., FRANKLIN, K. J., DANIEL, P. M., and PRITCHARD, M. M. (1947). *Studies of the Renal Circulation*, p. 126. Oxford: Blackwell Scientific.
VICK, J. A., CIUCHTA, H. P., and MANTHEI, J. H. (1965). *J. Pharmacol. exp. Ther.*, **150**, 382.
WOSORNU, J. L., and EASMON, C. O. (1970). *Brit. med. J.*, **1**, 723.
YOUNG, D. G., and CLARK, R. G. (1965). *Brit. J. Surg.*, **52**, 621.

DISORDERS OF MINERAL METABOLISM

Introduction

Mineral metabolism abounds with accounts which so intertwine the experimental data with the workaday clinical account that for most people the subject holds terrors which are quite unfounded.

You can be extremely competent at interpreting electrocardiograms and know almost nothing about muscle action potentials or intracellular metabolism, but you won't be much good at cardiograms if you don't know which are the PQRST waves on the electrocardiogram. Similarly in considering disorders of mineral metabolism certain facts must be remembered to make the thing intelligible.

1. Parathyroid hormone (PTH)
    i   Causes hypercalcaemia by mobilising calcium from bone
    ii Increases calcium and phosphorus reabsorption by the renal tubules
    iii Variably increases serum calcium by increasing absorption of calcium from the gut.
2. Vitamin D is absorbed from the diet (ergocalciferol) and formed in the skin (cholecalciferol). These substances are converted in the liver to 25-hydroxycholecalciferol and this is converted in the kidney to the metabolically active 1, 25-dihydroxycholecalciferol and/or the inactive metabolite 25, 26-dihydroxycholecalciferol.
3. The actions of 1, 25-dihydroxycholecalciferol are:
    i   Increased intestinal absorption of calcium
    ii Promotion of mineralisation of bone if mineralisation is deficient
    iii Promotion of resorption if bone mineralisation is already normal.
4. Vitamin D deficiency
    i   Causes reduced tubular reabsorption of phosphorus which returns to normal when normal doses of vitamin D are given *but* overdose with vitamin D does not cause excessive tubular reabsorption of phosphorus.
    ii Causes a myopathy
    iii Prevents the action of PTH on bone and gut.
5. Deficiency of PTH causes the effects of vitamin D deficiency because PTH is necessary for the conversion of vitamin D into its active metabolite 1, 25-dihydroxycholecalciferol.

Clinically the two commonest disorders of mineral metabolism encountered in adult general medicine are firstly an accidental finding of hypercalcaemia and secondly bone disease due to renal failure.

HYPERCALCAEMIA

The total serum calcium consists of three components: ionised calcium, protein-bound calcium and citrated calcium. It is the ionised calcium which is altered by Vitamin D and PTH. If the sources of error in estimating and interpreting levels of serum calcium are borne in mind the normal range of serum calcium is 8·9–10·3 mg/100 ml (2·2–2·6 mol/l). A number of factors influence the serum calcium other than changes due to bone disease.

Factors causing an increase in serum calcium:

1. Recent meal
2. Upright posture and exercise
3. Venous occlusion
4. Increase in plasma proteins particularly the serum albumin

Factors causing a decrease in serum calcium:

1. Recumbency
2. Precipitation of the proteins in the blood sample (e.g. by delay in performing the calcium estimations). For practical purposes therefore *if* the sample reaches the laboratory reasonably quickly and the serum calcium is reported as being in the normal range (particularly if it is at the lower end), one can be pretty certain that hypercalcaemia is not present.

So far as the serum phosphorus is concerned the levels are high in childhood, in renal failure and sometimes when bone is being rapidly destroyed. The symptoms and signs of hypercalcaemia are not often the presenting feature—it is no truism to say that the commonest presenting sign of hypercalcaemia is a raised serum calcium. The serum levels of phosphorus are otherwise of remarkably little value in adults except in rare instances of hypophosphataemic osteomalacia (see p. 442).

The only true physical sign of hypercalcaemia is corneal calcification which usually needs to be looked for very carefully and is often difficult to distinguish from arcus senilis—it is usually a thin band, best seen on the medial side and is separated from the conjunctiva by a clear band of cornea. However, if arcus is also present this clear band of normal cornea may not be present. The symptoms of hypercalcaemia are non-specific but certain of the symptoms are caused by the complications of hypercalcaemia e.g. hypertension, peptic ulceration, pancreatitis and renal calculi. Hypercalcaemia itself may cause polyuria, constipation, skin itching, headache, depression, generalised muscle weakness and almost any psychiatric disturbance.

The causes of hypercalcaemia are:

1. Osteolytic bone metastases
2. Non-metastatic bone resorption
   i Due to tumours producing a PTH-like polypeptide
   ii Due to production of vitamin D-like sterol by tumours
3. Hyperparathyroidism
4. Vitamin D ingestion
5. Paget's disease
6. Sarcoidosis
7. Thyrotoxicosis
8. Immobility
9. Addison's disease
10. Thiazide diuretics

Sorting out the Cause of Hypercalcaemia

1. The first step is to confirm that hypercalcaemia is in fact present by repeating the blood sample, taking all the correct precautions and using the correction factors for plasma protein levels and blood specific gravity.

2. A raised alkaline phosphatase will generally confirm that hypercalcaemia is probably present and that the hypercalcaemia is arising from bone destruction (thus usually excluding sarcoidosis, excess vitamin D ingestion, Addison's disease and diuretic ingestion). The level of alkaline phosphatase tends to be higher in hyperparathyroidism with predominantly bone involvement and less raised with renal involvement.

3. Estimation of the serum phosphorus contributes almost nothing. If persistently low it favours (but does not indicate) the diagnosis of hyperparathyroidism.

4. Skeletal radiology should come next. The purist will start only with the x-ray of the hands and skull. If subperiostial erosions of the distal phalanges and/or fragmentation of the cortices and a "pepperpot" skull are present the diagnosis of hyperparathyroidism is definite. In hyperparathyroidism more extensive skeletal radiology may reveal single or multiple lesions of osteitis fibrosa cystica or subperiostial erosions affecting the outer third of the clavicles, inner side of the neck of the femur or inner aspect of the upper tibia.

If hyperparathyroidism is not the cause of the hypercalcaemia skeletal radiology may reveal osteolytic bone secondaries, myeloma, reticulosis or leukaemia. If none of these is present radiologically and no other cause of hypercalcaemia is found a radio-isotope bone scan may reveal metastatic bone lesions which were not seen on the skeletal x-rays.

If sarcoidosis is present the gamma globulins should be raised and routine chest x-rays may show hilar adenopathy or parenchymal lung lesions. In sarcoidosis, bone lesions may be seen in the x-rays of the hands. If by this time sarcoidosis is seriously possible as the cause of hypercalcaemia a Kveim test should be performed.

5. By this stage the majority of cases of hypercalcaemia will have an established cause—however some will not. At this stage go back and take the history again particularly for ingestion of any tablets or tonics containing any form of vitamin D and also check the thyroid function and adrenal function.

6. If you are still struggling and by this time the problem is almost invariably:

    (a) Is it hyperparathyroidism? or

    (b) Is it a primary carcinoma with non-metastatic hypercalcaemia?

The next step is the *standard* hydrocortisone test. Hydrocortisone in a dose of 40 mg t.d.s. for 10 days will not affect the serum calcium levels in hyperparathyroidism but will reduce the serum calcium levels in other causes of hypercalcaemia. The *only exceptions* to this rule have been patients with hyperparathyroidism or metastatic bone lesions in whom the bony lesions have been diagnostic on the x-rays.

7. Estimation of the serum parathyroid hormone is available but should not usually be necessary to establish the cause of the hypercalcaemia. In a really difficult case it will be helpful but it is important to realise that PTH is measured by radio-immunoassay and that the immunologically active part of the polypeptide is not the same as the biologically active part. Further, some tumours produce a PTH-like hormone which, if present, will not distinguish between hyperparathyroidism and hypercalcaemia due to non-metastatic malignant disease which is producing an immunologically similar although not biologically identical polypeptide.

The main use of assaying the PTH level is to locate the site and side of the presumed parathyroid adenoma, having established that the cause of the hypercalcaemia is hyperparathyroidism.

HYPERPARATHYROIDISM

Primary hyperparathyroidism refers to excessive output of parathyroid hormone arising from spontaneously occurring parathyroid adenoma or hyperplasia. Secondary hyperparathyroidism refers to an excessive output of parathyroid hormone but the increased output is stimulated by a low level of serum calcium. Tertiary hyperparathyroidism refers to those cases of secondary hyperparathyroidism which go on to adenoma formation and uncontrolled and autonomous release of parathyroid hormone.

The majority of cases of primary hyperparathyroidism are due to a single adenoma although in about 5 per cent of cases there are two adenomas and in about the same number the affected parathyroid gland is situated in the mediastinum. For this reason it is sensible before exploring the neck to obtain venous samples by means of selective venous catheterisation of the innominate and jugular veins draining different parts of the lower neck, to measure the parathyroid hormone levels, so that the site of excess hormone production can be found. Selective venous catheterisation and sampling may not be necessary for first explorations of the neck, but in re-explorations it is mandatory. Re-exploration may be necessary if the hypercalcaemia is not cured by removal of an adenoma or if hypercalcaemia recurs.

Occasionally hyperparathyroidism is of familial origin or associated with multiple endocrine gland neoplasia. There are two types of multiple gland neoplasia:

Type 1 consists of adenomas of parathyroid, pituitary and pancreas glands

Type 2 consists of parathyroid adenoma, phaeochromocytoma, medullary thyroid carcinoma and Cushing's disease. This type is sometimes inherited as an autosomal dominant.

Patients with hyperparathyroidism are more likely to have renal stones than they are to have osteitis fibrosa but it is extremely unusual for the two to occur together in the same patient. The reason for this is quite unknown. Paradoxically patients who have osteitis fibrosa are likely to have a greater impairment of renal function than those with renal calculi because they often have nephrocalcinosis (but not renal stones).

Hyperparathyroidism accounts for about 5 per cent of renal calculi and about 15 per cent of recurrent calculi.

There are a few additional points which on occasions may be useful in the diagnosis of hyperparathyroidism.

(a) Phosphorus deprivation (with aluminium hydroxide) *sometimes* causes a rise in serum calcium in hyperparathyroidism especially if the routine calcium levels have been only equivocally raised.

(b) Patients with hyperparathyroidism have an aminoaciduria and sometimes a myopathy.

(c) Hydroxyproline excretion is increased but usually only if there is obvious bone involvement.

(d) Hyperparathyroidism causes a hyperchloraemic acidosis by decreasing the ability of the renal tubules to excrete hydrogen ion. The plasma chloride is therefore often marginally raised.

(e) The requirement for vitamin D is increased in hyperparathyroidism. Vitamin D given in the presence of hyperparathyroidism may re-mineralise the bones. Excessive rise in serum calcium can be prevented with a low-calcium diet and high phosphorus intake. It is usually worth doing this only if there is extensive pre-operative bone disease. This relative vitamin D deficiency in hyperparathyroidism is probably responsible for the occasional x-ray and histological appearance of osteomalacia in hyperparathyroidism.

Following parathyroidectomy the following points should be borne in mind (Dent, 1962):

1. The patient should be warned that symptoms of hypocalcaemia may occur and particularly that depression may occur after the operation.

2. Hypocalcaemia is worse when there is severe bone involvement pre-operatively.

3. The lowest calcium levels occur 4–10 days after operation. Tetany may precede hypocalcaemia.

4. The presence of hypocalcaemia should always be confirmed before treatment is started.

5. If hypocalcaemia occurs and provided that renal function is normal 20 ml of 20 per cent calcium gluconate should be given by *slow* intravenous injection daily.

6. If bone disease is severe pre-operatively vitamin D (2·0 mg/day) should be given for 2 months and then stopped. Vitamin D is not necessary if the hypocalcaemia is not causing symptoms.

7. The serum calcium and phosphorus levels should be followed twice weekly for the first 6 weeks. A return of serum calcium to pre-operative levels suggests that some tumour has been left behind. A rise in serum phosphorus means either hypoparathyroidism or the development of renal failure.

8. Alkaline phosphatase levels should also be monitored. A return to normal levels means that vitamin D can be stopped.

9. If tetany occurs and the serum calcium is normal the tetany is probably due to hypomagnesaemia. This is particularly likely if there is extensive bone disease.

URAEMIC BONE DISEASE (URAEMIC OSTEODYSTROPHY)

There are four principal manifestations of bone disease in chronic glomerular failure:

1. Osteomalacia, or rickets in children (bone pain and myopathy)
2. Osteitis fibrosa
3. Soft tissue calcification and osteosclerosis
4. Osteoporosis

TABLE VIII

MECHANISMS CAUSING THE CLINICAL MANIFESTATIONS OF CHRONIC RENAL FAILURE

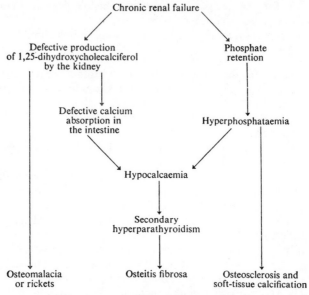

(By courtesy of Dr C. R. Patterson)

Table VIII shows the main mechanisms involved in the pathogenesis of these manifestations.

With progressive renal damage there is failure of the kidneys to convert circulating 25-hydroxycholecalciferol into the more active 1, 25-dihydroxycholecalciferol leading effectively to a deficiency of vitamin D and osteomalacia which can only be corrected by giving very large doses of vitamin D, hence the term "vitamin D resistance". Phosphorus retention in glomerular failure leads to hyperphosphataemia and hypocalcaemia and hence secondary hyperparathyroidism. The hyperphosphataemia may encourage excessive precipitation of calcium phosphate in soft tissues (leading to ectopic calcification) or in the bones (leading to osteosclerosis). Secondary hyperparathyroidism will lead to osteitis fibrosa and an autonomous adenoma may develop leading to tertiary hyperparathyroidism. The acidosis of renal failure also contributes to osteomalacia.

Following regular haemodialysis some patients develop osteoporosis. The incidence of this varies considerably and was particularly high in Newcastle and is sometimes known as Newcastle bone disease.

Management

Osteomalacia.—The main features are severe bone pain and muscle weakness (myopathy). Most patients with renal failure have hyperphosphataemia as well as malabsorption of calcium; the hyperphosphataemia is controlled with oral aluminium hydroxide (up to 20g/day) and the malabsorption of calcium, bone lesions and myopathy are treated with large doses of vitamin D. The two main problems with the administration of vitamin D are firstly that the effective dose may be variable even in the same patient and secondly that ectopic calcification may occur. It is therefore necessary to monitor the serum calcium and alkaline phosphatase levels frequently as well as the bone x-rays. Treatment is not necessary once the bone lesions and myopathy have healed. Vitamin D should be stopped if the serum calcium level rises to within the normal range. The serum alkaline phosphatase level should fall on treatment but the treatment should stop before the alkaline phosphatase reaches the normal range otherwise overdosage with vitamin D will occur—this may lead to renal calcification (nephrocalcinosis) which will worsen the renal failure and it may also lead to ectopic soft tissue calcification. It is customary to start treatment with 1·25 mg vitamin D_2 daily. Improvement in the myopathy and appetite occur early, the relief of bone pain and healing of osteomalacia take several weeks. The bone changes of any secondary hyperparathyroidism take several months to heal even on adequate doses of vitamin D. Vitamin D therapy should be *stopped immediately* if the serum calcium rises above 10·8 mg per cent, if anorexia, nausea or vomiting occur or if there is an unexplained rise in the blood urea. Once the myopathy and osteomalacia have healed it is customary to leave patients on a small dose of vitamin D (0·5 mg daily). It should be noted that the half-life of administered vitamin D in renal failure may be as much as six months. The administration of shorter-acting metabolites of vitamin D obviously has advantages over vitamin D itself.

Opinion is divided on the value of calcium supplements. Calcium absorption can be increased with oral calcium supplements and also a rise in serum phosphate may be prevented. However metastatic calcification can occur if the serum calcium phosphorus product is over 70.

Uraemic hyperparathyroidism is less common than osteomalacia and more difficult to treat. The secondary hyperparathyroidism may respond slowly to aluminium hydroxide, vitamin D therapy and if necessary haemodialysis with an adequate calcium concentration in the dialysate. However if osteitis fibrosa cystica and the radiological features of hyperparathyroidism in the fingers are severe or persistent or if metastatic calcification is increasing parathyroidectomy is indicated. Occasionally tertiary (autonomous secondary hyperparathyroidism) develops and this too should be treated with parathyroidectomy. Following parathyroidectomy in renal failure large doses of vitamin D are usually required.

OSTEOMALACIA AND RICKETS

Osteomalacia (adults) and rickets (children) occur when there is effectively a deficiency of vitamin D. Vitamin D is essential for the calcification of bone osteoid and the calcification of cartilage in growing bones. The causes of vitamin D deficiency are:

1. Inadequate dietary content.
2. Inadequate sunlight.
3. Malabsorption:
   Partial gastrectomy;
   Pancreatic disease;
   Biliary obstruction;
   Intestinal malabsorption.
4. Defective production of active metabolites of vitamin D:
   Renal failure;
   Liver disease;
   Anticonvulsant therapy.
5. "Resistance" to vitamin D due to renal tubular disorders:
   Generalised tubular damage (Fanconi syndrome);
   Isolated tubular defects;
   Renal tubular acidosis.

Biochemically osteomalacia and rickets are characterised by a low serum calcium and usually in adults a low phosphorus and a raised alkaline phosphatase. Urine calcium and phosphorus excretion are also correspondingly low. Radiologically the effects of rickets are seen on the growing parts of the long bones, i.e. the epiphyses; these are widened, the ends of the long bones are irregular (tufted) and also widened (splayed). These changes are due to the growing cartilage failing to become calcified. The increased cartilage at the epiphyses causes the swellings which may be seen at the ends of the ribs (rickety rosary). The skull may also be affected, being softer than normal and therefore misshapen. The associated vitamin D deficient myopathy may prevent the child's moving its head so that one particular part of the skull becomes flattened. The persistence of rickets during childhood causes the weight-bearing bones to become deformed causing either knock or bowed knees. Occasionally patients with rickets and osteomalacia get tetany but this is not common.

The radiological features of osteomalacia are the pathognomonic pseudo fractures and Looser's zones which are usually seen in characteristic sites e.g. neck of femur, upper ends of tibia, pubic ramus or clavicles. In the spine osteomalacia causes all the vertebrae to be soft and hence the intervertebral discs can push into the vertebrae, especially at their centres, causing the "codfish" spine. Osteoporosis tends to be patchy and causes individual vertebrae to collapse or become wedge-shaped. Sometimes osteomalacia is superimposed on osteoporosis e.g. in malabsorption or in liver disease.

Nutritional Rickets and Osteomalacia

There has to be a deficiency both of vitamin D in the diet and inadequate synthesis of vitamin D in the skin for nutritional rickets to occur. The condition is probably more frequent in Britain than is generally appreciated. It occurs particularly in immigrants in whom skin pigmentation or seclusion may prevent adequate exposure to what little sun there is. This is aggravated by the fact that many immigrants habitually eat food which is deficient in the vitamin. Nutritional vitamin D deficiency is also seen in the elderly in whom the skin becomes less effective in synthesising vitamin D. It may well be that subclinical osteomalacia is an important factor in the pathogenesis of fractures in the elderly.

Malabsorption of Vitamin D

Most vitamin D is absorbed in the duodenum so malabsorption is particularly likely if the duodenum has been by-passed. Bile salts are necessary for vitamin D absorption so that malabsorption of vitamin D is likely after prolonged biliary stasis or in the stagnant loop situation where bile salts are excessively deconjugated.

Defective Production of the Metabolites of Vitamin D (see p. 436)

Vitamin D Resistance (see p. 373)

OSTEOPOROSIS

Osteoporosis refers to the condition in which the collagen matrix of bone is reduced while the size of the bone remains normal. Along with a reduction in collagen there is also a reduction in the amount of bone salt. The biochemical structure of the bone matrix collagen and poly-saccharides in osteoporosis are probably normal.

There are three principal types of osteoporosis:

1. Senile.
2. Idiopathic juvenile.
3. Secondary.

With increasing age there is a generalised reduction in bone collagen and hence an increased incidence of osteoporosis. However, there is a group of patients who appear to have an accelerated and even localised form of the disease. In both forms the main symptoms are bone fractures, bone pain and loss of height. In the absence of these symptoms, which occur relatively late in the progression of the disease, the real problem lies in detecting the disorder before it has caused symptoms, particularly because at least 50 per cent of the bone mass must be lost before there is any demonstrable change in the density of the bones on x-ray.

There are available methods of refining the detection of osteoporosis in a preclinical stage although there is yet no convincing evidence that any useful purpose is served by large-scale screening programmes to detect the asymptomatic disease.

Methods of detecting preclinical osteoporosis:

1. Presence of unsuspected crush fractures of vertebrae (these are not always painful).

2. Thinning and reduction in trabecular pattern of bones—usually the vertebrae and femoral necks are the most common sites.

3. Sophisticated bone densitometry using known standards of bone density.

4. Cortical thickness indices; there is always a reduction in the cortical thickness of the bones in osteoporosis but this is not always easy to measure and is complicated by the fact that the cortical thickness depends on the height of the patient (and therefore the length of the long bones). Nevertheless there are available percentile charts for indices of cortical thickness related to the length of the bone which indicate whether at a given age the cortical thickness index falls within the normal range. The two commonest sites for measuring the cortical thickness are the right second metacarpal and the mid-point of the femur. There are other indices which measure the biconcavity of the vertebrae by comparing the height of the outside of the lumbar vertebrae with the height of the centre of the bone.

5. Bone biopsy.

It is usually part of the definition of osteoporosis that there are no detectable biochemical abnormalities such as abnormal serum calcium, phosphorus or alkaline phosphatase levels or urinary levels of calcium or hydroxyproline. By and large this is true, but it is most important to remember that a recent fracture (even asymptomatic crush fracture) may cause a rise in serum alkaline phosphatase which may remain elevated until the fracture heals; also immobilisation (such as may occur with severe pain or fracture) may cause a negative calcium balance so that 24-hour urinary calcium excretion may appear to be abnormally high. Calcium absorption may be reduced in juvenile idiopathic osteoporosis and there is a statistical tendency in a series of women for the serum calcium and the 24-hour urinary calcium to be higher after the menopause compared with pre-menopausal levels. There is now convincing evidence that in women senile osteoporosis begins at around the age of the menopause. Administered oestrogens can reduce the serum levels and urinary calcium excretion and delay the onset of osteoporosis. In tissue culture oestrogens block the action of parathyroid hormone on bone and also post-menopausal osteo-porosis is rare in hypoparathyroidism. These pieces of evidence suggest that post-menopausal osteoporosis is at least partially due to the increased action of parathyroid hormone on bone due to the absence of the protective effect of gonadal hormones. Nordin suggests that after the menopause most of the bone resorption occurs at night because calcium levels tend to fall at night and so slightly stimulate the para-thyroids. It is also suggested that in the elderly, minor and undetectable states of subclinical vitamin D deficiency are common and that conver-sion of vitamin D to its active metabolites may also be impaired in old age.

Other factors in the pathogenesis of osteoporosis may be fluoride deficiency and a high-protein diet which produces a mild acidosis that is partly buffered by bone minerals which are thereby depleted.

Management of Osteoporosis

One important rule in the management of osteoporosis is to avoid immobilisation and bed rest even if pain is quite severe. In the acute juvenile form of osteoporosis the symptoms and probably the whole disease process are episodic. Careful and continuous follow-up of cases of osteoporosis are necessary to detect the exacerbations.

All cases of symptomatic osteoporosis should have a series of 24-hour urinary calcium levels done and if there is evidence of excessive calcium excretion it is reasonable to try to reduce calcium excretion with a thiazide diuretic and phosphorus supplement. If urine calcium excretion is low it is reasonable to try to increase calcium absorption from the gut by giving a calcium supplement and small dose of vitamin D (0·25 mg/day, i.e. 10,000 iu). Once the urine calcium excretion has either risen to or fallen to the normal range it is probably wise to stop after about 3 months any calcium or phosphorus supplements and any vitamin D. It is now orthodox to prescribe oestrogens to women with post-menopausal osteoporosis and testosterone to men with senile osteoporosis.

Secondary Osteoporosis

It should not be forgotten that like hypertension the secondary causes of osteoporosis must be looked for because, although rare, most of them are treatable.

Causes of secondary osteoporosis:

1. Partial gastrectomy.
2. Malabsorption.
3. Cushing's disease.
4. Hypogonadism.
5. Acromegaly.
6. Hyperthyroidism.
7. Liver disease.
8. Scurvy.
9. Mast cell disease (urticaria pigmentosa).

HYPOCALCAEMIA

The main symptom of hypocalcaemia is tetany. The level of total calcium at which tetany occurs is extremely variable—some individuals can tolerate only a small fall in serum calcium; in others a much larger fall occurs before tetany develops. The development of tetany depends on the level of ionised calcium.

Hypocalcaemia may produce a wide variety of clinical features which include papilloedema and benign intracranial hypertension, epilepsy, "asthma" (due to laryngeal stridor), dementia, depression, dry skin, psoriasis, "pins and needles", constipation and moniliasis.

The main causes of hypocalcaemia are:

1. Hypoparathyroidism.
2. Vitamin D deficiency (nutritional or malabsorption).
3. Uraemic bone disease.
4. Acute pancreatitis.
5. Alkalosis.
6. Renal tubular disorders and relative resistance to vitamin D.
7. Hypomagnesaemia.
8. Anticonvulsant therapy.
9. Obstructive jaundice.
10. Medullary carcinoma of the thyroid.

HYPOPARATHYROIDISM

In hypoparathyroidism there is deficient secretion of parathyroid hormone which leads to hypocalcaemia and a raised serum phosphorus. Idiopathic hypoparathyroidism may be associated with pernicious anaemia, Addison's disease and malabsorption. Moniliasis appears most frequently in this variety of hypoparathyroidism.

A proportion of patients with idiopathic hypoparathyroidism have skeletal abnormalities which are not related to the hypocalcaemia, e.g. irregular length of the fingers, soft tissue calcification, short stature and tooth defects. These patients also have the biochemical abnormalities of hypoparathyroidism which however do not respond to injected parathyroid hormone; there is considered to be "end-organ resistance" to parathyroid hormone. This condition is called pseudohypoparathyroidism. A small number of patients have the same skeletal abnormalities without the biochemical disturbances—these patients are said to have pseudo pseudohypoparathyroidism. These conditions associated with skeletal abnormalities are much more frequently inherited than is idiopathic hypoparathyroidism.

The incidence of secondary hypoparathyroidism following thyroid surgery is low, but the reported incidences vary very much and several reputable authors have quoted incidences of up to 50 per cent—to some extent the incidence will depend on the criteria for hypoparathyroidism and the methods of assessment. Hypoparathyroidism has also been described following radioactive iodine therapy for hyperthyroidism. The treatment of hypoparathyroidism should be with dihydrotachysterol (DHT) which is an analogue of vitamin D and requires hydroxylation in the liver, but not in the kidney. It is suggested that calcium supplements may also increase the serum calcium in some patients with hypoparathyroidism and they are worth trying in an individual patient. DHT has the great advantage over vitamin D that it is much shorter-acting so that when stopped the toxic effects wear off much sooner.

RENAL TUBULAR DISORDERS

Disordered function of the renal tubules is commoner than is generally appreciated. Nearly all forms of acute or chronic renal damage produce impairment of tubular functions the most familiar being failure of water reabsorption in pyelitis and failure of sodium and chloride reabsorption in chronic renal failure. The functional defects associated with damage to the tubules will obviously relate to the normal functions of the tubules which are:

1. Reabsorption of calcium and phosphorus.
2. Reabsorption of glucose.
3. Reabsorption of some amino acids.
4. Excretion of potassium.
5. Excretion of hydrogen ion as ammonia, carbonic acid and dihydrogen sodium phosphate.

It follows that the features of renal tubular disorders will be related to any of the following:

1. Hypocalcaemia and hypophosphataemia.
2. Glycosuria.

3. Aminoaciduria.
4. Hypokalaemia.
5. Retention of hydrogen ion (acidosis).

Some of the tubular disorders are due to widespread damage from a toxic substance, either endogenous or exogenous. When tubular damage is due to a toxin all tubular functions are likely to be impaired although often to a varying degree. Isolated or single disorders of tubular function occur usually as a hereditary disorder which affects only one or only a few of the enzymes involved in the transporting of a substance normally reabsorbed or excreted. The name "Fanconi Syndrome" is applied to the *generalised* disorders of tubular function; in the Fanconi syndrome there is a generalised aminoaciduria because most or all the transport enzymes will be affected. Other forms of aminoaciduria occur either because there is an overproduction and hence high blood levels of an amino acid, e.g. phenylalanine, or because there is an isolated defect of one enzyme system responsible for reabsorption of one amino acid (e.g. cystinuria).

Causes of Fanconi Syndrome

1. Cystinosis.
2. Wilson's disease.
3. Myelomatosis.
4. Cadmium poisoning.
5. Ingestion of degraded tetracycline.
6. Glycogen storage disease.
7. Lead poisoning.
8. Neurofibromatosis and other benign fibromas of mesenchymal origin.

Besides the generalised tubular disorders there are a number of important disorders producing isolated tubular defects. The most important are:

1. Hypophosphataemic osteomalacia (excess loss of phosphorus).
2. Cystinuria (failure to reabsorb cystine and certain related amino acids).
3. Renal tubular acidosis (failure to excrete hydrogen ion).

HYPOPHOSPHATAEMIC OSTEOMALACIA

This condition occurs in two forms—one presents in childhood and is inherited, the other occurs in adult life and is sporadic. The inheritance of the childhood type is unusual in that it is inherited as a X-linked dominant which means that a female patient may pass the disease to half her sons and half her daughters and that a male patient may pass the disease to all his daughters but none of his sons. Males tend to have the disease more severely than females. A male patient must have inherited the conditions from his mother. A female patient is theoretically twice as likely to have inherited from her father as from her mother. The childhood form of the disease may remit spontaneously and re-occur later in life; however when this happens the stigmata of childhood rickets are always present. There are other differences between the sporadic adult type and the inherited childhood type (Dent and Stamp, 1971); for example, in the adult type the vertebrae appear to be much more severely affected by the osteomalacia, the myopathy is much more severe and frequently there is glycinuria. It is an important distinction because the adult type requires large doses of phosphate in addition to vitamin D whereas the childhood type does not require phosphate supplements.

The relative phosphaturia and hypophosphataemia result in rickets or osteomalacia. Unlike nutritional rickets in which there is nearly always radiological evidence of healing followed by relapses, the rickets of hypophosphataemia is constant. The disease usually remits in the teens although hypophosphataemia remains. Other members of the family may have hypophosphataemia or mildly raised alkaline phosphatase without having any other stigmata of the disease.

Cystinuria (see section on Renal Calculi, p. 448)

RENAL TUBULAR ACIDOSIS (RTA)

RTA is a cause of osteomalacia as well as causing renal calculi and nephrocalcinosis. The basic defect is an inability to excrete hydrogen ion. There is a tendency to excrete potassium instead of hydrogen ion which leads to hypokalaemia and muscle weakness. The rickets and osteomalacia are probably due to a combination of hypophosphataemia, acidosis and hypercalciuria which leads to hypocalcaemia and secondary hyperparathyroidism. This tends to cause phosphaturia in addition to the inherent tubular defect of phosphorus reabsorption.

Diagnosis of RTA

The condition should be considered in all cases of acidosis, nephrocalcinosis, renal calculi, hypokalaemia and osteomalacia. In the severe form there will be acidosis in the presence of alkaline urine; however the commonest variety ("incomplete RTA") does not have an acidosis unless the patient is given an acid load. This form can be detected by the short acid load test of Wrong and Davies (1959).

Varieties of RTA

The body, as a result of metabolism, produces about 2000 mEq per day of hydrogen ion. Most of this is excreted by forming carbonic acid which then forms CO_2 and water and is eliminated by the lungs. However about 70 mEq/day of hydrogen is excreted by the kidneys. This happens in three ways:

1. Formation of $NaH_2 Po_4$ from Na_2HPo_4.
2. Formation of HCO_3 some of which is excreted and some re-absorbed.
3. Formation of ammonia (NH_3).

The formation of ammonia is relatively fixed and is small at a urine pH around 7·4; it is higher at a lower urine pH. Around pH 6·5–7·4 hydrogen is predominantly excreted as phosphate; above 7·4 hydrogen ion is excreted mainly as bicarbonate. At lower urine pH there is little or no bicarbonate in the urine.

There are three ways in which the body may fail to eliminate hydrogen ion and in which the urine will be inappropriately alkaline when it should be acid.

1. Hydrogen ion release by tubular cells may be limited by the relative concentration of hydrogen ion in the cells and tubular lumen ("gradient failure").

2. Hydrogen ion release from tubular cells may be too slow ("rate failure").

3. Ammonia production may be reduced (in this type the urine may be acid but ammonia production at lower urine pH is reduced. Normally at low urine pH ammonia production is high). This type is diagnosed by finding a low urine ammonium.

Hydrogen ion *gradient* failure is known as Type I RTA; this disorder affects mainly the distal renal tubule. In this type the urine pH is fixed (because of the failure of hydrogen ion excretion), there is acidosis and hence a low plasma bicarbonate. However if the plasma bicarbonate is raised by infusion of bicarbonate the pH of the urine will rise, i.e. become more alkaline as more bicarbonate passes into the urine.

Hydrogen ion *rate* failure affects mainly the proximal tubule and the rate of hydrogen ion production is so slow that bicarbonate in the tubule is not neutralised and consequently is "wasted" and lost from the body. The urine pH is therefore high (alkaline) because it contains an excess of bicarbonate. However if the body is made very acidotic so that plasma bicarbonate falls and production of bicarbonate by the proximal tubule also falls, no excess bicarbonate appears in the urine; thus at very low plasma pH levels the urine can be acidified in the Proximal type of RTA whereas in the Distal type of RTA the urine cannot be acidified no matter how severe the acidosis. Also in the Proximal type of RTA more bicarbonate than should appears in the urine at all levels of plasma bicarbonate, i.e. hydrogen ion *rate* failure RTA is synonymous with "bicarbonate wastage".

Congenital RTA is generally Type I. It is commoner in women and presents in childhood with rickets, nephrocalcinosis, renal calculi, hypokalaemia and muscle weakness.

Acquired RTA is generally a mixture of Types I and II although occasionally it is Type II only. The causes of acquired RTA are:

1. Renal calculi.
2. Pyelonephritis.
3. Myeloma.
4. Hypergammaglobulinaemia.
5. Heavy-metal poisoning.
6. Outdated tetracycline.
7. Amphotericin B nephropathy.

The main complications of RTA are:

1. Osteomalacia (due to phosphaturia and hypophosphataemia, secondary hyperparathyroidism and acidosis).
2. Nephrocalcinosis or renal calculi (due to hypercalciuria, hyperphosphaturia and alkaline urine). There is a predisposition to urinary infection which may of course make the RTA worse. The renal stones which form may be triple phosphate stones (due to the urinary infection), calcium phosphate stones, or a mixture of these. In all cases of renal stone formation or nephrocalcinosis it is always worth looking for a complete or incomplete acidification defect of the urine. One of the main pitfalls in the diagnosis of incomplete RTA is the presence of urinary infection with urea-splitting organisms which produce ammonia and so may keep the urine alkaline despite adequate acidification by the tubules. It is therefore important to eliminate urinary tract infection before testing for RTA. It is also important to check plasma bicarbonate levels during the ammonium chloride acid load test to ensure that the plasma bicarbonate levels have been lowered sufficiently.

Treatment of RTA

The main treatment is with alkalis (sodium and potassium bicarbonate); this may heal the osteomalacia but usually vitamin D is required as well. The main danger of alkaline treatment is that the urine will be made more alkaline and so encourage renal infection and stone formation. The hypokalaemia and sodium depletion (if any) can be corrected with supplements.

RENAL CALCULI

Renal calculi consist either of relatively pure substances or mixtures of salts. Pure stones are generally due to a specific and recognisable disorder—unfortunately pure stones are the exception and the main problem with renal stones is to decide whether they are metabolic stones or whether they are due to infection or obstruction. The pure or metabolic stones with a rough indication of their percentage frequency of all stones are:

1. Calcium oxalate   (12 per cent).
2. Cystine   (3 per cent).
3. Uric acid   (3 per cent).

Stones which contain magnesium ammonium phosphate are almost always due to infection and most of these also contain varying amounts of calcium phosphate and calcium oxalate (triple phosphate stones). This group accounts for about 25 per cent of renal stones in this country.

The largest single group of stones (roughly a half) are those which contain a mixture of calcium phosphate and calcium oxalate. From a diagnostic point of view it is this group which provides the real problems because infection may be present coincidentally even though the stones are "metabolic" in origin. Hyperparathyroidism characteristically causes calcium phosphate (and calcium oxalate) stones although hyperparathyroidism in fact accounts for only about 5 per cent of renal calculi (about 15 per cent of recurrent calculi). A small proportion of stones consist of calcium oxalate but pure calcium phosphate stones are rare. Calcium phosphate is nearly always present either with calcium oxalate or magnesium ammonium phosphate.

Causes of Renal Calculi

Pure stones	i Uric acid
	ii Hyperoxaluria
	iii Cystinuria
Mixed stones (non-metabolic)	i Infection
	ii Obstruction
Mixed stones (metabolic)	i Hypercalciuria due to hypercalcaemia
	Hyperparathyroidism
	Vitamin D excess
	Sarcoidosis
	Immobilisation
	Milk alkali syndrome
	Carcinoma
	Hyperthyroidism

    ii Idiopathic hypercalciuria (largest single group)
   iii Renal tubular acidosis
   iv Medullary sponge kidney
    v Bowel disease (ulcerative colitis, ileostomies)

Some Factors in the Pathogenesis of Mixed Metabolic Stones

Calcium oxalate excretion in the urine is very nearly enough to cause a saturated solution so it is not surprising that any tendency to dehydration and low urine volume will produce stones consisting mainly of calcium oxalate. Calcium phosphate tends to precipitate in an alkaline solution hence calcium phosphate stones (with some calcium oxalate) will tend to occur in an alkaline urine (infection, RTA and other tubular disorders). In the absence of any obvious metabolic cause there must be other factors predisposing to renal stone formation; after all the majority of renal stones occur in the absence of any infective or metabolic cause. Other proposed mechanisms are:

1. Excess of nucleating substances. All stones contain a matrix consisting of mucoproteins—mucopolysaccharides which *in vitro* encourage precipitation of calcium salts.

2. Lack of an inhibitor to stone formation. Known inhibitors of crystal aggregation and accretion are pyrophosphate, cations (magnesium, zinc, etc) and polysaccharide inhibitor.

Uric Acid Stones

The most important factor in the formation of urate stones is an acid urine. Not all uric acid stone formers have hyperuricosuria. There appears to be a deficiency of ammonia production in many uric acid stone formers. Uric acid stones also occur in patients with leukaemia and polycythaemia particularly if there is a rapid response to anti-mitotic drugs. The treatment of uric acid stones is high fluid intake combined with alkalis (sodium bicarbonate 10g/day). At pH 7·0 uric acid is nearly 20 times as soluble as at pH5.

Xanthine stones occasionally occur particularly in the rare inborn error of metabolism xanthinuria. It is theoretically possible that the drug allopurinol which is a xanthine oxidase inhibitor could lead to xanthine stones by causing an accumulation of xanthine.

Pure Oxalate Stones

These usually occur in primary hyperoxaluria which is a rare and serious inborn error of metabolism associated with oxalate deposition in all the tissues of the body. It is usually fatal in childhood but more adult cases are being discovered.

Cystine Stones

Cystinuria is a tubular disorder in which there is a defect in reabsorption of cystine and the other related amino acids (lysine, arginine and ornithine). Cystine precipitates in an acid and concentrated urine. The treatment therefore consists of giving enough fluid (particularly at night) to keep the urine volume high. This will then prevent cystine stones forming and also dissolve any which are present. Cystine stones are not so radio-opaque as calcium-containing stones but if they are over 1 cm in diameter they can normally be seen on abdominal x-ray. The disease shows two forms of inheritance—recessive and incompletely recessive. In both forms the homozygotes have a high urinary cystine excretion whereas in the completely recessive form the heterozygotes have a normal cystine excretion and in the incompletely recessive form the heterozygotes have intermediate levels of cystine excretion. The same enzyme defect is present in the gut as in the renal tubule so that there is also a failure to absorb these amino acids from the gut.

Idiopathic Hypercalciuria

This is probably the most common single cause of metabolic renal stones and of nephrocalcinosis. Most normal people only absorb as much calcium from the diet as they need. Patients with idiopathic hypercalciuria absorb much more calcium from the diet than they need and the excess is excreted in the urine. When testing for the condition it is important to ensure that the patient is on a diet which contains enough calcium. If the dietary calcium is low even patients with idiopathic hypercalciuria may not excrete more than 300 mg calcium per 24 hours. Peaks of calcium oxalate excretion during the 24 hours are probably the initiating factors in stone formation in idiopathic hypercalciuria. The condition is much commoner in men and appears to become less frequent with increasing age. Treatment is with a low-calcium diet together with cellulose phosphate.

Renal Stones in Gut Disorders

Urate stones are liable to occur in patients with ileostomies and ulcerative colitis. All the reasons are not known but dehydration and low urine sodium excretion are partly responsible. Some patients with ileal dysfunction may form oxalate stones; this is probably because bile salts are not reabsorbed in the terminal ileum and together with the glycine to which they are conjugated they pass into the large gut where bacterial action removes the glycine which is then absorbed and excreted as oxalate. Normally bile salts are conjugated to taurine and not glycine but because of failure to reabsorb bile salts most taurine is lost from the body and the liver only has a limited ability to produce taurine.

Change in pH of the intestines also promotes glycine rather than taurine conjugation.

Management of Renal Stones

It is obviously essential that any stone or gravel passed should be examined—preferably by x-ray defraction crystallography. It may be necessary for stone formers always to pass urine through a net filter in order to have a specimen of the stone for examination. Any stone which contains triple phosphate is related to infection but whether this is primary or secondary will have to be determined. It is obviously important to measure 24-hour urine excretion of uric acid, calcium oxalate and cystine as well as amino acid chromatography of the urine. All the causes of hypercalcaemia and hypercalciuria should be excluded. Measuring the pH of the urine is important and if the urine is persistently alkaline in the absence of infection RTA should be excluded. It may also be necessary to test for other tubular disorders or evidence of tubular dysfunction; still the best screening test for tubular dysfunction is the urine concentration and dilution test.

Treatment of Mixed Metabolic Stones

1. Encourage high fluid intake.
2. Low calcium intake particularly in idiopathic hypercalciuria. It may be necessary for the patient to have a water softener. Cellulose phosphate will reduce calcium absorption and also increase urinary phosphate excretion.
3. If the stones contain a high proportion of calcium phosphate a reduced phosphate intake may be indicated. This can be achieved by giving aluminium hydroxide (Aludrox) which binds phosphorus in the gut.
4. If the stones contain a high proportion of oxalate a low-oxalate diet may be indicated.
5. Alkalis will obviously be indicated for the treatment of renal tubular acidosis and urate stones although in RTA care should be taken not to make the urine too alkaline.
6. Magnesium salts (magnesium oxide) have been found to be effective in some series.
7. Thiazide diuretics reduce urinary calcium excretion.

Nephrocalcinosis

This tends to be either cortical or medullary. Cortical calcium deposition occurs following renal cortical necrosis and sometimes after glomerulonephritis. Medullary calcium deposition occurs with any of the known causes of hypercalciuria. The medullary nephrocalcinosis of medullary sponge kidney tends to be localised.

MISCELLANEOUS DISORDERS

Magnesium Metabolism

Disturbances of magnesium metabolism play a small but occasionally significant part in disturbances of mineral metabolism. This is not particularly surprising because magnesium is the most abundant intracellular cation after potassium. About half the body magnesium is in the bone where it is involved in bone crystal architecture, although it is not part of the molecular crystal structure.

Hypomagnesaemia causes tetany, muscular weakness, depression and epilepsy, all of which may also occur with hypocalcaemia. The two sometimes co-exist particularly in malabsorption syndromes and in the presence of intestinal fistulae. The hypocalcaemia may not respond to vitamin D treatment until the hypomagnesaemia has been corrected. Hypomagnesaemia is fairly common in cirrhosis, particularly alcoholic cirrhosis; all the causative factors are not known, but the secondary aldosteronism and high gut ammonia probably play a part. The excess ammonia in the gut precipitates magnesium as insoluble magnesium ammonium phosphate, preventing its absorption. The same phenomenon is seen in cattle fed on grass fertilised with ammonium fertilisers; the resulting tetany is referred to as "grass staggers".

Serum magnesium may also be reduced in renal tubular disorders although in glomerular failure hypermagnesaemia occurs. There are now several reports of low magnesium excretion in some recurrent stone formers as well as reports of beneficial results in reducing stone formation by increasing magnesium intake. Magnesium excess produces muscle weakness leading eventually to peripheral and central nervous system depression and anaesthesia. Vasodilation also occurs.

The Significance of Calcitonin

Calcitonin is a calcium-lowering hormone produced by the C cells of the thyroid gland. It is however doubtful whether calcitonin plays a major part in normal calcium homeostasis. The only known disorder of calcitonin production is excess output due to medullary carcinoma of the thyroid, but even in this condition when calcitonin levels may be several hundred times the normal range no disorder of serum or urinary calcium occurs. Medullary carcinoma of the thyroid may be a familial disorder and is sometimes associated with phaeochromocytoma and parathyroid adenoma.

The main use of calcitonin is in the treatment of Paget's disease. The indications for treatment are: bone pain, hypercalcaemia, rapidly increasing bone deformity and increasing neurological compression due to the disease. Treatment has to be given by injection and has to be continued for at least six months. It is important to monitor the effects of treatment by sequential measurements of urinary hydroxyproline, serum alkaline phosphatase and serum calcium, particularly if this was elevated originally.

Diphosphonates

Diphosphonates are compounds which resemble pyrophosphate except that they are not susceptible to the action of the phosphatase enzymes in the body. They have many of the other properties of pyrophosphate and they can become bound to bone hydroxypatite crystals; if they do, the crystals cannot be dissolved by normal phosphatase enzymes. Diphosphonates may thus inhibit bone resorption and in higher doses they also inhibit bone mineralisation. They have therefore been used in a variety of conditions including Paget's disease in which prevention of mineralisation is likely to be beneficial. As diphosphonates become generally available they are likely to find a definite role in some disorders of mineral metabolism including Paget's disease; they are effective when given by mouth.

REFERENCES

DENT, C. E. (1962). *Brit. med. J.*, **3**, 1419 and 1495.

DENT, C. E., and STAMP, T. C. (1971). *Quart. J. Med.*, **40**, 303.

NORDIN, B. E. (1973). *Metabolic Bone & Stone Disease*. Edinburgh: Churchill-Livingstone.

PATTERSON, C. R. (1974). *Metabolic Disorders of Bone*, Oxford: Blackwell Scientific Publications.

WRONG, O. W., and DAVIES, H. E. (1959). *Quart. J. Med.*, **28**, 259

INDEX

Chromate poisoning, 138
Chronic bronchitis. *See* Bronchitis
Chvostek's sign, 160
Circle of Willis, 289
Cirrhosis, classification, 210
  pathophysiology, 203
Clubbing, causes of, 148
Coarctation, 37
  rib notching in, 37
Coeliac syndrome, 176
Cold agglutinins in viral pneumonias,
  227
Collagen disorders, 241
Coma, hyperosmolar, 358
Compliance of lung, 104
Condylomata lata, 327
Congenital adrenal hyperplasia, 363
Congenital heart disease, 71
Cone, foramen magnum pressure, 288
  tentorial pressure, 288
Coombs' test, 224
  in active chronic hepatitis, 201
Conn's syndrome, 81
Cord compression, 306
Corneal reflex, loss of, 282
Coronary, arteries, anatomy, 20
  artery disease, 20, 43
Cortical blindness, 269
Corticospinal tracts, 258
Corticosteroids, and gastric
  complications, 169
  in benign intracranial hypertension,
  289
  in diabetes mellitus, 354
  in erythema multiforme, 324
  in nephrotic syndrome, 391
  in sarcoidosis, 135
  in shock, 424
  in tuberculosis, 133
Cortisol, effects of, 352
  diurnal variation, 349
Costoclavicular syndrome, 308
Costophrenic angles, 97
Cranial nerves, 272
Creatinine clearance, 375
Creatinine phosphokinase, 51
Crepitations, 95
Cretinism, 320
Crigler-Najjar syndrome, 198
Crohn's disease, 179
  comparison with ulcerative colitis,
  180
  radiological findings, 180
  treatment, 180

Crossed hemiplegia, 257
Cryoglobulins, 228
Cryptogenetic fibrosing alveolitis, 122,
  123
Cushing's syndrome, 348, 364
  in bronchial carcinoma, 140
  treatment, 350
Cutaneous manifestations of malignancy,
  350
Cystic fibrosis, respiratory
  complications, 123
Cystinosis, 373
Cystinuria, 373, 442, 448
Cytomegalic inclusion disease,
  respiratory complications, 125

Damoiseau's S-shaped line in pleural
  effusion, 100
D.C. conversion, elective, 61
Deafness, 284
  in Paget's disease, 285
Dehalogenase, 320
Dehydration, clinical signs, 402
  in renal failure, 393
Delayed sensitivity reaction, 222
Delirium, 312, 313
Dementia, presenile, 314
Dermatitis. *See* Eczema
  herpetiformis, 325
Dermatology, classification of lesions,
  318
Dermatomyositis, 246
Dermatophagoides pteronyssinus in
  extrinsic asthma, 118
Descemet's membrane, 214
Desferrioxamine in treatment of
  haemochromatosis, 214
Dexamethasone suppression test, 350
Dextrans, use of, 420
Diabetes, 353–361
  and ischaemic heart disease, 144
  and renal infection, 381
  autonomic neuropathy in, 311
  causing diarrhoea, 188
  causing ketosis, 357
  causing nephrotic syndrome, 391
  causing neuropathies, 310
  causing pigmentation, 330
  latent, or pre-diabetes, 338
  treatment, 356
Diabetic coma, treatment of, 357
Dialysis, indications for, 397
  peritoneal, 397
Diaphragmatic hernia, 152

Renal tubular (*cont.*)
  disorders, 374, 441
  function, 372
Renogram, 81
Renin in Conn's syndrome, 81
Respiratory acidosis, 105
  causes, 107
  treatment, 107
Respiratory alkalosis, 105
  causes, 107
  treatment, 108
Respiratory centre, 106
Respiratory failure, definition, 114
Respiratory function tests, 100
Retina, 272
  central artery thrombosis, 275
  central vein thrombosis, 275
Retrobulbar neuritis, 273
  causes, 275
Retroperitoneal fibrosis, 409
  radiological appearances, 370
Reversed splitting, 12
Rheomacrodex in shock, 420
Rheumatic fever, 31
  prophylaxis, 32
  treatment, 32
Rheumatoid arthritis, 224, 236
  gold therapy, 239
  radiological findings, 234, 235
  treatment, 238
Rheumatoid factor, 224
Rhonchus, 95
Rib notching, 36
Riboflavin deficiency and skin disease, 326
Richter's hernia, 151
Rickettsiae in meningitis, 297
Rickets. *See* Osteomalacia
Riedel's lobe, 150
Riedel's thyroiditis, 341
Rinne's test, 285
Rolandic fissure, 262
Rombergism, 255
Rose-Waaler test, 236
Roth spots, in SBE, 41
Rotor syndrome, 198
"Rugger-jersey" spine, 233

Salicylate poisoning, metabolic effects, 408
  treatment, 409
Salicylates, in gastro-intestinal bleeding, 169
Sarcoidosis, 135

Sarcoidosis (*cont.*)
  cardiomyopathy, 90
  cutaneous manifestations, 326
  hypercalcaemia in, 431
  radiological findings, 234
Scabies, 324
Scalenus anterior syndrome, 308
Schilling test in malabsorption, 173
Schistosomiasis effects on liver, 202
Schmorl nodes, 233
Scintillation scan in thyroid disease, 335
Scleroderma, 149, 224, 326
  effects on heart, 90
Scrofulodermia, 328
Scurvy, cutaneous manifestations, 327
Seborrhoeic warts, 324
Secretin, 219
Seldinger technique, 30
Sengstaken tube, 205
Septicaemia, antibiotics in, 421
Serological tests for syphilis, 298
Serum lipids, 45
  in atheroma, 45
  in obstructive jaundice, 195
Serum proteins, 196
Serum sickness, 248
Shadows in chest X-rays, 98
Shock, causes, 411
  definition, 411
  management, 417
  pathophysiology, 414–416
Sick sinus syndrome, 62
Sickle-cell disease, renal infections in, 381
Sigmoidoscopy in ulcerative colitis, 182
Silicosis, 143
  radiological findings, 144
Sjögren's disease, prognosis, 238
  treatment, 238, 239
Skeletal scintiscanning, in osteomyelitis, 232
Skin, biopsy, 320
  classification of lesions, 318
  disease, 318
  histology, 319
  manifestations, of arterial insufficiency, 6
  of malignancy, 330
  of systemic disease, 325
"Sliding scale" in diabetes, 359
Smoking, and bronchial carcinoma, 138
  and peptic ulcer, 156
Sodium excretion in kidney, 390

Sore throat, 32, 33
Spastic colon, 187, 188
Spider naevi, causes of, 148
Spinal cord, anatomy, 255
blood supply, 293
Spongiosis, 320
Squint. *See* Strabismus, 279
Stabilisation of diabetes, 359
Stagnant loop syndrome, 177
Stamey's test in renal function, 81
Staphylococcal pneumonia, 123
Staphylococcal septicaemia, 123
Steatorrhoea, 172
Stein-Leventhal syndrome, 364
Steroids. *See* Corticosteroids
Stevens-Johnson syndrome, 149, 325
Still's disease, 235, 239
Stomal ulcer, 164
Strabismus, 279
Streptococcal infections, erythema
nodosum, 325
of the throat, 32
Streptomycin damage to auditory
nerve, 285
"String sign", 180
Subacute bacterial endocarditis. *See*
Bacterial endocarditis
Subarachnoid haemorrhage, 289
management, 292
Subclavian steal syndrome, 270
Subhyaloid haemorrhage, 275, 276
Sulphonylurea drugs, 356
Sydenham's chorea, 31, 303
Sylvian fissure, 262
Synalbumin, 355
Syphilis, 297
neurological manifestations, 300
serological tests, 298
Syringobulbia, 301
Syringomyelia, 301
clinical features of, 302
Systemic lupus erythematosus, 225, 246
drug-induced, 136, 248
skin lesions, 326
Systemic sclerosis, 244

Tabes dorsalis, 300
optic atrophy in, 301
Tachycardias, 58–60
treatment, 60
Takayasu's disease, 243
Temporal arteritis, 243
Temporal lobes, 268
Testicular atrophy, 207

Tetany, 440
after parathyroidectomy, 433
Thalamic syndrome, 259
Thalidomide in congenital heart disease,
71
Thiamin deficiency, cardiomyopathy in,
89
Thibierge-Weissenbach syndrome, 149,
245
Thomsen's disease. *See* Myotonia
congenita
Thrombo-angiitis obliterans. *See*
Buerger's disease
Thrombocytopenia in aspirin overdose,
409
Thrombolytic therapy, in pulmonary
embolism, 70, 127–128
in venous thrombosis, 69–70
Thyrocalcitonin, 432
Thyroid, antagonists, 342
carcinoma, 345, 346, 450
enzyme defects, 342
function tests, 333
gland, physiology, 332
Thyroidectomy complications, 339
Thyroiditis. *See* Hashimoto's disease
Thyrotoxicosis, classification, 336
confirmation of, 335
signs and symptoms, 336
treatment, 338
Thyroxine, 332
Tidal volume, 100
Tietze syndrome, 4
Tinker's disease, 332
Tonicity, 401
Toxoplasmosis, myocarditis in, 87
Tractus solitarius, 258
Transferrin, 213
Transient ischaemic attacks,
management, 271
Trasylol in pancreatitis, 218
Treponemal immobilisation test, 299
Tremor, 303
Tricuspid incompetence, 40
stenosis, 40
Trigeminal nerve, 282
neuralgia, treatment, 283
tracts of, 258
Tri-iodothyronine suppression test, 334
Trochlear nerve, 277, 278
Troisier's sign, 149
TSH-releasing hormone (TRH), 336
Tuberculin testing, 129
Tuberculosis, 128